Craniofacial Sutures

Frontiers of Oral Biology

Vol. 12

Series Editor

Paul Sharpe, London

Craniofacial Sutures

Development, Disease and Treatment

Volume Editor

David P. Rice, *London/Helsinki*

44 figures, 13 in color, and 10 tables, 2008

KARGER

Basel · Freiburg · Paris · London · New York · Bangalore · Bangkok · Singapore · Tokyo · Sydney

Frontiers of Oral Biology

David P. Rice
Senior Lecturer, Guy's Hospital
King's College, London SE1 9RT (UK)
and
Professor of Orthodontics
Institute of Dentistry and Helsinki University Central Hospital
Box 41, University of Helsinki
FIN-00014 Helsinki (Finland)

Library of Congress Cataloging-in-Publication Data

Craniofacial sutures : development, disease, and treatment / volume editor,
David P. Rice.
p. ; cm. – (Frontiers of oral biology, ISSN 1420-2433 : v. 12)
Includes bibliographical references and indexes.
ISBN 978-3-8055-8326-8 (hard cover : alk. paper)
1. Cranial sutures. 2. Craniosynostoses. I. Rice, David P. II. Series.
[DNLM: 1. Cranial Sutures–growth & development. 2. Craniosynostoses.
W1 FR946GP v.12 2008 / WE 705 C89083 2008]
QM105.C74 2008
612.8–dc22
2007048380

Bibliographic Indices. This publication is listed in bibliographic services, including Current Contents® and Index Medicus.

www.karger.com
Printed in Switzerland on acid-free and non-aging paper (ISO 9706) by Reinhardt Druck, Basel
ISSN 1420–2433
ISBN 978–3–8055–8326–8

Contents

Foreword

This epic-making book – *Craniofacial Sutures* – edited by David Rice together with his many research articles make him magister mundi of sutural biology. Elsewhere [1], I have discussed suture systems of the skull and their respective anatomic boundaries (table 1). Pruzansky [2] conceived of the skull as a community of bones separated by articulations, whereas Moffett [unpubl. manuscript] thought of the skull as a community of articulations separated by bones. Several different types of articulations were recognized by Moffett (table 2). The two views of Pruzansky and Moffett are actually complementary and simply represent different contexts in which to view development of the skull. This volume – *Craniofacial Sutures* – elegantly demonstrates both of these contexts.

The book is divided into 12 sections. David Rice himself is responsible for three of these: (a) Developmental Anatomy of Craniofacial Sutures; (b) Locate, Condense, Differentiate, Grow and Confront: Developmental Mechanisms Controlling Intramembranous Bone and Suture Formation and Function, and (c) Clinical Features of Syndromic Craniosynostosis. He has invited a number of world class biologists, geneticists, and clinicians to join him by writing intriguing chapters on a variety of different sutural topics. The molecular biology of craniosynostosis is advancing at a very rapid pace since my last reviews of the subject [3, 4].

I highly recommend this magnificent book to evolutionary biologists, craniofacial biologists, anthropologists, geneticists, craniofacial surgeons, plastic surgeons, oral and maxillofacial surgeons, orthodontists, and others with an interest in craniofacial and sutural biology.

Table 1. Suture systems

Sutures	Boundaries
Coronal	Separates anterior cranial segments from middle cranial segment
Lambdoid	Separates middle cranial segment from occipital bone
Sagittal	Divides skull into right and left halves
Craniofacial	Separates upper facial skeleton from anterior cranial region
Circummaxillary	Separates maxilla from adjacent facial bones

Table 2. Craniofacial articulations

Type of articulation	Example	Physiological function	Mechanical function	Remodeling response
Synovial	Temporomandibular joint	Jaw movement	Resists compression and shear to some extent	Limited, avascular
Cartilaginous	Cranial base synchondroses	Active growth	Resists compression	Limited, avascular
Fibrous	Cranial sutures	Allows passage through birth canal; passive growth secondary to brain enlargement	Respond to tension	Great, vascularized
	Facial sutures	Mastication	Sutures remain patent; shock absorbers for forces of mastication	Great, vascularized
	Periodontal fibers	Eruption of teeth; anchoring support of teeth	Responds to tension, compression and shear	Great, vascularized
Dental	Occlusal and interproximal articulations	Mastication and speech	Subject to compression and shear	None, acellular

David Rice is to be congratulated for spearheading this splendid volume.

M. Michael Cohen Jr.
Professor Emeritus of Pediatrics,
Dalhousie University, Halifax, N.S., Canada

References

1 Cohen MM Jr: Anatomic, genetic, nosologic, diagnostic, and psychosocial considerations; in Cohen MM, MacLean RE (eds): Craniosynostosis: Diagnosis, Evaluation, and Management. New York, Oxford University Press, 2000, chap 11, pp 119–143.

2 Pruzansky S: Clinical investigation of the experiments of nature. ASHA Rep 1973;8:62–94.

3 Cohen MM Jr: FGFs/FGFRs and associated disorders; in Epstein CJ, Erickson RP, Wynshaw-Boris A (eds): Inborn Errors of Development. New York, Oxford University Press, 2004, chap 33, pp 380–409.

4 Cohen MM Jr: Craniofacial anomalies; in Gilbert-Barness E (ed): Potter's Pathology of the Fetus, Infant, and Child. Philadelphia, Mosby, 2007, vol 1, chap 20, pp 885–918.

Preface

Craniofacial sutures are important sites of facial and calvarial bone growth. Sutures therefore contribute to differences in the shape, size and character of our face and skull and as a result in the way in which we perceive each other. Suture development, which occurs mainly during embryogenesis, has to be carefully synchronized with the development of the neighboring organs. These organs are primarily the brain, eyes, nose and mouth. If sutures close prematurely, a condition called craniosynostosis, further bone growth is not possible at the site of fusion. This results in uncoordinated compensatory craniofacial development and consequently produces deformity of the calvaria, orbits or face and may also result in dental malocclusion. This book brings together leading basic science researchers and clinicians to produce a review of craniofacial suture development and the clinical conditions that can result from abnormal suture development.

The book is broadly divided into five sections. First, there is a developmental biology section in which the developmental anatomy of both calvarial and facial sutures is described, and the key molecular mechanisms controlling intramembranous bone and suture formation are detailed. In addition, the factors controlling suture patency are discussed. Following this there is a chapter on how, from an evolutionary aspect, sutures form and why they form at specific locations and at specific times. The third section gives a synopsis of the major clinical conditions affecting craniofacial sutures, a comprehensive overview of human genetic mutations causing craniosynostosis, and evidence of genotype-phenotype correlations. In the fourth section the major molecular pathways involved in normal and abnormal suture development are described. It is intended that this section combined with the clinical sections provides an insight into the molecular etiology of sutural disorders. Finally, there is a review of current treatment philosophies and a look to the future.

David P. Rice, Helsinki
September 2007

Rice DP (ed): Craniofacial Sutures. Development, Disease and Treatment.
Front Oral Biol. Basel, Karger, 2008, vol 12, pp 1–21

Developmental Anatomy of Craniofacial Sutures

David P. Rice

Departments of Orthodontics and Craniofacial Development, King's College London, London, UK; Department of Orthodontics, University of Helsinki, Helsinki, Finland

Abstract

Sutures are fibrous joints in the vertebrate skull. They consist of two bone ends and intervening fibrous tissue which differentiates from embryonic mesenchyme. Sutures are not merely articulations between bones they are primary sites of osteogenesis mediating much of the growth of the face and skull vault. In this chapter the development of sutures will be described including the origin of sutural tissues, the determinants of suture location, and suture morphology. Also, the main functions of sutures will be explained.

Introduction: Definition of a Suture

Sutures are fibrous joints in the vertebrate skull (figs 1, 2). They consist of two bone ends and intervening fibrous tissue which differentiates from embryonic mesenchyme. Sutures are not merely articulations between bones they are primary sites of osteogenesis with osteoprogenitors proliferating, differentiating and functioning at the bone margins or osteogenic fronts. The bones that make up sutures are usually of intramembranous origin though not exclusively so, for example the frontoethmoidal suture is at the junction of an intramembranous bone and an endochondral bone.

The bones of the skull can be divided into the viscerocranium which supports the nasal passages, oral cavity and the pharynx and forms the face, and the neurocranium which surrounds the brain. The neurocranium can be subdivided into the base of the skull and the calvaria (skull vault). The bones of the skull base are formed by endochondral ossification and the cartilaginous joints

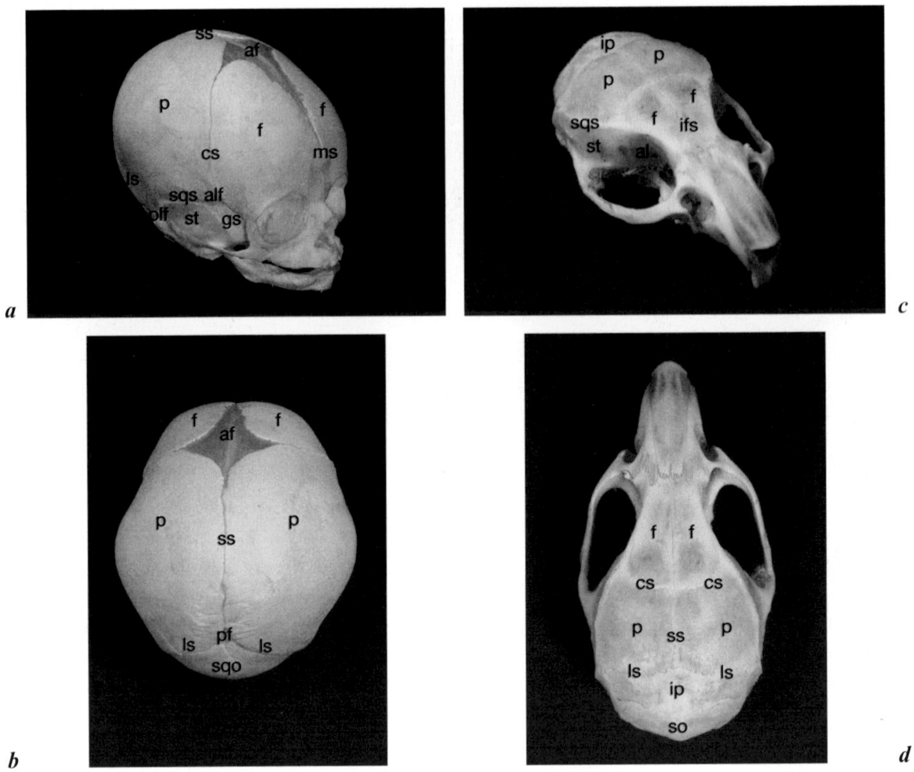

Fig. 1. Calvarial bones, sutures and fontanelles. ***a***, ***b*** Neonate human. ***c***, ***d*** Mature mouse. Mice make a good mammalian model for studying craniofacial bones and sutures. They essentially have the same bones and joints, only the shape, size and orientation varies. af = Anterior fontanelle; alf = anterior lateral fontanelle (sphenoidal); al = alisphenoid bone; cs = coronal suture; f = frontal bone; gs = greater wing of sphenoid bone; ifs = interfrontal suture; ip = interparietal bone; ls = lambdoidal suture; ms = metopic suture (interfrontal); p = parietal bone; pf = posterior fontanelle; plf = posterolateral fontanelle (mastoid); so = supraoccipital bone; sqo = squamous part of occipital bone; sqs = squamosal suture; ss = sagittal suture; st = squamous part of temporal bone.

between the bones are called synchondroses. The bones of the calvaria and face are primarily formed by intramembranous ossification.

Fontanelles are located in the calvaria where three or more bones converge. At birth fontanelles are larger than sutures but as the calvarial bones continue to grow after birth their size rapidly diminishes. At birth sutures and fontanelles are reasonably robust but flexible structures that allow for the temporary compression of the calvaria during childbirth.

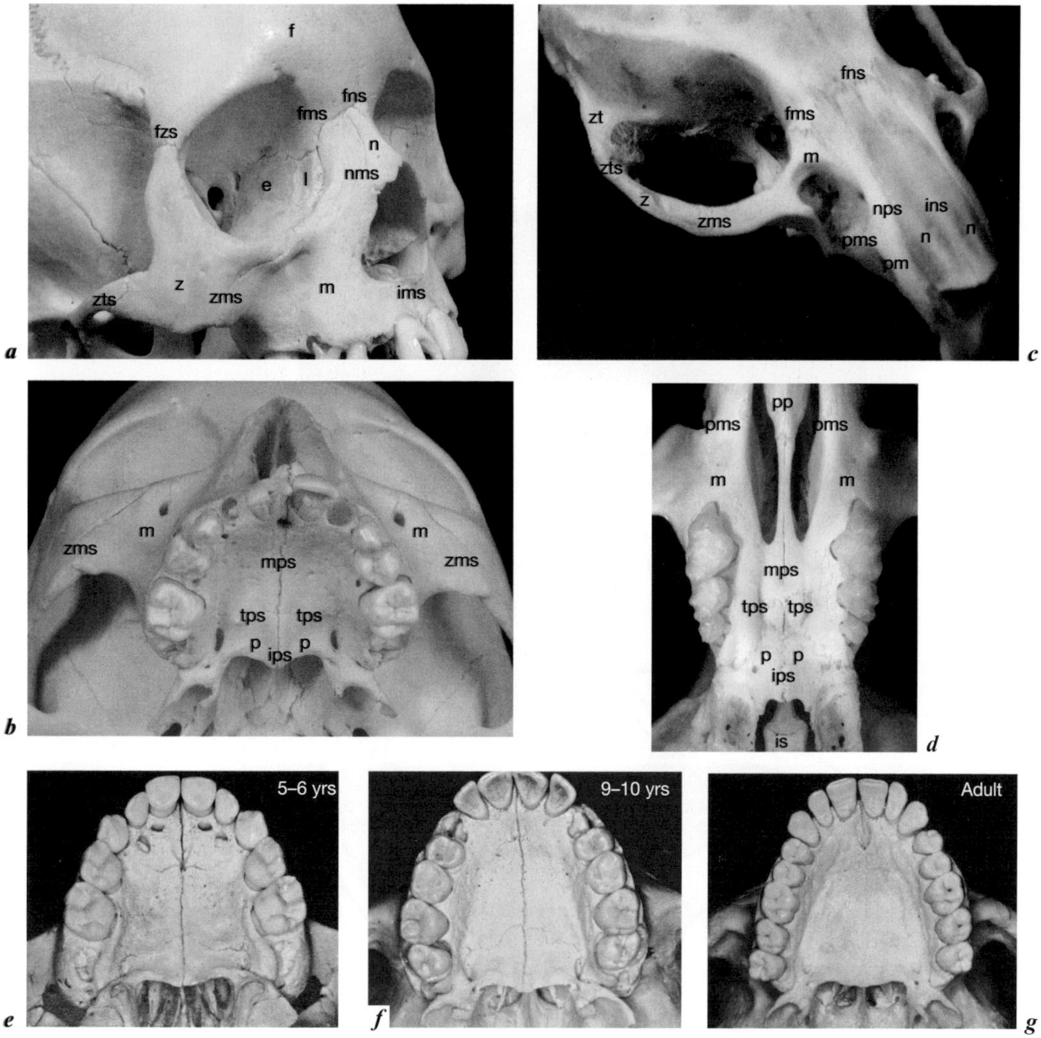

Fig. 2. Selected facial osteology and sutures. ***a***, ***b*** 7-year-old human. ***c***, ***d*** Mature mouse. ***e–g*** Closure of the human median palatine (intermaxillary suture). Growth at the median palatine suture continues until approximately 17 years. The suture fuses between 30 and 35 years. e = Ethmoid bone; f = frontal bone; fms = frontomaxillary suture; fns = frontonasal suture; fzs = frontozygomatic suture; ims = intermaxillary suture; ins = internasal suture; ips = interpalatine suture; is = interphenoidal synchondrosis; l = lacrimal bone; m = maxilla; mps = median palatine suture; n = nasal bone; nms = nasomaxillary suture; nps = nasopremaxillary suture; p = palatine bone; pm = premaxilla; pms = premaxilla maxillary suture; pp = palatine process of premaxilla; tps = transverse palatine suture; z = zygomatic bone; zms = zygomaticomaxillary suture; zt = zygomatic process of temporal bone; zts = zygomaticotemporal suture.

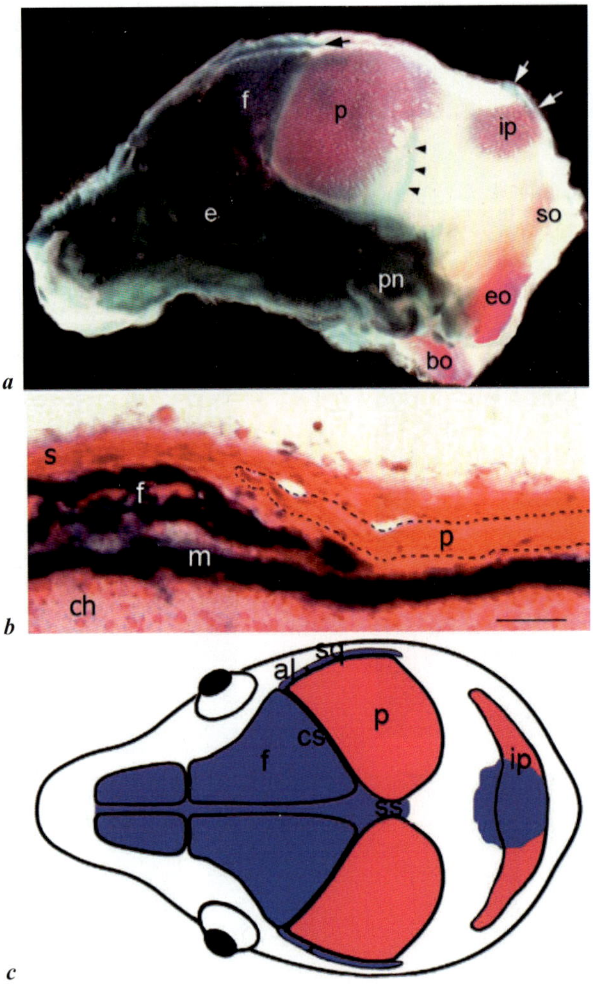

Fig. 3. Tissue origin of the craniofacial bones. Mouse head E17.5. ***a*** *Wnt1-Cre/R26R* head stained with X-gal (blue-green) to show transgene-expressing neural crest-derived tissue and alizarin red to show bone mineral. The facial bones and sutures express the transgene as do the frontal bones, the alisphenoid, the squamous part of temporal bone, the central section of the interparietal region (white arrows), and the meninges under the frontal and parietal bones (arrowheads). Also the internasal, frontonasal, interfrontal, coronal sutures and most of the sagittal suture (black arrow) are X-gal-positive. ***b*** The boundary of neural crest and mesodermal-derived calvarial tissue at the coronal suture. Section through the coronal suture of a *Wnt1-Cre/R26R* head stained with X-gal (blue-green) and fast red. The frontal bone and meninges are X-gal-positive. The parietal bone (dotted outline) is X-gal-negative. ***c*** Tissue origin of the calvaria. Neural crest is shown in blue, mesoderm in red. bo = Basioccipital; ch = cerebral hemisphere; e = eye; eo = exoccipital;

The Origin of the Craniofacial Skeleton

The skeletal elements of the skull are derived from embryonic mesoderm and cranial neural crest (CNC). CNC cells originate from the neural epithelium in the neural folds. These cells undergo epithelial-to-mesenchymal transition, and migrate to their final destinations in the neck and craniofacial regions [1]. In avians, quail-chick chimaeras have allowed detailed studies of the fate of CNC cells [2–4]. In mouse, CNC cell destinations have been studied by histological analysis of early embryos, transplantation, vital dye labeling experiments, and more recently by the analysis of transgenic mice in which CNC cells are permanently labeled [5–10]. These studies have demonstrated that in both avians and mammals the facial skeleton and anterior cranial base are entirely of CNC origin, and that the posterior cranial base skeleton is derived from paraxial and somitic mesoderm.

The contribution of neural crest cells to the different elements of the calvaria has been studied in mice, birds and frogs. Analysis of the *Wnt1-Cre/R26R* transgenic mouse, which carries a permanent neural crest cell lineage marker has shown that the frontal bone, alisphenoid bone, part of the interparietal bone and the squamous part of the temporal bone, and the interfrontal and coronal suture mesenchyme are of CNC origin [8] (fig. 3). A tongue of neural crest-derived tissue from the interfrontal suture extends posteriorly to contribute to the early sagittal suture mesenchyme between the parietal bones, although at later stages it does not constitute the whole of the sagittal suture mesenchyme [11]. The dura mater covering the developing cerebral hemispheres (forebrain) underneath the frontal and parietal bones is of neural crest origin. The parietal bones themselves and the meninges covering the mid- and hindbrain are of mesodermal origin. Thus in mouse, calvarial tissue layers caudal to the frontal bones arise from mesoderm with the exception of the meninges underneath the parietal bones. Although this work gives an indication of the contribution of neural crest cells to different calvarial elements it does not exclude the possibility of the mesoderm also contributing to these tissues.

In birds, using quail-chick chimaeras Couly et al. [3] found that the neural crest contributes to both the frontal and parietal bones, and to the sutures between these bones. Also using quail-chick chimaeras and more recently cell tracing experiments where either CNC or paraxial mesodermal cells were

m = meninges; pn = pinna of ear; s = skin. Other labels see figure 1. Scale: 1 mm (***a***), 100 μm (***b***). Images reproduced from Jiang et al. [8] and Morriss-Kay and Wilkie [11] with kind permission of the authors and Elsevier Science and The Anatomical Society of Great Britain and Ireland.

infected with β-galactosidase-encoding replication-incompetent retroviruses, Noden [12], Evans and Noden [13] and Le Lievre [14] found conflicting results that in birds the calvarial neural crest territory is restricted to the supraorbital region of the frontal bone. In avians, this rostral section of the frontal bone arises from a different ossification center to that which forms the more caudal section of the frontal bone, with which it later fuses. Humans also have a similar secondary frontal bone ossification center which gives rise to the nasal spine of the frontal bone (table 1). Both Couly et al. [3] and Noden [12] and Evans and Noden [13] found that the avian dura mater is derived from CNC cells.

Frogs have a single frontoparietal bone and neural crest contributes to this bone as well as to the parasphenoid and squamosal bones in the calvaria [15].

Apparent differences in the position of the neural crest-mesoderm boundary in the calvaria are possibly due to variation in technique and analysis but may also reflect inaccurate nomenclature of the bones and/or a lack of accurate homology between mammals, avians and amphibians in the frontal, parietal and interparietal region [8, 16]. Also, it has been suggested that the neural crest-mesodermal boundary might have shifted location during vertebrate evolution [15, 16].

It is also worth noting that vertebrate calvaria are made up of multiple independent ossification centers. Some bones are formed by the fusion of two or more made ossification centers while other bones are formed from a single ossification center. Whether ossification centers fuse or not can alter the apparent boundary between the bones that finally result and as a consequence may appear to change the crest-mesoderm boundary. In summary, either the crest-mesoderm boundary could have shifted during evolution or the boundary remained fixed in place but the frontal and parietal bones have been identified differently [15].

Importance of Tissue Origin

Does the tissue origin matter? As far as the calvaria is concerned osteoblasts can differentiate and function normally and sutures can maintain patency whether they are of neural crest or mesodermal origin. Osteoblasts that develop from either CNC or mesoderm are functionally indistinguishable. What may be more important, than cellular origin, is the local milieu in which CNC cells or mesodermal cells find themselves. Both CNC cells and mesodermal cells possess a high degree of plasticity, and given the correct inductive signals can be patterned by the environment [17].

The origin of the tissue becomes important when deficiencies in neural crest cell formation, migration or proliferation occur resulting in abnormality.

Table 1. Ossification of selected human craniofacial bones

Bone	Number of ossification centers and ossification timing and sequence	Ossification type	Notes
Calvarial bones			
Frontal	Two centers in 8th week One each side of midline, located at frontal tuberosity Two secondary centers in 10th week for nasal spine	Intramembranous	Right and left halves fuse across metopic suture after birth
Parietal	Two centers in 8th week One positioned apically to the other, these fuse early	Intramembranous	Occasionally suture formed between the two centers
Occipital	Upper squamous part (equivalent to interparietal bone in mouse): two centers, one on each side of midline in 8th week Lower squamous part (equivalent to supra-occipital bone in mouse): two centers in 7th week Lateral parts: two centers for each in 8th week Basilar part: one center in 7th week	*Combination* Upper squamous part: intramembranous Lower squamous, lateral and basilar parts: endochondral	Upper and lower squamous parts fuse after 12th week Lateral, basilar and occipital parts fuse by year 4
Sphenoid	Presphenoidal part: six centers in 8th to 9th week One center in each lesser wing, then two centers in presphenoidal body, then later one center in each sphenoidal concha Postsphenoidal part: eight centers in 8th week One center in basal cartilage of each greater wing One center in upper part of each greater wing Two centers in sella turcica One center in each medial pterygoid plate One center in each lingula	*Combination* Greater wings (upper sections), medial pterygoid plate except hamulus, lateral pterygoid plate: intramembranous Lesser wings, greater wings (basal sections), body, conchae: endochondral	Presphenoidal and postsphenoidal parts fuse in 8th month Intramembranous ossification spreads from the greater wings into lateral pterygoid plates
Temporal	Squamous part: one center in 8th week Petromastoid part: up to fourteen centers in 20th to 24th week Tympanic part: one center in 12th to 16th week Styloid part: two centers, one starts before birth and one after birth	*Combination* Squamous and tympanic parts: intramembranous Petromastoid and styloid parts: endochondral	

Table 1. (continued)

Bone	Number of ossification centers and ossification timing and sequence	Ossification type	Notes
Facial bones			
Maxilla	One center in 7th week	Intramembranous	There is not a separate ossification center in the premaxilla region ossification from the single maxillary center spreads anteriorly to fill this area
Nasal	One center in 9th to 10th week	Intramembranous	
Palatine	One center in 8th week	Intramembranous	
Zygomatic	One center in 8th week	Intramembranous	

Based on *Gray's Anatomy*, ed 38 and 39 [26–29].

A good example of this is in the pathogenesis of Treacher Collins syndrome. Treacher Collins syndrome is thought to be caused by a reduction in the numbers of neural crest cells and this results in multiple craniofacial defects, including malar/zygomatic and mandibular hypoplasia [18].

Maintenance of the boundary between CNC and mesodermal cells is also important. The CNC and mesodermal boundary at the coronal suture is established and maintained by ephrin-Eph signaling. Abnormalities in this signaling caused by loss-of-function mutations in *EFNB1* result in craniofrontonasal syndrome characterized by coronal suture synostosis [19]. In mice coronal suture synostosis exhibited by *Twist1*$^{+/-}$ mice is accompanied by abnormal ephrin-Eph signaling and abnormal mixing of CNC and mesodermal cells in the coronal suture [20].

Ossification of the Craniofacial Skeleton and the Establishment of Sutures

Ossification of the craniofacial skeleton begins with condensation of neural crest or mesodermally derived cells into tightly packed masses. Within these centers cells differentiate into either chondroblasts which form cartilage or osteoblasts which form bone. In comparison, endochondral ossification involves the formation of a cartilage template or scaffold which is later removed prior to its replacement by bone formed by osteoblasts. During intramembranous ossification osteoblasts secrete osteoid which then calcifies with no cartilage anlagen. The process of condensation formation and the control of cell fate in determining whether chondroblasts or osteoblasts are formed will be discussed in more detail by Rice and Rice [pp. 22–40]. During intramembranous ossification bones develop in a layer, or 'membrane', of mesenchymal tissue which is often in contact with the dermal layer of the skin. Hence the term dermal bone is applied. In the calvaria, this mesenchymal layer is also in contact with the underlying dura mater covering the brain. Signaling from both the skin and the dura has been shown to regulate intramembranous bone development and also suture closure [21, 22].

Craniofacial intramembranous bones grow mainly by ossification at the sutures and also by modeling and remodeling of their other surfaces. For example, an increase in maxillary width is accomplished by growth at the median palatal suture as well as bone appositional growth on the external surfaces and resorption on the internal surfaces to allow the maxillary air sinus to development form. Also, when the maxillary teeth develop and erupt, the alveolar section of the maxilla forms by modeling and remodeling around the teeth. In the calvaria there is a co-ordinated balance between osteoblast-driven apposition which occurs mainly on the ectocranial surface and osteoclast-driven resorption which occurs mainly on the endocranial surface [23, 24]. These synchronized processes control bone thickness and are important in shaping individual bones [25].

In the human embryonic skull, cartilage formation begins in the body of the sphenoid bone and the basilar part of the occipital bone at crown-rump (CR) length 11–14 mm equivalent to approximately the 7th week of gestation [26]. Ossification of the human skull begins in the face with the first signs starting in the mandible and the maxilla between 15 and 20 mm CR (7th week) (table 1). Ossification begins in the palatine and nasal bones between 25–30 mm CR (8th week) and 33–38 mm CR (9th to 10th week), respectively [26]. Ossification commences slightly later in the calvaria than the face. The frontal bone ossification centers appear between 25 and 30 mm CR (8th week) while those of the parietal, upper and lower squamous parts of the occipital bone appear between 30 and 37 mm CR (8th to 9th week).

It has been previously suggested that like other vertebrates humans have a premaxilla (os incisivum) and that this arises from two ossification centers in the premaxillary region [30]. However, there is good evidence that this is not the case and that ossification from the main maxillary center spreads anteriorly to fill this region [31]. There may be an unmineralized defect which corresponds to where a premaxillary suture would be, which is referred to as the interalveolar suture of Farmer. This is visible at birth as a cleft anterior in the palate from the incisive foramen laterally.

In the mouse, facial and calvarial bone formation starts at embryonic day 12.5 (E12.5) [32]. The frontal bone has two centers of ossification one on each side of the midline. Like its human equivalent, the two elements of the mouse frontal bone fuse postnatally across interfrontal suture in the midline. Each parietal bone and the interparietal bone (termed the upper part of the squamous occipital bone in humans) both have two ossification centers which fuse together to make each separate the definitive bone [33].

In the mouse viscerocranium the ossification centers of the premaxilla and the maxilla are the first to be seen at E12.5. In addition to the main ossification center in the maxilla several other centers arise and these later amalgamate. These additional centers are located close to the upper first molar tooth anlagen, in the lateral margins of the palatal shelves, and in the periorbital region both lateral and inferolateral to the nasal capsule. Interestingly, the maxilla and mandible have been described as originating from a single mesenchymal condensation from which presumably individual ossification centers arise [34].

In the chick, facial bone formation starts at E7.5 and calvarial bone formation at E8.5 [34, 35]. In the calvaria, bone matrix deposition starts in the lateral parts of the frontal and squamosal bones and ossification spreads medially. Then at E13 the parietal bones start to ossify [35].

Craniofacial Bone Position and Identity, and Suture Location

With the exception of the coronal suture the site where a suture forms is determined by the relative growth of adjacent craniofacial bones [11, 36–38]. Some investigators have also suggested that the dura mater can influence or even dictate where a calvarial suture is formed, and that this is in response to tension in the dura, as a result of neurocranial expansion, directed via the basicranial processes [39, 40].

Where bony margins meet to form a suture is determined not only by factors stimulating or inhibiting bone growth but also by the position and number of skeletogenic condensations and subsequently the centers of ossification that make up each bone. In the axial and appendicular skeleton anterior-posterior patterning and positional identity of bones are determined at a molecular level by the Hox code. Homeobox genes act at the early stages of condensation formation; they are important in determining the timing, position and shape of skeletogenic condensations and therefore have a fundamental influence on axial and appendicular skeletogenesis [41, 42]. Hox genes are not expressed in the major part of the craniofacial region. Indeed, for the majority of the craniofacial skeleton it is essential to stay *Hox*-negative during development [43]. Ectopic expression of *Hoxa2* in the craniofacial mesenchyme in mice results in an inhibition of craniofacial bone development [44]. The only Hox genes that do contribute to the craniofacial skeleton are those expressed in the occipital somites and the 2nd branchial arch. Therefore, the Hox code contributes to the posterior cranial base, the stapes bone, the styloid process and part of the hyoid bone only.

Although we are starting to understand what controls osteoblast differentiation and function and that ossification centers arise from osteogenic condensations, in the mammalian skull we know relatively little about what controls the initiation of osteogenesis at a particular time and location, that is to say the regulation of where and when individual skull bones develop.

In the brachial arches, it is known that Dlx homeobox-containing transcription factors regulate the proximodistal identity of the maxillary and mandibular processes [45]. The 6 *Dlx* genes are genomically linked and (uniquely) expressed in a nested pattern in the developing branchial arch mesenchyme. They provide a combinatorial code such that they are responsible for the development, pattern and subsequent morphology of the skeletal elements formed in the jaws. Using intricate mouse genetics it has been shown that a complex combination of *Dlx* genes control branchial identity, such that loss of function of multiple *Dlx* genes in different allelic combinations results in distinct morphological differences in facial development. $Dlx5^{-/-}$; $Dlx6^{-/-}$ double mutants are particularly interesting. When the function of both *Dlx5* and *Dlx6* are lost there is a homeotic transformation in which the maxilla is replicated in the mandibular arch. Despite this major disruption upper and lower incisors occasionally develop and when they do they usually develop without their respective alveolar bones. Also, a second set of palatine and pterygoid bones develop in conjunction with the ectopic maxilla. In addition, $Dlx5^{-/-}$; $Dlx6^{-/-}$ mice also have no frontal or parietal bones implicating a role for *Dlx5* and *Dlx6* in calvarial bone development. The fact that $Dlx5^{-/-}$; $Dlx6^{-/-}$ mutants exhibit a duplicate maxilla instead of merely a loss of the mandibular structures suggests that there is a higher level of patterning (position and identity) which governs skeletogenesis in the branchial arches. The source of this may well be FGF8 from the ectoderm. *FGF8* expression is maintained in $Dlx5^{-/-}$; $Dlx6^{-/-}$ mutants and loss of *FGF8* specifically in the ectoderm covering the branchial arches results in a loss of most first branchial arch structures except those that develop from the most distal region including the lower incisors [46]. FGF8 is important for the survival, proliferation and possibly attraction of the CNC cells into the facial region. In the avian embryo, exogenous FGF8 can largely rescue the absent facial development caused by the excision of the anterior *Hox*-negative neural crest. Interestingly, excision of the anterior *Hox*-negative neural crest results in a downregulation of *FGF8* in the 1st branchial arch ectoderm, suggesting that not only epithelium to mesenchyme signaling but also mesenchyme to epithelium signaling controls facial skeletal development [47]. The factors

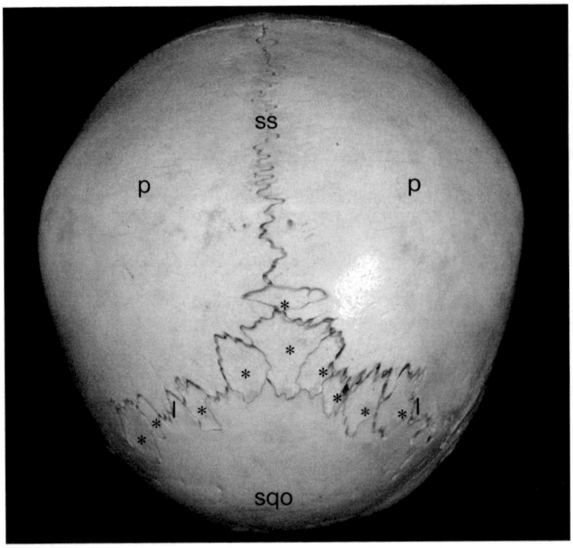

Fig. 4. Wormian bones. Multiple wormian or intrasutural bones in the human lambdoid suture (asterisks). l = Lambdoid suture; p = parietal bone; sqo = squamous part of occipital bone (interparietal); ss = sagittal suture.

regulating the initiation of skull skeletogenesis and patterning are discussed further from an evolutionary stand point by Depew et al. [pp. 57–78].

Wormian Bones

Wormian or sutural bones are small calvarial bones that develop from additional ossification centers in the sutures or fontanelles (fig. 4). They develop some distance from the calvarial bones within the calvarial mesenchyme, so that ossification centers are initiated de novo, osteoblasts differentiate and lay down bone matrix. In the human, wormian bones most commonly occur in the lambdoid suture. They are seen in a number of conditions including cleidocranial dysplasia, all types of osteogenesis imperfecta, hydrocephalus, hypothyroidism and lateral meningocele syndrome.

Suture Morphology

In the mouse, most sutures including the interfrontal, sagittal and lambdoidal sutures are formed when bone fronts, that are initially far apart, approximate

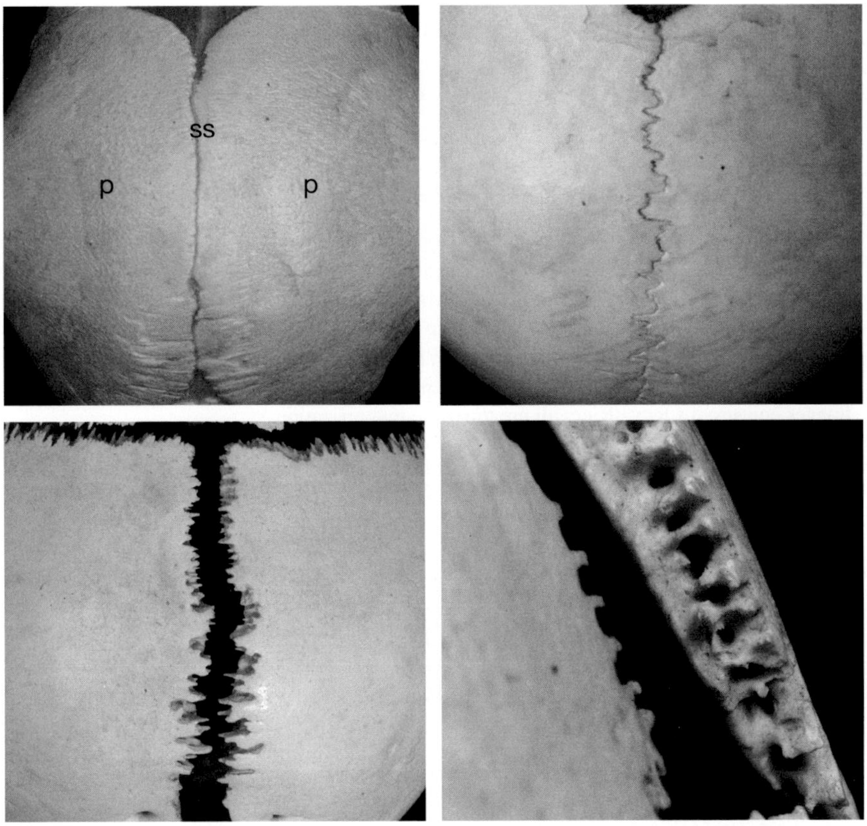

a b c d

Fig. 5. Sagittal suture morphology. ***a–d*** The human sagittal suture develops from a simple straight end-to-end butt joint into an interlocking joint with increasingly complex interdigitation. p = Parietal bone; ss = sagittal suture.

each other relatively late in embryonic development. The initial osteogenic condensations of the frontal and parietal bones form close to the skull base, sandwiched between the developing eye and brain [32]. Osteogenesis then proceeds in an apical direction with the bones confronting each other in interfrontal and sagittal sutures. At first, the sagittal suture lies in a sulcus between the two cerebral hemispheres with the osteogenic fronts turned endocranially towards the meninges. However, shortly after birth butt joints are formed with the osteogenic fronts confronting each other 'head on' [48]. Postnatally the morphology of the sagittal suture changes from a simple butt joint to one with multiple interlocking projections (fig. 5).

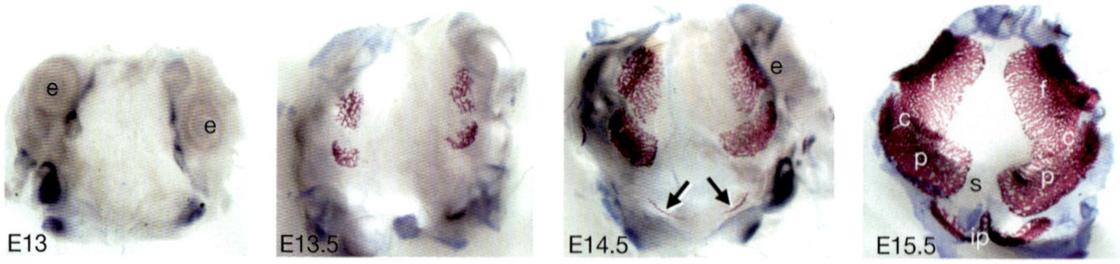

Fig. 6. Calvarial bone and suture development. Skeletal stain by alizarin red (mineralized bones) and alcian blue (cartilages) in calvarial explants. Calvarial bones start developing from osteogenic condensations at E12–E13. Mineralized frontal (f) and parietal (p) bones are visible by E13.5. By E14 the interparietal (ip) bone is visible as two separate ossification centers (arrows). By E15 the sagittal suture (s) between the opposing parietal bone plates has formed, as have the coronal sutures (c) between the frontal and parietal bone plates. e = Eye. (Images courtesy of Ritva Rice; all are the same magnification.)

The development of the coronal suture is different in that the osteogenic fronts of the frontal and parietal bones approximate and overlap each other very early during suture morphogenesis (fig. 6). This is, in part, due to the osteogenic condensations of the frontal and parietal bones being initially closer together than those of the two frontal or two parietal bones. In addition, the overlap of the frontal and parietal bones is set early in development. The coronal suture lies at the junction of neural crest-derived and mesoderm-derived tissue which is established at E9 when the two cell populations meet. Even at this early stage the mesodermal (parietal) tissue lies external to the neural crest (frontal)-derived tissue and this relationship is maintained thereafter [8]. Once the coronal suture has been established on the inferior lateral aspect of the calvaria, suture formation then progresses medially, toward the midline, in a zipper-like fashion. This morphogenesis is reflected in the histological maturation of the suture with a more advanced degree of maturation being exhibited laterally than medially [36].

As we have seen the bones of a suture can meet end-on in a butt joint (e.g. sagittal and median palatine sutures), or can overlap to form a beveled joint (e.g. coronal and squamosal sutures), or meet in a 'tongue and groove' relationship where a ridge of one bone fits into a groove of its neighbor. This specialized suture is called a schindylesis (e.g. vomerosphenoidal suture).

In all sutures, once the osteogenic fronts have approximated, the intervening mesenchymal tissue increases in thickness to form a highly cellular 'blastema'. Finally, a fibrous central zone appears between the two opposing bones, heralding the 'mature' suture [49].

Secondary Cartilages and Chondroid Bone

Accumulations of cartilage can occur in the mesenchyme of developing sutures [49]. These are generally transient, eventually being transformed back into fibrous tissue, fibrocartilage or into bone. Rarely, such cartilages may be found stenosing a suture [50]. These are often referred to as secondary cartilages having not been derived from the 'primary' cartilaginous skeleton [51]. If a cartilage develops close to the sagittal suture, it may take the form of a rod, elliptical in cross section. The cartilage tends to reside in the endocranial sector of the mesenchyme above the sagittal venous sinus. It may be present just prior to birth and then disappear shortly postpartum [38, 52]. Pritchard et al. [38] suggested that in the rodent this cartilage may be a forward extension of the tectal region of the chondrocranium. 'Chondroid tissue' has also been described at the sutural edge, notably in the metopic/interfrontal suture, where it has been linked to sutural fusion [53, 54].

It is known that stimuli such as mechanical stress, ischemia and anoxia can enhance mesenchymal cell differentiation into chondroblasts, while mechanical tension, an adequate blood supply and hyperoxia can favor differentiation into osteoblasts [55]. These factors may be of importance in determining which route an uncommitted mesenchymal cell takes.

Suture Function and Dysfunction

The main functions of sutures are to act as: (1) sites of bone growth, (2) articulations, holding the constituent elements of the skull together while allowing deformation of the skull during child birth and thereafter minor movements, and (3) mechanical stress absorbers, thus protecting the sutural osteogenic tissue [56]. The skull is made up of numerous separate bony elements and this permits growth to occur at the edges of the bones for as long as the skull is required to enlarge around the developing brain, eyes, ears, nose and dentition. Bone growth occurs by intramembranous osteogenesis at the bone margins in sutures, and continued growth is dependent on maintaining the space between the opposing bone margins so that they do not unite. Such a fusion would stop any further growth at that location.

The mammalian calvaria undergoes most of its growth during the embryonic and early postnatal periods. In contrast, the facial skeleton undergoes most of its rapid growth later. As a consequence calvarial sutures are most active relatively early in development while facial sutures are most active later, during adolescence.

Growth of the bones that make up a suture occurs in broadly equal amounts in each bone and is usually at right angles to the suture line. However, data from studies where metal implants have been placed on either side of a suture, and growth monitored, indicate that growth is not necessarily equal on both sides of a suture [56]. For example, in the frontonasal suture, apposition on the frontal bone side is 5-fold greater than that on the nasal bone side. Greater bone growth on one side of a suture compared to the other is sometimes seen in response to craniosynostosis. Compensatory growth in response to the premature fusion at one suture can occur at other sutures and this reaction may be asymmetric with apposition at one bone end greater than at its partner [57].

Also, in relation to each other, bones may either slide, as is seen in the nasopremaxillary suture in rats, or rotate about a sutural line. The two maxillary bones rotate in all three dimensions in relation to each other and in an anterior posterior plane [58, 59]. In median palatal suture, there is more growth in the posterior section than in the anterior section which results in the two maxillary bones rotating in relation to each other in the transverse plane.

Once a suture has been established either apposition or resorption can occur at the bone ends as the demands of each situation befit. This permits adjustments in the size, shape and spatial orientation of the contiguous parts of the craniofacial skeleton during development and growth [24, 60]. Sutures can also adapt to pathological disturbances such as hydrocephalus, in which the calvaria expands secondary to an increased intracranial pressure. Thus, the growth of the calvaria and the underlying brain are highly co-ordinated.

Sutures are tightly regulated structures that must stay patent to function. When this regulation is not appropriately controlled and a suture closes prematurely (synostosis), deformity can result. This may take the form of local ridging of the affected individual suture or have more widespread and serious effects. Once two facial or calvarial bones have fused across a suture further growth is restricted at that location. As the head continues to develop and grow, the lack of bone growth at this site may be compensated for by extra growth at another location. However, restricted growth at one or more sutures combined with compensatory growth elsewhere will result in deformity. Deformity caused by premature suture closure is illustrated in figure 6 and discussed more by Hukki et al. [pp. 79–90], Rice [pp. 91–106] and Wan et al. [pp. 209–230]. Craniosynostosis can also affect sutures in the face.

Another example of disrupted sutural growth leading to deformity is seen when growth is restricted in the palatal suture. Sutural growth is one of the main contributors to overall facial growth in all three dimensions [58, 61]. Growth in the median palatal suture continues until approximately 17 years and is the most important factor contributing to the width of the maxilla. Of secondary importance is appositional remodeling of the outer aspects of the maxilla [58, 61]. If growth in the median palatal suture is defective a narrow maxilla will result with possible malocclusion of the upper molar and premolar teeth with their lower

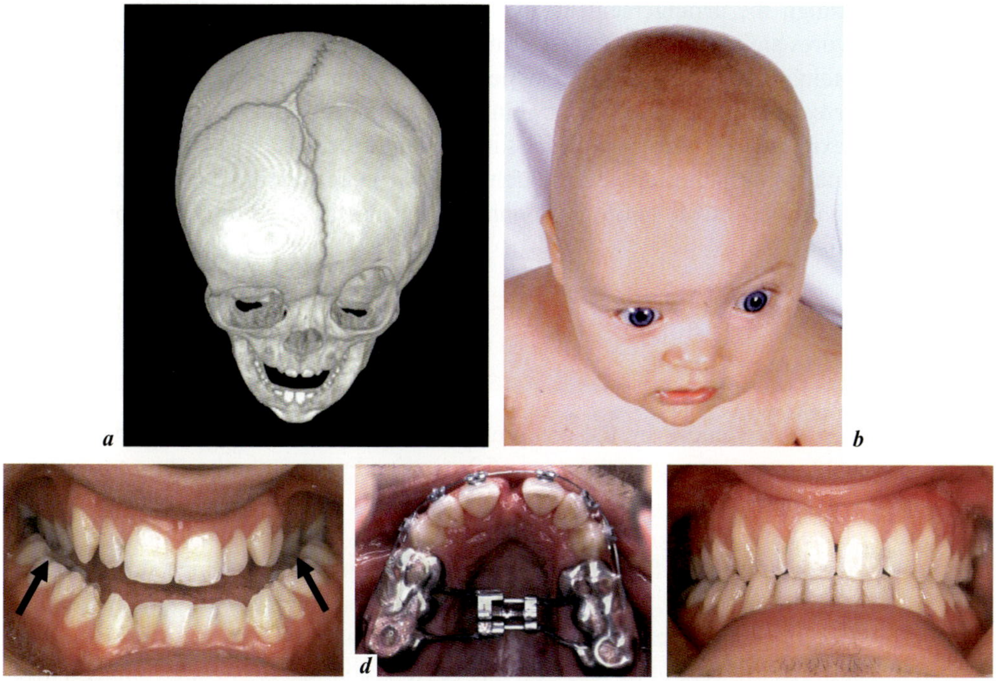

Fig. 7. Suture function and pathology. ***a***, ***b*** 3-Dimensional computed tomogram and clinical photograph of child, aged 6 months, with unilateral (left) coronal suture synostosis. Sutures are osteogenic growth sites and have to remain patent to function. If they fuse before the development of the head is complete growth is constrained at the affected suture. Compensatory osteogenesis at other sutures can occur, however this can lead to deformity, as seen in this child with an asymmetric distortion of the forehead and orbital regions. (Images courtesy of Jyri Hukki.) ***c–e*** Growth of the median palatal suture. ***c*** The upper dental arch is normally slightly broader than the lower dental arch resulting in the upper teeth occludingslightly lateral to the corresponding lower arch teeth. Lack of growth in the median palatine suture can lead to a dental cross-bite: a malocclusion between the upper and lower posterior teeth where the upper molars and premolars occlude more medially with the lower teeth (arrows). ***d***, ***e*** This can be corrected with orthodontic appliances, where the expansion in the upper dental arch is in part due to increased sutural growth [71]. ***d*** Expansion of the maxillary arch with orthodontic appliances, viewed from below. ***e*** The upper teeth now occlude slightly lateral to and overlap the lower teeth.

counterparts. Instead of the maxillary teeth occluding laterally to the mandibular teeth they will occlude more medially resulting in dental cross-bite (fig. 7).

Under normal conditions, mechanical stress on craniofacial sutures results from masticatory forces. Sutures are specially organized to resist strain, notably through the arrangement and structure of sutural fibers. Although calvarial sutures are not as strong under bending, they absorb more energy under impact loading when compared to bone without sutures. Also, energy absorption increases with increased sutural interdigitation [62]. Interestingly, sutural complexity and the number of intrasutural bones increase with intentional cranial vault deformation applied though external head binding [63]. The mechanical influences on suture development and patency are discussed by Herring [pp. 41–56].

Suture Closure

As evidenced by the compression of the skull during childbirth, sutures and fontanelles posses a degree of flexibility. For structural and protective reasons sutures loose this limited mobility and become more rigid. This is accomplished by interdigitation of the opposing bony margins and ultimately fusion across the suture (fig. 5). Except for the metopic suture, which starts to close after the first year, after a period of major broadening of the forehead, and is obliterated by 7 years of age, most calvarial sutures start to fuse in adult life between the ages of 25 and 30 years [64]. In contrast to calvarial sutures, most facial sutures remain patent until late adulthood. For example the frontomaxillary, nasomaxillary and zygomaticomaxillary sutures do not start to fuse until the 7th or 8th decade of life [65]. This is presumably due to mechanical strain applied through masticatory forces on the upper part of the face. The exception is the intermaxillary suture which starts to fuse between the age of 30 and 35 years [66].

In the mouse, all calvarial sutures, except for the posterior section of the interfrontal suture, remain patent. The posterior section of the interfrontal suture fuses between 25 and 45 days postnatal, and it does this in an anterior to posterior manner [67]. The Sprague-Dawley rat exhibits a similar pattern with posterior section of the interfrontal suture fusing between 12 and 30 days postnatal. Here fusion starts on the endocranial side and progresses outwards [68–70]. However, in the rat, localized areas of synostosis, especially in the sagittal suture, can occur at any time after the 21st postnatal day [38].

Acknowledgements

I am very grateful to Dr. Ritva Rice and Professor Gillian Morriss-Kay for their help with this chapter.

References

1 Trainor P, Nieto MA: Jawsfest: new perspectives on neural crest lineages and morphogenesis. Development 2003;130:5059–5063.
2 Noden DM: Origins and patterning of craniofacial mesenchymal tissues. J Craniofac Genet Dev Biol Suppl 1986;2:15–31.
3 Couly GF, Coltey PM, Le Douarin NM: The triple origin of skull in higher vertebrates: a study in quail-chick chimeras. Development 1993;117:409–429.
4 Huang R, Zhi Q, Patel K, Wilting J, Christ B: Contribution of single somites to the skeleton and muscles of the occipital and cervical regions in avian embryos. Anat Embryol (Berl) 2000;202:375–383.
5 Nichols DH: Neural crest formation in the head of the mouse embryo as observed using a new histological technique. J Embryol Exp Morphol 1981;64:105–120.
6 Serbedzija GN, Bronner-Fraser M, Fraser SE: Vital dye analysis of cranial neural crest cell migration in the mouse embryo. Development 1992;116:297–307.
7 Chai Y, Jiang X, Ito Y, Bringas P Jr, Han J, Rowitch DH, Soriano P, McMahon AP, Sucov HM: Fate of the mammalian cranial neural crest during tooth and mandibular morphogenesis. Development 2000;127:1671–1679.
8 Jiang X, Iseki S, Maxson RE, Sucov HM, Morriss-Kay GM: Tissue origins and interactions in the mammalian skull vault. Dev Biol 2002;241:106–116.
9 Pietri T, Eder O, Blanche M, Thiery JP, Dufour S: The human tissue plasminogen activator-Cre mouse: a new tool for targeting specifically neural crest cells and their derivatives in vivo. Dev Biol 2003;259:176–187.
10 Tan SS, Morriss-Kay GM: Analysis of cranial neural crest cell migration and early fates in postimplantation rat chimaeras. J Embryol Exp Morphol 1986;98:21–58.
11 Morriss-Kay GM, Wilkie AO: Growth of the normal skull vault and its alteration in craniosynostosis: insights from human genetics and experimental studies. J Anat 2005;207:637–653.
12 Noden DM: The control of avian cephalic neural crest cytodifferentiation. I. Skeletal and connective tissues. Dev Biol 1978;67:296–312.
13 Evans DJ, Noden DM: Spatial relations between avian craniofacial neural crest and paraxial mesoderm cells. Dev Dyn 2006;235:1310–1325.
14 Le Lievre CS: Participation of neural crest-derived cells in the genesis of the skull in birds. J Embryol Exp Morphol 1978;47:17–37.
15 Hanken J, Gross JB: Evolution of cranial development and the role of neural crest: insights from amphibians. J Anat 2005;207:437–446.
16 Noden DM, Trainor PA: Relations and interactions between cranial mesoderm and neural crest populations. J Anat 2005;207:575–601.
17 Schneider RA: Neural crest can form cartilages normally derived from mesoderm during development of the avian head skeleton. Dev Biol 1999;208:441–455.
18 Dixon J, Dixon MJ: Genetic background has a major effect on the penetrance and severity of craniofacial defects in mice heterozygous for the gene encoding the nucleolar protein Treacle. Dev Dyn 2004;229:907–914.
19 Twigg SR, Kan R, Babbs C, Bochukova EG, Robertson SP, Wall SA, Morriss-Kay GM, Wilkie AO: Mutations of ephrin-B1 (EFNB1), a marker of tissue boundary formation, cause craniofrontonasal syndrome. Proc Natl Acad Sci USA 2004;101:8652–8657.
20 Merrill AE, Bochukova EG, Brugger SM, Ishii M, Pilz DT, Wall SA, Lyons KM, Wilkie AO, Maxson RE Jr: Cell mixing at a neural crest-mesoderm boundary and deficient ephrin-Eph signaling in the pathogenesis of craniosynostosis. Hum Mol Genet 2006;15:1319–1328.
21 Tyler MS, Hall BK: Epithelial influences on skeletogenesis in the mandible of the embryonic chick. Anat Rec 1977;188:229–239.
22 Opperman LA, Sweeney TM, Redmon J, Persing JA, Ogle RC: Tissue interactions with underlying dura mater inhibit osseous obliteration of developing cranial sutures. Dev Dyn 1993;198:312–322.
23 Ford EH: The growth of the foetal skull. J Anat 1956;90:63–72.
24 Rice DP, Kim HJ, Thesleff I: Detection of gelatinase B expression reveals osteoclastic bone resorption as a feature of early calvarial bone development. Bone 1997;21:479–486.

25 Enlow DH, Hunter WS: A differential analysis of sutural and remodeling growth in the human face. Am J Orthod 1966;52:823–830.
26 Lemire R: Embrylogy of the skull; in Cohen MJ, Maclean R (eds): Craniosynostosis, Diagnosis, Evaluation, and Management. Oxford, Oxford University Press, 2001, chap 3.
27 Standring S: Gray's Anatomy, the Anatomical Basis of Clinical Practice, ed 39. Oxford, Elsevier Churchill Livingstone, 2005.
28 Williams P: Gray's Anatomy, ed 38. Edinburgh, Churchill Livingstone, 1995.
29 Berkovitz B, Holland G, Moxham B: Oral Anatomy, Embryology and Histology, ed 3. Edinburgh, Mosby, 2002.
30 Woo JK: Ossification and growth of the human maxilla, premaxilla and palate bone. Anat Rec 1949;105:737–761.
31 Wood NK, Wragg LE, Stuteville OH, Oglesby RJ: Osteogenesis of the human upper jaw: proof of the non-existence of a separate premaxillary centre. Arch Oral Biol 1969;14:1331–1339.
32 Rice DP, Rice R, Thesleff I: Molecular mechanisms in calvarial bone and suture development, and their relation to craniosynostosis. Eur J Orthod 2003;25:139–148.
33 Kaufman M, Bard J: The Anatomical Basis of Mouse Development. London, Academic Press, 1999.
34 Dunlop LL, Hall BK: Relationships between cellular condensation, preosteoblast formation and epithelial-mesenchymal interactions in initiation of osteogenesis. Int J Dev Biol 1995;39: 357–371.
35 Holleville N, Quilhac A, Bontoux M, Monsoro-Burq AH: BMP signals regulate Dlx5 during early avian skull development. Dev Biol 2003;257:177–189.
36 Johansen VA, Hall SH: Morphogenesis of the mouse coronal suture. Acta Anat (Basel) 1982;114:58–67.
37 Moss ML: Growth of the calvaria in the rat; the determination of osseous morphology. Am J Anat 1954;94:333–361.
38 Pritchard JJ, Scott JH, Girgis FG: The structure and development of cranial and facial sutures. J Anat 1956;90:73–86.
39 Moss ML: Functional anatomy of cranial synostosis. Childs Brain 1975;1:22–33.
40 Smith DW, Tondury G: Origin of the calvaria and its sutures. Am J Dis Child 1978;132:662–666.
41 Hall BK, Miyake T: All for one and one for all: condensations and the initiation of skeletal development. Bioessays 2000;22:138–147.
42 Carapuco M, Novoa A, Bobola N, Mallo M: Hox genes specify vertebral types in the presomitic mesoderm. Genes Dev 2005;19:2116–2121.
43 Creuzet S, Couly G, Vincent G, Le Douarin NM: Negative effect of Hox gene expression on the development of the neural crest-derived facial skeleton. Development 2002;129:4301–4313.
44 Kanzler B, Kuschert SJ, Liu YH, Mallo M: Hoxa-2 restricts the chondrogenic domain and inhibits bone formation during development of the branchial area. Development 1998;125:2587–2597.
45 Depew MJ, Simpson CA, Morasso M, Rubenstein JL: Reassessing the Dlx code: the genetic regulation of branchial arch skeletal pattern and development. J Anat 2005;207:501–561.
46 Trumpp A, Depew MJ, Rubenstein JL, Bishop JM, Martin GR: Cre-mediated gene inactivation demonstrates that FGF8 is required for cell survival and patterning of the first branchial arch. Genes Dev 1999;13:3136–3148.
47 Creuzet S, Schuler B, Couly G, Le Douarin NM: Reciprocal relationships between Fgf8 and neural crest cells in facial and forebrain development. Proc Natl Acad Sci USA 2004;101:4843–4847.
48 Decker JD, Hall SH: Light and electron microscopy of the new born sagittal suture. Anat Rec 1985;212:81–89.
49 Markens IS: Embryonic development of the coronal suture in man and rat. Acta Anat (Basel) 1975;93:257–273.
50 Kokich V: The biology of sutures; in Cohen MJ (ed): Craniosynostosis: Diagnosis, Evaluation and Management. New York, Raven Press, 1986, chap 4.
51 Schaffer J: Die Stützgewebe; in von Möllendorf W (ed): Handbuch der mikroskopischen Anatomie des Menschen. Berlin, Julius Springer, 1930, pp 338–350.
52 Vinkka H: Secondary cartilages in the facial skeleton of the rat. Proc Finn Dent Soc 1982;78(suppl 7): 1–137.

53 Manzanares MC, Goret-Nicaise M, Dhem A: Metopic sutural closure in the human skull. J Anat 1988;161:203–215.
54 Sahar DE, Longaker MT, Quarto N: Sox9 neural crest determinant gene controls patterning and closure of the posterior frontal cranial suture. Dev Biol 2005;280:344–361.
55 Hall BK: Cellular differentiation in skeletal tissues. Biol Rev Camb Philos Soc 1970;45:455–484.
56 Persson M: The role of sutures in normal and abnormal craniofacial growth. Acta Odontol Scand 1995;53:152–161.
57 Jane J, Persing J: Neurosurgical treatment of craniosynostosis; in Cohen MJ, Maclean R (eds): Craniosynostosis Diagnosis, Evaluation, and Management. Oxford, Oxford University Press, 2001, chap 18.
58 Bjork A, Skieller V: Growth of the maxilla in three dimensions as revealed radiographically by the implant method. Br J Orthod 1977;4:53–64.
59 Bjork A, Skieller V: Facial development and tooth eruption. An implant study at the age of puberty. Am J Orthod 1972;62:339–383.
60 Rice D: Molecular Mechanisms in Calvarial Bone and Suture Development; PhD thesis. Helsinki, Helsinki University Press, 1999.
61 Bjork A: Sutural growth of the upper face studied by the implant method. Acta Odontol Scand 1966;24:109–127.
62 Jaslow CR: Mechanical properties of cranial sutures. J Biomech 1990;23:313–321.
63 Anton SC, Jaslow CR, Swartz SM: Sutural complexity in artificially deformed human *(Homo sapiens)* crania. J Morphol 1992;214:321–332.
64 Todd T, Lyon D: Cranial suture closure. Its progress and age relationship. II. Ectocranial closure in adult males of white stock. Am J Phys Anthropol 1925;8:23–45.
65 Miroue M, Rosenberg L: The Human Facial Sutures: A Morphometric and Histologic Study of Age Changes from 20 to 95 Years. Masters thesis. Seattle, University of Washington, 1975.
66 Persson M, Thilander B: Palatal suture closure in man from 15 to 35 years of age. Am J Orthod 1977;72:42–52.
67 Bradley JP, Levine JP, Roth DA, McCarthy JG, Longaker MT: Studies in cranial suture biology. IV. Temporal sequence of posterior frontal cranial suture fusion in the mouse. Plast Reconstr Surg 1996;98:1039–1045.
68 Opperman LA, Nolen AA, Ogle RC: TGF-beta 1, TGF-beta 2, and TGF-beta 3 exhibit distinct patterns of expression during cranial suture formation and obliteration in vivo and in vitro. J Bone Miner Res 1997;12:301–310.
69 Moss ML: Fusion of the frontal suture in the rat. Am J Anat 1958;102:141–165.
70 Roth DA, Longaker MT, McCarthy JG, Rosen DM, McMullen HF, Levine JP, Sung J, Gold LI: Studies in cranial suture biology. I. Increased immunoreactivity for TGF-beta isoforms (beta 1, beta 2, and beta 3) during rat cranial suture fusion. J Bone Miner Res 1997;12:311–321.
71 Skieller V: Expansion of the midpalatal suture by removable palates, analysed by the implant method. Rep Congr Eur Orthod Soc 1964;40:143–158.

Dr. David P. Rice
Professor of Orthodontics
Institute of Dentistry and Helsinki University Central Hospital
Box 41, University of Helsinki
FIN–00014 Helsinki (Finland)
E-Mail David.Rice@helsinki.fi

Rice DP (ed): Craniofacial Sutures. Development, Disease and Treatment.
Front Oral Biol. Basel, Karger, 2008, vol 12, pp 22–40

Locate, Condense, Differentiate, Grow and Confront: Developmental Mechanisms Controlling Intramembranous Bone and Suture Formation and Function

David P. Rice, Ritva Rice

Departments of Orthodontics and Craniofacial Development, King's College London, London, UK; Department of Orthodontics, University of Helsinki, Helsinki, Finland

Abstract

The key mechanisms controlling where and when craniofacial bones and hence sutures form are discussed in this review. These include the formation and growth of skeletogenic condensations, tissue to tissue interactions between the epithelium, skeletogenic mesenchyme and the underlying dural and neural tissues. Also discussed are the key processes determining intramembranous bone growth, namely osteoblastogenesis and osteoclastogenesis.

Mesenchymal Skeletogenic Condensations

Condensation formation is a fundamental stage in skeletogenesis. Osteogenic condensations not only determine when and where a bony element will form but also influence the final size and shape of many bones. The first morphological sign of bone formation, whether it is through intramembranous or endochondral ossification, is the establishment of a condensation of cells. Cellular condensation is the first step in the morphogenesis of most (mesodermally) mesenchymally derived organs.

Condensation occurs following the migration of cells to a specific location and then stimulation to start the condensation process for example through epithelial-mesenchymal tissue interaction. Dispersed cells begin to aggregate, this cell population expands and then differentiates into a single cell type, either chondroblasts or osteoblasts in the case of skeletogenic condensations (fig. 1). Condensations can be visualized morphologically as a tightly packed mass of

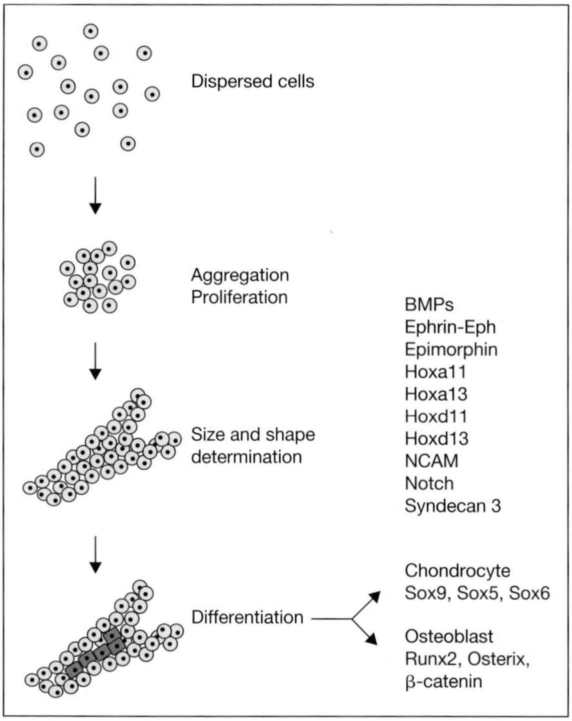

Fig. 1. Skeletogenic condensation formation. Once mesenchymal cells are at the correct location and have received the inductive signals to start skeletogenesis, dispersed morphologically indistinct cells begin to aggregate into a cluster of cells. The cell population expands by proliferation and the mass/condensation begins to take on (resemble) the same shape as the final skeletal element. Cells in the center of this cell mass then differentiate into osteoblasts or chondroblasts.

cells. Chondrogenic condensations can be observed with peanut agglutinin lectin histochemistry [1] and osteogenic and chondrogenic condensations can be localized by their ability to transiently express *Thrombospondin-4*, a glycoprotein. Mouse skeletogenic condensations express also other molecular markers including *aggrecan*, *type I collagen* and a splice variant of *type II collagen*, *αI*, that is not specific to chondrocytes. The key stages and processes of condensation formation and function are (1) the initiation of cells to aggregate into a tightly packed mass, (2) boundary determination, (3) the control of cell turnover, (4) cell adhesion, (5) cell differentiation and function, and (6) the regulation of condensation growth. The processes of osteogenic condensation formation and function during embryogenesis, to form the first bony elements, are directly comparable with the processes of cell aggregation, proliferation, differentiation and function that occur in the osteogenic fronts of established craniofacial intramembranous bones. Thus data from the suture model can be used to help us understand the developmental processes occurring in osteogenic condensations. Conversely information from condensation models can be applied to the developing suture to help study its function and dysfunction.

Initiation

Condensations are initiated by location-specific signals. Although the source and nature of these signals are largely unknown, it is known that cues from the adjacent epithelium can stimulate the process. Mesenchymal cells then react by a combination of enhanced cell turnover, aggregation toward a focus and failure to disperse away from that focus [2]. A variety of extracellular matrix and cell surface molecules including syndecans, neural cell adhesion molecule (NCAM) and neural cadherin (N-cadherin) are all thought to be important in mesenchymal condensate formation [3]. NCAM is known to mediate cell adhesion and is thought to play a role in the initiation of the condensation process. Tgfβs regulate the glycoprotein fibronectin which in turn regulates NCAM [3–5].

Other growth factors involved in the initiation process include the bone morphogenetic proteins (BMPs). Misexpression of the BMP antagonist Noggin in the avian limb leads to an absence of skeletal elements with mesenchymal cells not aggregating into prechondrogenic condensations [6]. Notch signaling may act at multiple stages during osteoblast and chondroblast development. Notch appears to be a negative regulator of the early stages of prechondrogenic condensation formation, with loss-of-function experiments in limb micromass culture promoting the initiation of prechondrogenic condensations [7].

During vertebral bone formation the extracellular factor Epimorphin is involved in the earliest initiation stages, promoting cell aggregation and cell sorting in prechondrogenic condensations. *Epimorphin* expression is regulated by SHH from the notochord and mediated by Sox9 [8]. Sox9 is a transcription factor that acts at multiple steps during skeletogenesis. It is essential for chondrocyte differentiation but also has a role in condensation initiation as inactivation of *Sox9* from the mesenchyme of limb buds prior to condensation formation results in a complete absence of bone and cartilage.

Condensation Boundary, Size and Shape Determination

The size and shape of a condensation are, in part, determined by the factors regulating the boundary between the condensation and the surrounding tissue.

Ephrin-Eph signaling is important in many developmental systems in controlling cell sorting, cell movement and boundary formation. An example of this is the establishment and maintenance of the boundary between the cranial neural crest and mesodermally derived tissues in the developing calvaria [9]. This boundary occurs at the coronal suture with abnormalities in ephrin-Eph signaling resulting in defects in cell segregation and ultimately synostosis across the suture.

Both Eph receptors and ephrin ligands can activate downstream signaling cascades simultaneously thus permitting bidirectional signaling. Signaling through the membrane-bound ephrin ligands is called reverse signaling and through the Eph receptors, forward signaling. Ephrin-Eph signaling can respond to environmental cues which are important in the initial stages of skeletogenesis. Taken together, ephrin-Ephs are excellent candidates for a role in the setting up of the boundaries around skeletogenic condensations and controlling their size and shape.

The *Hox* family of genes encode transcription factors which control regional identity and cell fates in the body axis and limbs. Genes at the 5′ end of the *Hox* clusters, *Hoxa9–13* and *Hoxd9–13*, control the timing, position, size and shape of the individual bones in the limb and they appear to do this by acting at the mesenchymal condensation stage as well as later in skeletogenesis. This regulation is mediated through hedgehog, BMP and ephrin-Eph signaling [10, 11].

Misexpression of *Hoxa13* in the avian limb results in cartilage homeotic transformations and a reduction in bone length. Specifically, *Hoxa13* controls cartilage size by regulating cell-to-cell adhesiveness during the prechondrogenic condensation stage [12]. *Hoxd11* also acts at the initial stages of cartilage condensation with misexpression in the hind limb producing two phalanges instead of one [13]. *Hoxa13* controls limb skeletal morphogenesis through BMP and ephrin-Eph signaling. Hoxa13 directly binds to BMP2 and BMP7, and the expression of *BMP2* and *BMP7* is reduced in *Hoxa13*$^{-/-}$ mutant mice. Also, exogenous application of BMP2 or BMP7 partially rescues the digit abnormalities seen in *Hoxa13*$^{-/-}$ mice.

Loss of *EphA7* expression correlates with loss of cell adhesion and chondrogenic capacity in *Hoxa13*$^{-/-}$ mouse limbs [10]. In addition, blocking EphA7, with neutralizing antibodies, inhibits the capacity of *Hoxa13*$^{+/-}$ cells to condense and form chondrogenic nodules. However, the expression of *EphA7* in *Hoxa13*$^{-/-}$ mice is not completely abolished, which suggests that other proteins may also regulate *EphA7*. An obvious candidate for this is the paralogous group 13 Hox protein, Hoxd13, which has an overlapping gene expression profile with that of *Hoxa13*. Also, *Hoxa13*$^{-/-}$ and *Hoxd13*$^{-/-}$ mice have overlapping phenotypes with malformations in the same skeletal tissues observed in both mice. As predicted Hoxd13 upregulates *EphA7*, and *EphA7* is a direct target of both Hoxa13 and Hoxd13 [11]. *Hoxa13*$^{-/-}$;*Hoxd13*$^{-/-}$ mice exhibit a more severe phenotype than the single knockout mice, showing an almost complete lack of limb skeletogenic condensation formation.

The functional cooperation of paralogous *Hox* genes at the condensation stage of skeletogenesis is also demonstrated by *Hoxa11*$^{-/-}$;*Hoxd11*$^{-/-}$ mice which have smaller condensations than controls [14]. That said, the major limb defects exhibited by *Hoxa11*$^{-/-}$; *Hoxd11*$^{-/-}$ mice appear to be due to later defects in chondrocyte maturation rather than an early disruption in condensation formation.

The heparan sulphate proteoglycan syndecan 3 has been implicated in regulating condensation boundary and size [2]. Syndecans are (single-pass) integral cell membrane components that act as co-receptors for growth factors and activate signal transduction via their cytoplasmic domains. They form an integral part in mediating BMP, fibroblast growth factor (FGF) and hedgehog (HH) signaling during skeletogenesis [15]. Syndecan 3 is known to interact with FGF2/FGFR signaling during early limb development. FGFs produced in the apical ectodermal ridge, a morphologically distinct region at the growing tip of the developing limb bud, mediate the outgrowth of the limb by stimulating proliferation in the underlying mesodermal cells. This development is dependent on syndecan 3 with disruption of syndecan 3 function resulting in an inhibition of FGF-driven outgrowth. Indeed, FGF2 upregulates *syndecan 3*. During avian development syndecan 3 is localized to the cell layer surrounding prechondrogenic limb condensations. This localization together with its localization in the mesodermal cells in the developing limb and also in the proliferative zone in the growth plate is consistent with a role in restricting mitotic activity to specific locations and with regard to skeletogenic condensations, controlling their size and growth rate. Heparan sulfate proteoglycans, including syndecan 3, have been shown to modulate the activity of BMPs available for signaling during cartilage differentiation in limb micromass culture [16]. As BMPs have been shown to play a role in mesenchymal proliferation and differentiation, this may have implications for condensation proliferation as well as cell fate determination. Also, the transcription factor Pax2, which is regulated by BMP7, controls condensation size.

It is known that syndecan 3 binds to fibronectin to disrupt cell adhesion via the inactivation of NCAM. Tenascin-C and tenascin-W are extracellular glycoproteins that bind to syndecans and regulate cellular responses to fibronectin. In cell culture, tenascin-C antagonizes the adhesive effects of fibronectin and blocks cell cycle progression of anchorage-dependent fibroblasts on fibronectin through inhibition of syndecan-4. Tenascin-C and tenascin-W have similar expression patterns in the developing bones and may be able to functionally compensate for one another as the *tenascin-C*$^{-/-}$ mouse does not have a bony phenotype [17]. Taken together, the combined function of syndecans and tenascins appears to regulate cell proliferation and prevent cell spreading which regulates the perimeter of the condensation and condensation size.

Cell Adhesion

Cell to cell and cell to matrix adhesion is known to be important at many stages during skeletogenic condensation formation and function. We have already seen how NCAM, fibronectin and extracellular proteoglycans and glycoproteins interact with growth factors to regulate condensation initiation, help set up the condensation boundaries and regulate condensation size. Cadherins are integral cell membrane glycoproteins that are important in anchoring adherens junctions (intercellular junctions) to the actin cytoskeleton via multiprotein complexes that include α-catenin and β-catenin and plakoglobin [18]. As β-catenin also binds to Tcf/Lef transcription factors to regulate canonical Wnt growth factor signaling, β-catenin can act as a convergence point in the control of cell to cell adhesion as well as Wnt signaling. The extent of adherens junction formation, mediated by N-cadherin in chondrogenic micromass cultures, can modulate Wnt-induced nuclear activity of β-catenin [19]. Destabilization of the β-catenin association may increase the transcriptionally active pool of β-catenin, thus lowering the threshold for Wnt signaling [18]. Taken together, caherins can modulate Wnt signal transduction which is known to control skeletogenic cell fate [20].

Through loss-of-function antibody or transfection studies and also gain-of-function studies it has been possible to show that N-cadherin promotes the early stages of condensation formation. In addition, N-cadherin needs to be downregulated for chondrocyte differentiation to progress, probably by stabilizing cell to cell adhesion and/or increasing the threshold for Wnt signaling. Although important, N-cadherin appears not to be essential for chondrogenesis as limbs taken from *N-cadherin*$^{-/-}$ mice, which normally die prior to the start of skeletogenesis at E10, can form cartilage in organ culture [21]. The authors of this study suggest that cadherin11 might functionally compensate for N-cadherin during the condensation phase of chondrogenesis.

In contrast to chondrogenesis where *N-cadherin* is lost as chondrocytes differentiate, during osteogenesis *N-cadherin* and *cadherin11* expression are maintained but the expression of *R-cadherin (cadherin 4)* is downregulated. N-cadherin and E-cadherin mediate early human calvaria osteoblast differentiation promoted by BMP2 [22]. Transgenic expression of a dominant negative, truncated form of N-cadherin targeted to osteoblasts results in a delay in osteoblast differentiation and a switch of cell fate with more adipose cells forming rather than osteoblasts from multipotent mesenchymal cells. As a consequence bone mineral density is reduced. This phenotype can be rescued by transcriptional overactivation β-catenin [23].

FGF signaling is important in regulating osteogenesis and mutations in *FGFRs* cause several craniosynostosis syndromes, characterized by abnormal osteogenesis in the calvaria [24] [see Passos-Bueno et al., pp. 107–143 and

Hajihosseini, pp. 160–177]. FGF2 increases cell to cell adhesion and *N-cadherin* expression in calvarial cell cultures and the effect on cell adhesion is blocked by application of neutralizing antibodies to N-cadherin. The S252W mutation in FGFR2 confers a gain-of-function which results in Apert syndrome craniosynostosis. S252W mutant osteoblasts show increased N-cadherin but not NCAM mRNA and protein levels. The mutation leads to increased cell to cell adhesion and increased osteoblast marker gene activation. Effects that are suppressed by neutralizing antibodies to N-cadherin, but not NCAM [25].

Cell Differentiation

Once mesenchymal condensations reach a critical threshold size cells in the center of the condensation stop proliferating and differentiation is initiated [26]. For cell differentiation into a chondrogenic or osteoblastic lineage to occur firstly condensation promoting genes must be downregulated and then chondroblastic or osteoblastic-specific genes must be upregulated [2].

Wnt growth factor signaling through β-catenin has key roles at multiple stages of osteoblast and chondroblast differentiation [20]. β-Catenin negatively regulates the differentiation of multipotent mesenchymal cells into a skeletogenic precursor, common to osteoblasts and chondroblasts. High levels of β-catenin and upregulation of the transcription factor Runx2 are associated with differentiation into a precursor cell which still has both osteo- and chondrogenic potential with final commitment into an osteoblastic lineage dependent on the transcription factor Osterix [27]. Conversely, downregulation of β-catenin and upregulation of the transcription factors Sox9 and later Sox5 and Sox6 is required to send mesenchymal cells down a chondroblastic lineage [20]. Wnt signaling through Wnt10b and the co-receptor Lrp5 positively control the expansion of the population of committed osteoblastic precursors and Axin2, a scaffold protein which promotes the degradation of β-catenin, suppresses this proliferation. *Axin2*$^{-/-}$ mutants exhibit craniosynostosis [28].

Tissue Interactions

Calvarial bones grow in close contact with dura mater which is the outermost layer of the meninges covering the brain. Interactions between dural cells and the calvarial mesenchyme have been shown to be important in the regulation of osteogenesis within a suture and thus in the control of suture patency. These interactions are required to maintain rodent coronal and sagittal sutures open with fusion occurring if the dura mater is removed [29, 30]. Conversely, the dura mater has also been shown to regulate suture closure. The posterior frontal (PF) suture in mice and rats fuses postnatally (25–45 and 12–30 days, respectively), while all other calvarial sutures remain open long into adulthood. By placing different-sized mesh and other barriers between the dura and suture it has been established that soluble factors rather than cell-cell or cell-matrix interactions control this regulation [31]. Placement of a silicone sheet between the dura mater and the PF suture, which prevents signaling between the two layers, results in delayed suture fusion [32].

Location-specific cues from the dura mater also regulate suture patency. Experiments involving the surgical removal and translocation of the sagittal and PF sutures, so that the sagittal suture sits over the dura of the PF suture and the PF suture sits over the sagittal suture dura, result in the abnormal fusion of the sagittal suture and the PF suture remaining patent. Increased levels of Tgfβ1 and Fgf2 proteins are produced in the dura mater underlying the PF suture just prior to and during the fusion while the patent sagittal suture produces only low levels of these growth factors [33]. Greenwald et al. [34] targeted an adenoviral construct of secreted form of Fgf2 to PF or coronal dura mater in vivo to demonstrate that Fgf2 was responsible for the increased proliferation, extracellular matrix molecule synthesis, and for the synthesis of Tgfβ1. They also showed that a similar targeting of a truncated form of Fgfr1, which blocks Fgf signaling, caused infected PF sutures to stay patent. This elegant study showed that Fgf signaling regulates postnatal suture fate. Differential signaling through Tgfβ isoforms produced by the dura mater have been shown to control calvarial suture patency. Tgfβ2 has a role in promoting suture fusion while Tgfβ3 is required to help keep sutures patent [35]. In humans mutations in *TGFβ receptors 1* and *2*, which are proposed to confer a gain-of-function, cause craniosynostosis [24]. This correlates well with the loss of *Tgfβr2* studies in mice which result in an absence of frontal bone and a delay in parietal bone development [36].

Unlike calvarial sutures, facial sutures are not in contact with the dura mater. So do other external cues regulate facial suture morphogenesis, function and patency in a similar way to those signals originating in the dura which control calvarial sutures? It has been hypothesized that other tissues in the face play an equivalent signaling role to that of the dura. And it has been shown that the nasal capsular cartilages, which develop adjacent to the median palatal suture, regulate suture patency, with the rat median palatal suture fusing if it is not cocultured with the nasal cartilages [37].

Interaction of cranial neural crest cells with the epithelium is known to influence skeletogenesis over a critical period during development. Outgrowth of the mandible is controlled by epithelial mesenchymal interactions. The growth factor endothelin 1 (ET1) is produced in the branchial arch epithelium and signals through its receptor endothelin A (ETA) which is located in the underlying mesenchyme. Ablation of either ET1 or ETA results in a severe truncation of the mandible [38].

Intramembranous Bone Formation and Growth

The majority of the bones of the face and calvaria form by intramembranous ossification. During this process bones develop within a 'membranous' sheet of mesenchyme with osteoblastic precursors condensing, proliferating and then differentiating directly into functioning osteoblasts. This is in contrast to endochondral ossification, which occurs in the cranial base and the majority of the bones of the appendicular and axial skeleton, where firstly a cartilagenous scaffold is made which is subsequently removed by chondro/osteoclasts and finally replaced by bone formed by osteoblasts.

Osteoblastogenesis

Osteoblast differentiation, at a transcriptional level, is controlled by the runt domain-containing protein Runx2 (Cbfa1), the zinc finger-containing protein Osterix (Osx) and β-catenin [20, 39].

Runx2 is a transcriptional activator of osteoblast differentiation which activates most osteoblastic markers including osteocalcin, bone sialoprotein and collagen α1(I) [40]. It is one of a three-member family of closely related genes that encode the α-chain DNA binding components of the heterodimeric core binding factor complex (Cbf). Several isoforms of RUNX2 have been isolated which bind to an osteoblast *cis*-acting element in the osteocalcin promoter [41]. Haploinsufficiency of RUNX2 in humans results in cleidocranial dysplasia (OMIM 119600) which is characterized by delayed ossification of the calvarial sutures and fontanelles, dental anomalies including supernumerary and unerupted teeth, hypoplastic or missing clavicles and short stature [24].

Runx2$^{-/-}$ mice exhibit a dramatic phenotype with an almost complete absence of osteoblasts. *Runx2*$^{-/-}$ mice also have defects in chondrocyte differentiation and maturation. Core-binding factor beta (Cbfβ) heterodimerizes with Runx2 before activating transcriptional targets. Using conditional approaches which rescue the midgestation lethality of *Cbf*β$^{-/-}$ mice due to defective hematopoiesis, several groups have shown that Cbfβ is required for Runx2 function during skeletal development [42]. *Cbf*β$^{-/-}$ mice exhibit a delay in endochondral and intramembranous ossification with a similar, but less severe, skeletal phenotype to that seen in *Runx2*$^{-/-}$ *mice.*

Runx2 is regulated by phosphorylation and several transcription factors including Stat1 (signal transducer and activator of transcription 1) and Twist1. Stat1 interacts with Runx2 in its latent form, not in the nucleus but in the cytoplasm. This inhibits nuclear localization of Runx2 and consequently its nuclear transcriptional activity. *Stat1*-deficient mice exhibit accelerated osteoblast differentiation which results in increased bone mass. Runx2 is also inhibited by the Twist1 protein through direct binding to the Twist box sequence [43]. As might be predicted loss-of-function mutations in *TWIST1* do not cause cleidocranial dysplasia but result in craniosynostosis, with excessive osteogenesis of the calvarial bones [24]. *Twist1* is expressed by early osteoprogenitors but not by mature osteoblasts and has been suggested to act as a negative regulator of osteogenesis [44, 45]. Double heterozygotes for *Twist1* and *Runx2* deletion show a partial rescue of the widened calvarial sutures seen in *Runx2*$^{+/-}$ mice [43].

Osterix is genetically downstream of Runx2 as *Runx2* expression is maintained in *Osx*$^{-/-}$ mice, but *Osx* is not expressed in *Runx*2$^{-/-}$ mice [27]. *Osx*$^{-/-}$ mice exhibit a similar phenotype to that of *Runx2*$^{-/-}$ mice with a complete lack of differentiated osteoblasts. Mesenchymal condensations are generated in *Osx*$^{-/-}$ mice and in addition to expressing *Runx2*, *Osx*$^{-/-}$ osteoblastic precursors also express chondrocyte marker genes. This suggests that *Runx2*-positive cells still possess chondrocyte/osteoblast bipotential. It has been speculated that Osx may act as a negative regulator of chondrocyte differentiation by inhibiting *Sox9* and *Sox5* [27].

Canonical Wnt signaling is important during osteoblast differentiation with the transcriptional regulator β-catenin playing a key role. Wnt ligands bind to frizzled receptors and LRP5 and LRP6 co-receptors. Signal transduction is then induced which involves the stabilization of β-catenin (dephosphorylation) which enables β-catenin to form a transcription activation complex involving TCF/LEF proteins. Gain of *LRP5* function results in increased bone mass caused by increased bone formation resulting in increased bone density, enlarged mandible and the bony outgrowth torus palatinus [46]. Conversely, loss of *LRP5* function results in reduced bone mass. Conditional deletion of *β-catenin* in cranial neural crest cells (Wnt1-Cre) causes a total absence of facial and calvarial bones, except for the interparietal bone which is of mesodermal origin [47]. A total blockade of osteoblast differentiation with calvarial mesenchymal cells differentiating into chondrocytes instead of osteoblasts is seen in mice carrying a conditional deactivation of *β-catenin* in mesenchymal progenitors (Dermo1-Cre and Prx1-Cre) [20, 48, 49]. Axin2 forms part of a destruction complex that aids β-catenin phosphorylation and therefore deactivation. *Axin2*$^{-/-}$ mice exhibit increased calvarial osteoblastic progenitor proliferation, which results in craniosynostosis [28].

Other transcription factors which have nonessential roles in osteoblast differentiation include Msx1, Msx2, Dlx5, Atf4, AP1(Fos/Jun), Krox20 and Sp3 [39, 50].

Taken together, Runx2, Osterix and β-catenin are all essential for osteoblast differentiation. Runx2 functions at multiple stages, firstly directing multipotent mesenchymal cells into a skeletogenic chondrocyte/osteoblast cell fate. Following this Runx2, Osterix and β-catenin direct cells down an osteoblastic lineage and at the same time inhibit them from differentiating into

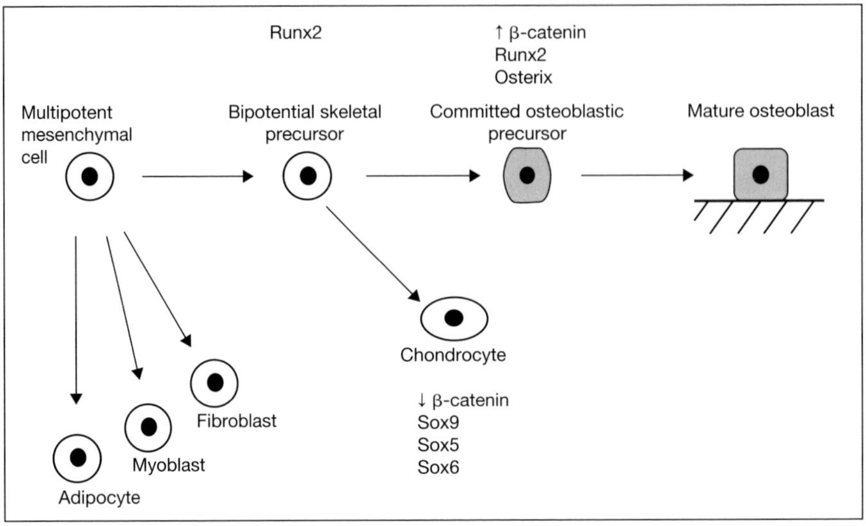

Fig. 2. Transcriptional control of osteoblast differentiation. Osteoblasts differentiate from multipotent mesenchymal cells. Runx2 is known to promote initial differentiation into skeletogenic cells with potential to develop into either osteoblasts or chondrocytes. Following this the combined action of Runx2, elevated β-catenin and the osteoblastic commitment factor Osterix result in differentiation into a committed osteoblastic progenitor. A reduced level of β-catenin and elevated levels of Sox9, Sox5 and Sox6 result in the bipotential progenitors following a chondrocytic lineage.

chondrocytes (fig. 2). In addition, Runx2 is thought to play a role in limiting the terminal differentiation of osteoblasts into osteocytes, thus maintaining the active osteoblastic population [51].

Wnts are not the only growth factors to play key roles during osteoblast development. BMP, FGF, HH, TGFβ and insulin growth factor signaling are all active [52]. Ihh is essential for osteoblast differentiation in bones that form by endochondral ossification, with bones of the axial and appendicular skeleton devoid of Runx2-positive osteoblasts in *Ihh*$^{-/-}$ mice. However, intramembranous bone development continues, with *Ihh*$^{-/-}$ mutants forming calvarial bones [53]. It is anticipated that crosstalk between different signaling pathways during osteoblast development will occur at multiple levels. One example of this is between HH and Wnt-β-catenin signaling which are integrated during the early stages of long bone osteoblast development [49].

Although BMP2, BMP4, BMP6 and BMP7 are known to promote osteogenesis in vitro, using mouse genetics it has not been possible to demonstrate a direct role for these BMPs in osteoblast differentiation [52]. However,

BMP3$^{-/-}$ mice do have a bony phenotype which has confirmed its role as a negative regulator of osteogenesis [54]. Indirect evidence through the analysis of transcription factors that are regulated by BMPs, namely Msx1, Msx2, Foxc1 and Alx4, and the analysis of BMP inhibitors such as noggin have demonstrated roles for BMPs during calvarial bone and suture development [29, 55–58]. Through the analysis of *FGF18*$^{-/-}$ mice, FGF18 has been shown to be a positive regulator of osteoblastic proliferation and differentiation and a negative regulator of chondrogenesis [59]. BMP, FGF and TGFβ signaling pathways will be discussed at length in relation to suture development and function later in this book.

Osteoclastogenesis and the Crosstalk between Osteoblasts and Osteoclasts

Intramembranous bone development is not just about bone formation (osteoblast differentiation and function) but also about bone resorption in the form of modeling newly formed bone and later remodeling. The cells responsible for bone resorption are osteoclasts and in the developing calvaria osteoclasts appear relatively early during bone development, at E16.5 in the mouse, only 3 days after bone development has commenced [60]. Although some osteoclasts are located in the sutures, where they have a role in the maintenance of suture patency, most resorption occurs on the endocranial surface of the developing calvarial bones. This is balanced by apposition on the ectocranial surfaces so that the calvaria expands in unison with the developing brain. Thus bone development is a co-ordination of bone formation and degradation.

Osteoclasts develop from hematopoietic progenitor cells. Much of our knowledge of the regulation of osteoclast differentiation comes from the study of mutant mice with osteopetrotic phenotypes, characterized by increased bone density caused by reduced osteoclast numbers or activity. The transcription factor PU.1 is responsible for the earliest step in osteoclast differentiation. *PU.1*$^{-/-}$ mice lack not only osteoblasts but also macrophages, which share a common progenitor. *PU.1*$^{-/-}$ mice do however have monocytes and the phenotype can be rescued by bone marrow transplantation which tells us that PU.1 acts at a level after the monocytic lineage has been established but before the division of the macrophage/osteoclast lineage (fig. 3). After commitment to an osteoclastic lineage, progenitors require macrophage colony-stimulating factor (M-CSF) for further differentiation. Osteopetrotic mice, *op/op*, that lack *M-CSF* form macrophages but not osteoclasts. The inability of marrow transplantation to cure this phenotype indicates that M-CSF is produced by cells external to the hematopoietic system [39].

Nuclear factor κB (NFκB) is a family of dimeric transcription factors composed of various combinations of structurally related proteins: p50 (NFκB1),

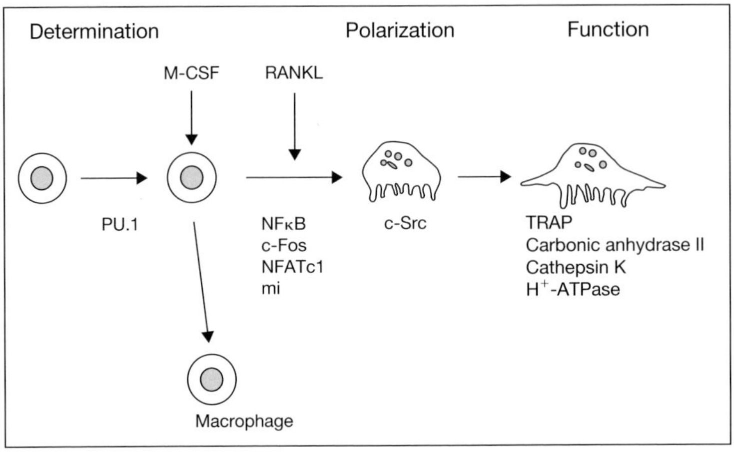

Fig. 3. Osteoclast differentiation. The transcription factor PU.1 is the first to direct multipotent hematopoietic cells into a macrophage/osteoclast lineage. Thereafter the secreted factors M-CSF and RANKL, produced by osteoblasts and stromal cells, and the transcription factors NFκB, c-Fos, NFATc1 and mi act to control osteoclast differentiation. Mice lacking the non-receptor tyrosine kinase, c-Src, can form multifunctional osteoclastic cells but these are nonfunctional. Osteoclast function including dissolution of mineral and collagen is regulated by the enzymes TRAP, carbonic anhydrase II, H^+-ATPase and cathepsin K.

p52 (NFκB2), p65 (RelA), C-Rel (Rel) and RelB. Mice lacking both *p50* and *p52* subunits exhibit a severe osteopetrotic phenotype, but here osteoclast differentiation is affected at a slightly later stage compared to the mice described above. This inability to form osteoclasts is contrasted by the ability of $p50^{-/-}$; $p52^{-/-}$ mice to form nonfunctional macrophages [61].

NFκB is activated by RANK (receptor activator of NFκB)/RANK ligand (RANKL) signaling, as are several other transcription factors critical for osteoclast differentiation. These include the activator protein 1 protein c-Fos and NFATc1 (nuclear factor of activated T cells, cytoplasmic, calcineurin-dependent 1). *c-Fos* null mice exhibit an osteopetrotic phenotype. Embryonic stem cells which can differentiate into osteoclasts in response to RANKL fail to differentiate into osteoclasts if *NFATc1* is deactivated. c-Fos appears to act upstream of NFATc1. c-Fos is required for *NFATc1* expression and in the presence of RANKL, NFATc1 rescues osteoclastogenesis in precursors lacking c-Fos [62].

Osteopetrotic mice that have normal numbers of osteoclasts but whose osteoclasts are unable to resorb bone demonstrate that tartrate-resistant acid phosphatase (TRAP), calcitonin, carbonic anhydrase II and cathepsin K, as well as others, are important for osteoclast function (fig. 3) [52].

Appropriate communication between osteoclasts and osteoblasts is central to co-ordinated bone development and growth as well as many other processes including the maintenance of suture patency, fracture repair and calcium homeostasis. Two growth factors, M-CSF and RANKL, are necessary and sufficient to drive osteoclastogenesis and are integral to the crosstalk between osteoclastic progenitors and other cells, notably stromal cells and osteoblasts [63]. RANKL, a tumor necrosis factor-related protein, is bound to the surface of many cell types including osteoblasts and stromal cells. RANKL activates its receptor RANK, a transmembrane receptor expressed by osteoclastic precursors. Underlining the importance of this direct cell-to-cell communication both $RANKL^{-/-}$ and $RANK^{-/-}$ mice have an identical osteopetrotic phenotype with a complete lack of osteoclasts [63].

Osteoprotegerin (OPG) is a secreted receptor that lacks a transmembrane domain. OPG acts in a dominant negative manner to inhibit osteoclastogenesis by competing with RANK for RANKL binding sites. Overexpression of *OPG* leads to osteopetrosis whereas deletion of *OPG* causes enhanced osteoclastic activity resulting in osteoporosis [52]. In a regulatory feedback mechanism, OPG is produced by osteoblasts in response to estrogens, TGFβs and BMPs. Taken together, osteoblasts/stromal cells co-ordinate modeling and remodeling by stimulating the local differentiation and activation of osteoclasts through direct RANKL/RANK signaling. This process is tempered by OPG.

Intramembranous Bone Growth

Craniofacial intramembranous bones develop from initial ossification centers and these expanding bones will either confront each other and form a suture, or merge to create a single bony unit [see Rice, pp. 1–21]. Growth occurs at the leading edges or osteogenic fronts of the immature bones and when these bony fronts converge a suture is formed. Intramembranous bone growth not only occurs at the two osteogenic fronts of each suture but also in the periosteum. In the developing calvaria this appositional growth occurs mainly on the ectocranial surfaces to increase the bone thickness. Bone development and growth are not just about osteoblastic apposition but a coordinated process of formation and destruction. In the developing calvaria, synchronized appositional and resorptive activity allows expansion of the underlying brain while maintaining bone thickness and suture patency. In the face, the balance between osteoblastic apposition and osteoclastic resorption has a large effect on determining the final shape and size of each bony element.

Presumably agonists and antagonists of the Tgfβ superfamily, FGF, HH and Wnt signaling pathways control the growth of intramembranous bones from initial condensation to their final size, but we know relatively little about this process. We do know however that this enlargement is regulated by the

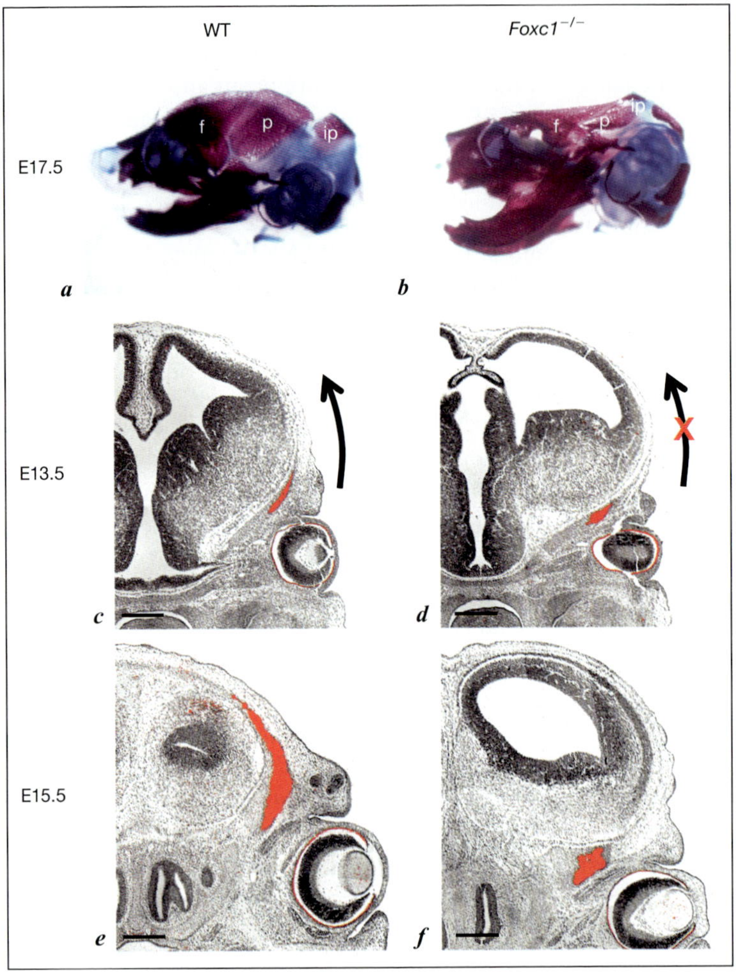

Fig. 4. Calvarial bone growth. The progression of calvarial bone development requires the regulation of *Msx2* and *Alx4* by Foxc1. *Foxc1*$^{-/-}$ mice exhibit a lack of calvarial bone growth with the frontal and parietal bones staying rudimentary in size and location. ***a***, ***b*** Alizarin red and alcian blue staining. ***c–f*** E13.5 and E15.5 frontal tissue sections; mineralized bone is visualized by *bone sialoprotein* expression. Scale bars: 200 μm. f = Frontal bone; ip = interparietal bone; p = parietal bone. (Images reproduced from Rice et al. [56] with kind permission of the authors and Elsevier Science.)

forkhead/winged transcription factor Foxc1 (fig. 4). Mice lacking *Foxc1* have calvarial bones that do not grow beyond a rudimentary size and remain at the sites of the initial osteogenic condensations. Foxc1 regulates BMP-mediated osteoprogenitor proliferation specifically at the leading edge of the developing calvarial bones thus restricting bony expansion. Foxc1 does this by regulating the BMP targets *Msx2* and *Alx4* [56]. In both humans and mice, loss of function mutations in *Msx2* and *Alx4* result in similar 'hole in the head' phenotypes to those exhibited by *Foxc1*$^{-/-}$ mutant mice [58, 64, 65].

References

1 Miyake T, Cameron AM, Hall BK: Stage-specific onset of condensation and matrix deposition for Meckel's and other first arch cartilages in inbred C57BL/6 mice. J Craniofac Genet Dev Biol 1996;16:32–47.

2 Hall BK, Miyake T: All for one and one for all: condensations and the initiation of skeletal development. Bioessays 2000;22:138–147.

3 Hall BK, Miyake T: Divide, accumulate, differentiate: cell condensation in skeletal development revisited. Int J Dev Biol 1995;39:881–893.

4 Chimal-Monroy J, Diaz de Leon L: Expression of N-cadherin, N-CAM, fibronectin and tenascin is stimulated by TGF-beta1, beta2, beta3 and beta5 during the formation of precartilage condensations. Int J Dev Biol 1999;43:59–67.

5 Hall BK, Miyake T: The membranous skeleton: the role of cell condensations in vertebrate skeletogenesis. Anat Embryol (Berl) 1992;186:107–124.

6 Pizette S, Niswander L: BMPs are required at two steps of limb chondrogenesis: formation of prechondrogenic condensations and their differentiation into chondrocytes. Dev Biol 2000;219: 237–249.

7 Fujimaki R, Toyama Y, Hozumi N, Tezuka K: Involvement of Notch signaling in initiation of prechondrogenic condensation and nodule formation in limb bud micromass cultures. J Bone Miner Metab 2006;24:191–198.

8 Oka Y, Sato Y, Tsuda H, Hanaoka K, Hirai Y, Takahashi Y: Epimorphin acts extracellularly to promote cell sorting and aggregation during the condensation of vertebral cartilage. Dev Biol 2006;291:25–37.

9 Merrill AE, Bochukova EG, Brugger SM, Ishii M, Pilz DT, Wall SA, Lyons KM, Wilkie AO, Maxson RE Jr: Cell mixing at a neural crest-mesoderm boundary and deficient ephrin-Eph signaling in the pathogenesis of craniosynostosis. Hum Mol Genet 2006;15:1319–1328.

10 Stadler HS, Higgins KM, Capecchi MR: Loss of Eph-receptor expression correlates with loss of cell adhesion and chondrogenic capacity in Hoxa13 mutant limbs. Development 2001;128: 4177–4188.

11 Salsi V, Zappavigna V: Hoxd13 and Hoxa13 directly control the expression of the EphA7 Ephrin tyrosine kinase receptor in developing limbs. J Biol Chem 2006;281:1992–1999.

12 Yokouchi Y, Nakazato S, Yamamoto M, Goto Y, Kameda T, Iba H, Kuroiwa A: Misexpression of Hoxa-13 induces cartilage homeotic transformation and changes cell adhesiveness in chick limb buds. Genes Dev 1995;9:2509–2522.

13 Goff DJ, Tabin CJ: Analysis of Hoxd-13 and Hoxd-11 misexpression in chick limb buds reveals that Hox genes affect both bone condensation and growth. Development 1997;124:627–636.

14 Boulet AM, Capecchi MR: Multiple roles of Hoxa11 and Hoxd11 in the formation of the mammalian forelimb zeugopod. Development 2004;131:299–309.

15 Pacifici M, Shimo T, Gentili C, Kirsch T, Freeman TA, Enomoto-Iwamoto M, Iwamoto M, Koyama E: Syndecan-3: a cell-surface heparan sulfate proteoglycan important for chondrocyte proliferation and function during limb skeletogenesis. J Bone Miner Metab 2005;23:191–199.

16 Fisher MC, Li Y, Seghatoleslami MR, Dealy CN, Kosher RA: Heparan sulfate proteoglycans including syndecan-3 modulate BMP activity during limb cartilage differentiation. Matrix Biol 2006;25:27–39.

17 Scherberich A, Tucker RP, Samandari E, Brown-Luedi M, Martin D, Chiquet-Ehrismann R: Murine tenascin-W: a novel mammalian tenascin expressed in kidney and at sites of bone and smooth muscle development. J Cell Sci 2004;117:571–581.

18 Stains JP, Civitelli R: Cell-cell interactions in regulating osteogenesis and osteoblast function. Birth Defects Res C Embryo Today 2005;75:72–80.
19 Modarresi R, Lafond T, Roman-Blas JA, Danielson KG, Tuan RS, Seghatoleslami MR: N-cadherin mediated distribution of beta-catenin alters MAP kinase and BMP-2 signaling on chondrogenesis-related gene expression. J Cell Biochem 2005;95:53–63.
20 Hartmann C: A Wnt canon orchestrating osteoblastogenesis. Trends Cell Biol 2006;16:151–158.
21 Luo Y, Kostetskii I, Radice GL: N-cadherin is not essential for limb mesenchymal chondrogenesis. Dev Dyn 2005;232:336–344.
22 Hay E, Lemonnier J, Modrowski D, Lomri A, Lasmoles F, Marie PJ: N- and E-cadherin mediate early human calvaria osteoblast differentiation promoted by bone morphogenetic protein-2. J Cell Physiol 2000;183:117–128.
23 Castro CH, Shin CS, Stains JP, Cheng SL, Sheikh S, Mbalaviele G, Szejnfeld VL, Civitelli R: Targeted expression of a dominant-negative N-cadherin in vivo delays peak bone mass and increases adipogenesis. J Cell Sci 2004;117:2853–2864.
24 Rice DP: Craniofacial anomalies: from development to molecular pathogenesis. Curr Mol Med 2005;5:699–722.
25 Lemonnier J, Hay E, Delannoy P, Lomri A, Modrowski D, Caverzasio J, Marie PJ: Role of N-cadherin and protein kinase C in osteoblast gene activation induced by the S252W fibroblast growth factor receptor 2 mutation in Apert craniosynostosis. J Bone Miner Res 2001;16:832–845.
26 Cottrill CP, Archer CW, Wolpert L: Cell sorting and chondrogenic aggregate formation in micromass culture. Dev Biol 1987;122:503–515.
27 Nakashima K, Zhou X, Kunkel G, Zhang Z, Deng JM, Behringer RR, de Crombrugghe B: The novel zinc finger-containing transcription factor osterix is required for osteoblast differentiation and bone formation. Cell 2002;108:17–29.
28 Yu HM, Jerchow B, Sheu TJ, Liu B, Costantini F, Puzas JE, Birchmeier W, Hsu W: The role of Axin2 in calvarial morphogenesis and craniosynostosis. Development 2005;132:1995–2005.
29 Kim HJ, Rice DP, Kettunen PJ, Thesleff I: FGF-, BMP- and Shh-mediated signalling pathways in the regulation of cranial suture morphogenesis and calvarial bone development. Development 1998;125:1241–1251.
30 Opperman LA, Sweeney TM, Redmon J, Persing JA, Ogle RC: Tissue interactions with underlying dura mater inhibit osseous obliteration of developing cranial sutures. Dev Dyn 1993;198:312–322.
31 Opperman LA, Passarelli RW, Nolen AA, Gamper TJ, Lin KYK, Ogle RC: Dura mater secretes soluble heparin-binding factors required for cranial suture morphogenesis. In Vitro Cell Dev Biol Animal 1996;32:627–632.
32 Roth DA, Bradley JP, Levine JP, McMullen HF, McCarthy JG, Longaker MT: Studies in cranial suture biology. II. Role of the dura in cranial suture fusion. Plast Reconstr Surg 1996;97: 693–699.
33 Most D, Levine JP, Chang J, Sung J, McCarthy JG, Schendel SA, Longaker MT: Studies in cranial suture biology: up-regulation of transforming growth factor-beta1 and basic fibroblast growth factor mRNA correlates with posterior frontal cranial suture fusion in the rat. Plast Reconstr Surg 1998;101:1431–1440.
34 Greenwald JA, Mehrara BJ, Spector JA, Warren SM, Fagenholz PJ, Smith LE, Bouletreau PJ, Crisera FE, Ueno H, Longaker MT: In vivo modulation of FGF biological activity alters cranial suture fate. Am J Pathol 2001;158:441–452.
35 Opperman LA, Adab K, Gakunga PT: Transforming growth factor-beta 2 and TGF-beta 3 regulate fetal rat cranial suture morphogenesis by regulating rates of cell proliferation and apoptosis. Dev Dyn 2000;219:237–247.
36 Ito Y, Yeo JY, Chytil A, Han J, Bringas P Jr, Nakajima A, Shuler CF, Moses HL, Chai Y: Conditional inactivation of Tgfbr2 in cranial neural crest causes cleft palate and calvaria defects. Development 2003;130:5269–5280.
37 Adab K, Sayne JR, Carlson DS, Opperman LA: Nasal capsular cartilage is required for rat transpalatal suture morphogenesis. Differentiation 2003;71:496–505.
38 Clouthier DE, Hosoda K, Richardson JA, Williams SC, Yanagisawa H, Kuwaki T, Kumada M, Hammer RE, Yanagisawa M: Cranial and cardiac neural crest defects in endothelin-A receptor-deficient mice. Development 1998;125:813–824.

39 Kobayashi T, Kronenberg H: Minireview: transcriptional regulation in development of bone. Endocrinology 2005;146:1012–1017.
40 Ducy P, Zhang R, Geoffroy V, Ridall AL, Karsenty G: Osf2/Cbfa1: a transcriptional activator of osteoblast differentiation. Cell 1997;89:747–754.
41 Ducy P, Karsenty G: Two distinct osteoblast-specific *cis*-acting elements control expression of a mouse osteocalcin gene. Mol Cell Biol 1995;15:1858–1869.
42 Yoshida CA, Furuichi T, Fujita T, Fukuyama R, Kanatani N, Kobayashi S, Satake M, Takada K, Komori T: Core-binding factor beta interacts with Runx2 and is required for skeletal development. Nat Genet 2002;32:633–638.
43 Bialek P, Kern B, Yang X, Schrock M, Sosic D, Hong N, Wu H, Yu K, Ornitz DM, Olson EN, Justice MJ, Karsenty G: A twist code determines the onset of osteoblast differentiation. Dev Cell 2004;6:423–435.
44 Rice DP, Aberg T, Chan Y, Tang Z, Kettunen PJ, Pakarinen L, Maxson RE, Thesleff I: Integration of FGF and TWIST in calvarial bone and suture development. Development 2000;127: 1845–1855.
45 Yousfi M, Lasmoles F, Marie PJ: TWIST inactivation reduces CBFA1/RUNX2 expression and DNA binding to the osteocalcin promoter in osteoblasts. Biochem Biophys Res Commun 2002;297:641–644.
46 Boyden LM, Mao J, Belsky J, Mitzner L, Farhi A, Mitnick MA, Wu D, Insogna K, Lifton RP: High bone density due to a mutation in LDL-receptor-related protein 5. N Engl J Med 2002;346: 1513–1521.
47 Brault V, Moore R, Kutsch S, Ishibashi M, Rowitch DH, McMahon AP, Sommer L, Boussadia O, Kemler R: Inactivation of the beta-catenin gene by Wnt1-Cre-mediated deletion results in dramatic brain malformation and failure of craniofacial development. Development 2001;128: 1253–1264.
48 Day TF, Guo X, Garrett-Beal L, Yang Y: Wnt/beta-catenin signaling in mesenchymal progenitors controls osteoblast and chondrocyte differentiation during vertebrate skeletogenesis. Dev Cell 2005;8:739–750.
49 Hu H, Hilton MJ, Tu X, Yu K, Ornitz DM, Long F: Sequential roles of Hedgehog and Wnt signaling in osteoblast development. Development 2005;132:49–60.
50 Komori T: Regulation of osteoblast differentiation by transcription factors. J Cell Biochem 2006;99:1233–1239.
51 Kanatani N, Fujita T, Fukuyama R, Liu W, Yoshida CA, Moriishi T, Yamana K, Miyazaki T, Toyosawa S, Komori T: Cbfbeta regulates Runx2 function isoform-dependently in postnatal bone development. Dev Biol 2006;296:48–61.
52 Karsenty G, Wagner EF: Reaching a genetic and molecular understanding of skeletal development. Dev Cell 2002;2:389–406.
53 St-Jacques B, Hammerschmidt M, McMahon AP: Indian hedgehog signaling regulates proliferation and differentiation of chondrocytes and is essential for bone formation. Genes Dev 1999;13:2072–2086.
54 Daluiski A, Engstrand T, Bahamonde ME, Gamer LW, Agius E, Stevenson SL, Cox K, Rosen V, Lyons KM: Bone morphogenetic protein-3 is a negative regulator of bone density. Nat Genet 2001;27:84–88.
55 Liu YH, Tang Z, Kundu RK, Wu L, Luo W, Zhu D, Sangiorgi F, Snead ML, Maxson RE: Msx2 gene dosage influences the number of proliferative osteogenic cells in growth centers of the developing murine skull: a possible mechanism for MSX2-mediated craniosynostosis in humans. Dev Biol 1999;205:260–274.
56 Rice R, Rice DP, Olsen BR, Thesleff I: Progression of calvarial bone development requires Foxc1 regulation of Msx2 and Alx4. Dev Biol 2003;262:75–87.
57 Warren SM, Brunet LJ, Harland RM, Economides AN, Longaker MT: The BMP antagonist noggin regulates cranial suture fusion. Nature 2003;422:625–629.
58 Antonopoulou I, Mavrogiannis LA, Wilkie AO, Morriss-Kay GM: Alx4 and Msx2 play phenotypically similar and additive roles in skull vault differentiation. J Anat 2004;204:487–499.
59 Liu Z, Xu J, Colvin JS, Ornitz DM: Coordination of chondrogenesis and osteogenesis by fibroblast growth factor 18. Genes Dev 2002;16:859–869.

60 Rice DP, Kim HJ, Thesleff I: Detection of gelatinase B expression reveals osteoclastic bone resorption as a feature of early calvarial bone development. Bone 1997;21:479–486.
61 Franzoso G, Carlson L, Xing L, Poljak L, Shores EW, Brown KD, Leonardi A, Tran T, Boyce BF, Siebenlist U: Requirement for NF-kappaB in osteoclast and B-cell development. Genes Dev 1997;11:3482–3496.
62 Matsuo K, Galson DL, Zhao C, Peng L, Laplace C, Wang KZ, Bachler MA, Amano H, Aburatani H, Ishikawa H, Wagner EF: Nuclear factor of activated T-cells (NFAT) rescues osteoclastogenesis in precursors lacking c-Fos. J Biol Chem 2004;279:26475–26480.
63 Boyle WJ, Simonet WS, Lacey DL, Osteoclast differentiation and activation. Nature 2003;423: 337–342.
64 Satokata I, Ma L, Ohshima H, Bei M, Woo I, Nishizawa K, Maeda T, Takano Y, Uchiyama M, Heaney S, Peters H, Tang Z, Maxson R, Maas R: Msx2 deficiency in mice causes pleiotropic defects in bone growth and ectodermal organ formation. Nat Genet 2000;24:391–395.
65 Wilkie AO, Tang Z, Elanko N, Walsh S, Twigg SR, Hurst JA, Wall SA, Chrzanowska KH, Maxson RE Jr: Functional haploinsufficiency of the human homeobox gene MSX2 causes defects in skull ossification. Nat Genet 2000;24:387–390.

Dr. David P. Rice
Professor of Orthodontics
Institute of Dentistry and Helsinki University Central Hospital
Box 41, University of Helsinki
FIN–00014 Helsinki (Finland)
E-Mail David.Rice@helsinki.fi

Rice DP (ed): Craniofacial Sutures. Development, Disease and Treatment.
Front Oral Biol. Basel, Karger, 2008, vol 12, pp 41–56

Mechanical Influences on Suture Development and Patency

Susan W. Herring

University of Washington, Seattle, Wash., USA

Abstract

In addition to their role in skull growth, sutures are sites of flexibility between the more rigid bones. Depending on the suture, predominant loading during life may be either tensile or compressive. Loads are transmitted across sutures via collagenous fibers and a fluid-rich extracellular matrix and can be quasi-static (growth of neighboring tissues) or intermittent (mastication). The mechanical properties of sutures, while always viscoelastic, are therefore quite different for tensile versus compressive loading. The morphology of individual sutures reflects the nature of local loading, evidently by a process of developmental adaptation. In vivo or ex vivo, sutural cells respond to tensile or cyclic loading by expressing markers of proliferation and differentiation, whereas compressive loading appears to favor osteogenesis. Braincase and facial sutures exhibit similar mechanical behavior and reactions despite their different natural environments.

Introduction

Sutures are a part of the craniofacial skeleton and share its mechanical loads. At the same time sutures are obviously less stiff than the bones they join. This flexibility is the key to the particular mechanical roles played by sutures, which accommodate deformations of the skull that include distortions during birth (important for humans but probably less so for other species), distensions caused by internal pressures, cyclic loading from muscle activity, and traumatic impacts.

Like all components of the musculoskeletal system, sutures respond to mechanical loading. Indeed, the adaptability of sutures to their environment has been evident for decades, if not centuries. Although early workers analogized sutures to cartilaginous growth plates and assumed an independent growth capacity [1], most information since then has underscored the fact that sutural morphology and growth are easy to modify. This, of course, does not prove that the signal is a mechanical one, but it does point our attention to the local environment and phenomena that affect it. The study of mechanically induced transcription and expression in sutures is made complex by their compound nature, consisting of a variety of extracellular matrix zones, many different cell types, and a well-developed vasculature. Essentially all of these elements are known to respond to mechanical stimuli in isolation [2–7]. Thus, although it is no surprise to find that sutures also respond [8], it is difficult to sort out which cells are responsible. The same problem characterizes the very similar periodontal ligament, which is basically a suture between alveolar bone and the bone-like cementum that surrounds dental roots.

Although there is a large literature relating mechanics to suture biology, it is highly focused. Most studies have dealt with artificial loading of rodent vault or palatal sutures either in vitro or in vivo, with a smattering of rabbit and primate studies. Interest in these models centers around the identification of mechanically responsive transcription and expression. By comparison, understanding of how sutures actually behave under loading, i.e., their mechanical properties and what loads they receive in vivo, is less advanced. In this review an attempt will be made to synthesize these diverse areas. Readers are also referred to other recent reviews on the biology and mechanobiology of sutures [9–16]. For present purposes, sutures are considered to be the fibrocellular tissues that join membrane bones, but it is recognized that some of the most important aspects of suture biology concern the bone fronts rather than the sutures per se.

Mechanical Properties of Sutures

As explained in several current textbooks [17, 18], the engineering parameter most germane to suture biology is strain, technically defined as a change in length divided by original length, often expressed as a percentage. When forces place loads on solid objects, both stress and strain arise. Strain is thought to be the property sensed by cells, and in any case strain, in contrast to stress, is measurable. In elastic solids, stress divided by strain is a constant, the elastic modulus, roughly equivalent to stiffness.

In some nonmammalian vertebrate taxa, sutures are movable joints, contributing to range of movement rather than force transmission [19, 20]. In mammals, however, perhaps because of the requirements of forceful mastication, sutures are constructed for relatively efficient transmission of loads. They often feature interdigitating and/or overlapping bony fronts. Mature sutures are distinguished by well-developed fiber systems that not only unite the bone fronts, but also can resist deformation in tension, compression, or both [21, 22]. Sutures that show marked adaptation for force transmission can rival the strength of the bones they join [23, 24]. Nevertheless, sutures are zones of flexibility and energy absorption that undergo much greater deformations than the rigid bones of the skull regardless of rate or direction of loading [25–27].

The energy-absorbing qualities of sutures are related to their viscoelasticity, itself a result of their extracellular matrix of collagen fibers, proteoglycans, and water [28]. Thus their mechanical properties are nonlinear and influenced by loading rate and duration as fluid is forced out of the sutural space and collagen fibers are rearranged [29]. Probably because the fibers are usually organized to resist either predominantly compression or tension, mechanical properties can be quite different depending on the direction of loading [27]. As might be anticipated from the variety of bony morphologies and fiber arrangements, different sutures vary in their mechanical properties, with more interdigitated sutures typically showing higher elastic moduli [30].

The best studied aspect of sutural mechanical properties is their change with age. Force-bearing sutural ligaments that unite the bones are poorly, if at all, developed in fetal and early postnatal skulls [31]. Bony interdigitation is also a late-developing feature [32]. These changes imply that infant sutures should be less stiff and also less capable of energy absorption than older sutures, a finding supported by several studies [33–35]. Despite the fact that site-specific morphologies are not yet distinct, mechanical properties vary among different infant sutures. In week-old rats the posterior interfrontal suture was weaker and less stiff than the coronal or sagittal sutures [36]; interestingly, the posterior interfrontal suture is the only suture that fuses in this species [13].

Strain Regimes in Relation to Mechanical Properties

In life, the skull and its sutures are subjected to three types of strain regimes radically different in pattern and magnitude. The first type is impact loading from sudden forces produced accidentally from falls or foreign objects or produced intentionally by fighting. The latter are usually thought of in association with head-butting conflicts in horned ungulates, but also include human fighting styles such as boxing. Typically the magnitude of impact loads is high, as is the rate of loading. It seems unlikely that sutures could be adapted for unpredictable impact loading other than having a reasonable safety factor in mechanical properties. The most significant mechanical properties for resisting impacts are energy absorption capacity and ultimate strength.

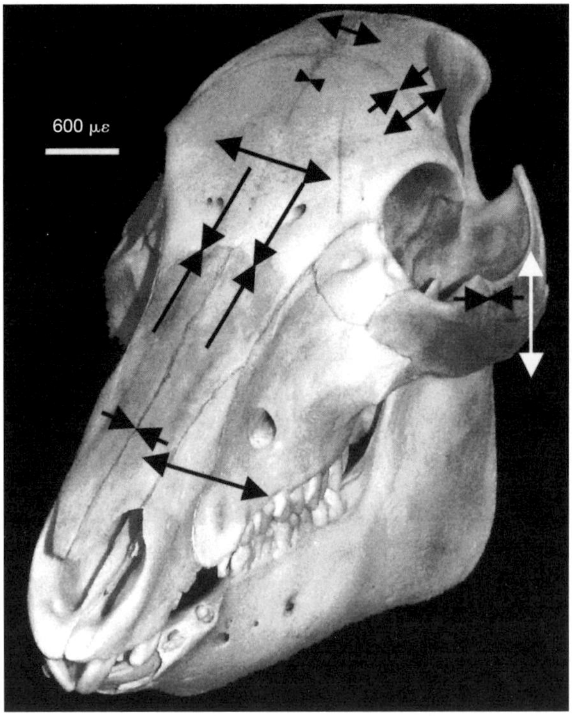

Fig. 1. Typical sutural strains measured during cyclic mastication in miniature pigs [21, 38, 53, 55]. Arrows pointing away from the suture (premaxillary-maxillary, anterior interfrontal, interparietal, horizontal part of zygomatic) indicate tensile strain. Arrows pointing toward the suture (internasal, nasofrontal, posterior interfrontal and vertical part of zygomatic) indicate compressive strain. The coronal suture is individually variable and may be tensile, compressive or both [21]. Modified from Herring and Ochareon [51].

The second strain regime encountered by the skull and sutures is cyclic loading from function or from the pulsations of blood vessels [37]. Feeding (including ingestion, mastication and swallowing) is probably the major source of large-magnitude cyclic loading, but the skull also receives transmitted stresses from postcranial bones, for example during locomotion. Feeding loads result from muscle contraction, either directly (temporalis muscle pulling on parietal bone) or indirectly (reaction forces at the teeth or jaw joints). Cyclic functional loading produces fairly high strain rates. For example, rats typically chew at 5 Hz, and the jaw closing muscles are active for no more than 50% of the cycle; thus, maximum loading would be achieved in 100 ms or less. Cyclic functional loading also features variable, but often high magnitudes of strain. As illustrated in figure 1, mastication in pigs can strain sutures up to 2,000 $\mu\varepsilon$, either in compression (nasofrontal) or tension (zygomatic, premaxillary-maxillary) [22, 38]. Stiffness, viscoelasticity and fatigue resistance would all affect the ability of a suture to deal with cyclic loads.

The third strain regime is quasi-static strain arising from the presence of adjacent tissues. Because the skull is generally conceived as an exoskeleton, these are usually interpreted as tensile strains caused by pressure from, or especially growth of, internal organs. For example, intracranial pressure from increasing brain volume has been calculated to produce quasi-static tensile strains on the order of 300 $\mu\varepsilon$, which could either act directly on the suture [34] or indirectly through mechanotransduction by the dura mater [39]. An analog for facial sutures might be the cranial base cartilages and nasal septum, the growth of which could cause tension in the outer lying sutures. In the case of facial sutures any effect of strain must be direct, as there is no equivalent for the dura mater. Quasi-static strains can also come from external structures. For example, indentation of the braincase could be caused by stresses from enlarging musculature external to a suture. The weight of the head resisted by the vertebral column also constitutes a quasi-static load. Quasi-static strains are presumed to be low in magnitude and, of course, slow. Viscoelastic properties would be of special importance for sutural performance under such a strain regime.

Sutures in situ: Normal Strain Environments

Sutures do not exist until the osteogenic fronts of adjoining bones approximate each other, a comparatively late ontogenetic event. Mechanical loading, strictly speaking, is not possible until the structure exists. Nevertheless, the dramatic regional enlargements that characterize fetal development mean that quasi-static strains must be present in the future suture area. Such strains, which may cause ossification centers to separate in space, may have a role in suture positioning [40].

Once a suture has formed, loading is possible. Impact loading is not an element of normal development, and cyclic loading does not begin until muscles become active relatively late in mammalian ontogeny. However, quasi-static strains resulting from differential growth are probably very significant for sutures during fetal and infant life. Experimental alterations of intracranial pressure clearly do change suture morphology. Hydrocephaly modifies fiber orientation in the rat coronal suture from a compression-resisting to a tension-resisting architecture, whereas microcephaly thickens the bones without affecting the compression-resisting fibrous architecture [41]. Growth also seems to be affected, with tensile strain elongating bones at suture margins and compressive strain leading instead to thicker bones. Osteogenesis at the bone front tends to be greater at the attachment of fibers, i.e., tension sites [42]. Skulls from infants with hydrocephalus are thin but enlarged to house the increased intracranial contents [15]. In contrast, reduction of intracranial pressure by microcephaly produces small thick skulls with frequent synostosis. Mooney et al. [43] have summarized animal studies documenting suture stenosis in relation to microcephaly and shunting of hydrocephaly, which presumably reduce intracranial pressure levels and thus reduce tension (or increase compression) in sutures.

Cyclic strains from muscle contraction originate before birth as fetal jaw movements become coordinated [reviewed by 44] but paralysis apparently has no effect on developing sutures [45]. Postnatal muscle function acting on more mature sutures, however, does have an influence, as argued many years ago by Moss [46]. Suture strain resulting from muscle contraction can be tensile, compressive, or both, depending on the particular suture and the particular muscle, and magnitudes are typically an order of magnitude larger than strain on the adjacent bones [21, 22], reflecting the fact that sutures are much less stiff than bones. Increased jaw muscle force is associated with increased interdigitation and decreased tensile stiffness of the mouse sagittal suture [47], while a soft diet leads to simpler, narrower, and sometimes obliterated facial sutures in rats [48]. The toothless and therefore nonmasticating osteopetrotic *(op/op)* mouse shows similar changes in both facial and vault sutures, as well as poorly developed sutural ligaments [49, 50].

Although the absence of masticatory strain retards sutural growth, the growth rates of different sutures in normal animals are not correlated with the polarity of masticatory strain [51]. Sutural morphology, however, does show a specific relationship with the polarity of cyclic strain. Both in pigs and in fish, it has been reported that compressed sutures are more highly interdigitated [51, 52] than tensed sutures. In pigs it is clear that the prominent interdigitations are necessary for the fibers to be arranged in a compression-resistant orientation (fig. 2) [21, 53]. Furthermore, an ontogenetic change in strain from compression to tension in the posterior interfrontal suture is associated with a simplification of the osteogenic fronts [54]. Another characteristic of sutures under cyclic compression is the presence of chondroid tissue or cartilage, which may permit rapid growth in a relatively anoxic environment [55].

There are no longitudinal or experimental studies evaluating the role of impact loading on sutures. Male wild sheep have more interdigitated sutures, particularly in the braincase, than females [56], but in addition to impact loading this could reflect quasi-static loading from heavier horns or higher-magnitude cyclic loading from larger muscles.

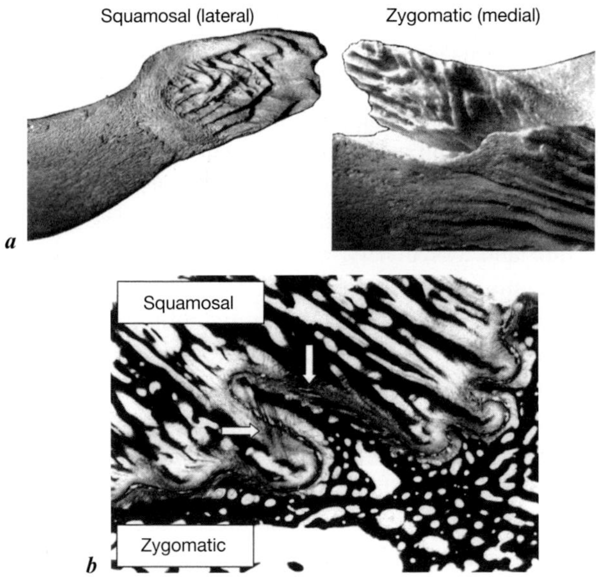

Fig. 2. Morphology of the pig zygomatic suture (vertical part), which undergoes cyclic compression during mastication. ***a*** The chevron-shaped interdigitating bony processes on the lateral surface of the left squamosal bone and the medial surface of the left zygomatic bone are shown. ***b*** The processes from the squamosal fitting into valleys of the zygomatic are shown. The sutural ligaments (white arrows) are arranged obliquely so that fibers will be stretched when the bones are forced together by the compressive load.

Artificial Strain Environments in Intact Animals

Quasi-Static Tension: Elongated Osteogenic Fronts and Widened Sutures

Although study of the natural mechanics of sutures is difficult, it is comparatively easy to impose an extrinsic force such as an orthodontic spring on sutures of the braincase and palate, and much of our knowledge comes from such experiments. Such loads fall into the quasi-static category. Most studies used tensile loads, because of the therapeutic potential of tension to grow bone (also used in distraction osteogenesis), but a few employed compression. The virtue of artificial strain regimes is the availability of sham controls, allowing some confidence that cell and molecular reactions to the imposed strains can be identified. In addition, in some cases similar strain regimes can be applied to organ cultures (see below), enabling a comparison of in vivo and in vitro responses.

Quasi-static tensile loads have been applied in vivo to the sagittal suture of rats and mice [29, 57–59], the internasal suture of rabbits [60], and the interpremaxillary and intermaxillary sutures of rats and macaques [61–65]. The latter imitates a common orthodontic treatment, rapid palatal expansion. Another clinical modality, a reverse head-gear appliance, has been used to apply tensile strain to multiple facial sutures in rats and macaques [66, 67]. In terms of morphology and cell activity, this strain regime reliably produces increases in suture width, proliferation rate and vascularity, accompanied by increased matrix production and mineralization at the bone fronts [60, 62, 67]. Sutural ligament fibers and cells are frequently elongated in the direction of tension [57], and type III collagen, which is associated with adaptation to mechanical stress, is induced [58]. The rat midpalatal suture, which normally contains cartilage, is transformed to a ligamentous connection and expresses collagen I instead of collagen II, a response shown to be mediated by upregulation of β_1 integrin and the reorganization of the cytoskeleton [61]. As might be expected, expansion lowers sutural stiffness [29]. Stretching mouse sagittal sutures for 2 weeks caused the upregulation of not only type I collagen, but also alkaline phosphatase and osteopontin, probably by osteoblasts [59]. Thus the defect that results from the widened suture is rapidly ossified and the end result is elongated bone fronts [63]. Interestingly, the association between angiogenesis and osteogenesis may be more than a correlation, based on evidence that vascular pericytes are a major source of the expanded osteoprogenitor population [64, 65]. Several of these studies compared different magnitudes of tensile loading, usually finding that increased loading resulted in a greater osteogenic response [57].

Quasi-Static Compression: Thicker Bones, Narrower Sutures

As mentioned above, there are comparatively few studies on sutures using quasi-static compressive loads in vivo. Head-gear appliances, which are assumed to compress multiple facial sutures, have been used in macaques [68], and miniplates have been placed across the coronal suture of fetal lambs, presumably causing compression as the bony fronts attempt to elongate [69]. Intrauterine constraint is usually considered as placing most sutures under compression [70, 71]. Positional lambdoid suture plagiocephaly in humans may also be an example of quasi-static compression [72], as may artificial deformation of human or animal skulls, although in these cases compression at one suture may lead to tension at others [73, 74]. The results of these disparate compression studies were essentially identical. The osteogenic fronts lengthened less, but the bones thickened. The sutures were narrowed, but in most studies did not fuse. In the monkey study some 'osteogenic' fronts actually became resorptive [68], and in human positional plagiocephaly, affected sutures showed heightened levels of TGF-β_3 [72], a growth factor implicated in preserving suture patency [75]. However, intrauterine constraint was associated with cartilage formation and occasional synostotic bridging of the human sagittal suture and the mouse squamosal and coronal sutures [70, 71].

Cyclic Strain: Anabolic Regardless of Polarity

Probably the most interesting experiments involving externally imposed loads are the recent series of papers by Mao and colleagues [76–79] in which cyclic forces were used. For these procedures animals were typically anesthetized each day for a short period of controlled loading. Although the loading was not physiological, its frequency and magnitude were roughly in the ranges for masticatory loading. Particularly informative was a comparison of two rabbit facial sutures, the nasofrontal and premaxillomaxillary, which were respectively shown to receive strong compression and mild tension when the incisor teeth were loaded [78]. In addition to a sham control, some animals received 'static' loading for 10 min/day – basically a single cycle, not equivalent to the sustained quasi-static loads discussed above. In another set of experiments, compressive cycles were imposed on rat incisors, although the strain regime on the sutures may have been tensile (gauges were evidently placed parallel to the suture rather than across it) [77, 79]. In all cases, the cyclically loaded sutures showed sutural widening with increased cells, followed in longer-term studies [78] by bone elongation. Bone thickness was not assessed, but additional observations on the rat sutures indicated that osteoclastic as well as osteoblastic activity was increased [79] and that the expression of MMP-2, a gelatinase possibly associated with mineralization [80], was upregulated, at least in the posterior frontal suture [77]. The remarkable finding of this work is the apparently identical reaction of sutures to cyclic compression and cyclic tension. Insofar as comparisons are possible, cyclic loading in either direction resembles quasi-static tension, producing a general growth response at the sutures. This result is quite different from the narrowing and stasis associated with quasi-static compression, but conforms with in vivo work showing that cyclic compression associated with mastication is perfectly consistent with vigorous suture growth [51].

Sutures Strained in vitro: Gene Expression and Growth Factor Signaling

Bones and sutures grown in culture are removed from the intrinsic strain regimes of the animal, resulting in different morphology. For example, in the absence of an expanding brain, osteogenic fronts that would approximate each other in vivo may form an overlapping suture instead [16]. Biologically, the systems are different as well, because in vitro preparations lack a blood supply (hence the very significant angiogenic reaction and pericyte invasion associated with in vivo quasi-static tension [64, 65] is eliminated) and can be examined with or without tissue layers such as the dura mater. In addition to the simpler (if not always realistic) biology, loads applied in vitro can be simpler as well, and thus better controlled. These preparations thus lend themselves to molecular analysis more easily than studies on intact animals.

As in vivo, quasi-static tension of mouse and rat sagittal sutures in vitro over a period of hours to days widened the sutures, stimulated proliferation of both osteoblastic and fibroblastic sutural cells, and led to elongation of the osteogenic fronts [4, 8, 81]. Striking changes in gene expression occurred almost immediately. After only 5 min, stretched sutures released FGF-2 and demonstrated increased permeability and intracellular Ca^{2+} [82]. Other immediate events observed by various authors were the appearance of MMP-9, another gelatinase associated with mineralization [83], at stressed bone locations [14] and upregulation of TBX2, a probable inhibitor of osteogenesis, in the central part of the suture [84]. Within 90 min, the expression of IGF-1 and its receptor was increased in both sutural fibroblasts and osteoblasts [81]. By 3 h α-adaptin C, which is associated with endocytosis, was induced in central suture fibroblasts [8] and BMP-4 was expressed by osteoprogenitors [4]; by 6 h, Cbfa1 was upregulated as well [4].

A model in which 30 min of quasi-static tension/day was applied to rat calvaria has been exploited to clarify the interaction of loading and the dura mater [85]. FGFs were noted to be produced by the dura mater, and in the absence of the dura, normally patent sutures fused. Tensile strain was found to delay or prevent the fusion of posterior interfrontal sutures, which were distinguished from unloaded (fusing) controls by the presence of FGFR1 at the osteogenic fronts and FGFR2 in the central area. The implication of these studies is that applied forces may work by influencing FGF signaling between the dura mater and the suture [85].

An in vitro cyclic compression regime (cited as unpublished observations by Ignelzi et al. [86]) was found to produce mouse sagittal suture fusion, not because the bones were pushed together but because of a general osteogenic response. This effect appeared to involve soluble factors manufactured by the loaded tissues, because cocultured unloaded sutures also showed osteogenesis and fusion. The osteogenic fronts in this loaded model were more cellular and showed more collagen than unloaded controls, but the faster-growing bone tissue was less mineralized [86].

Table 1. Summary of suture responses to strain regimes

	Compression		Tension	
	quasi-static	cyclic	quasi-static	cyclic
Examples				
Intrinsic	Weight of head	Feeding	Brain enlargement	Feeding
Extrinsic	Uterine constraint	In vitro loading	Palatal expansion	In vitro loading
Suture				
Width	Narrower	Wider	Wider	Wider
Tissue	Cartilage common	Cartilage common	More fibrous More vascular	More fibrous
Proliferation	Less	More	More	More
Fibers	Less prominent	Oblique	Straight	Cruciate/straight
Bone fronts				
Growth	Less	More	More	More
Morphology	Thicker	Interdigitating Chondroid common	Thinner	Flat

Although sutures also receive impact loads, their consequences are unknown. Because these responses are qualitatively similar in braincase and facial sutures, in vivo and in vitro, neither the dura mater nor a functioning vascular system appears to be required.

Conclusions

Sutures are viscoelastic structures that in vivo receive quasi-static, cyclic, and impact loads of various magnitudes, frequencies and directions. The load-bearing elements consist of the collagenous fibers of the sutural ligament supplemented by bound water. The compliance of sutures renders them far more deformable than the bones they join, and they are locations of energy absorption for the skull as a whole.

Sutures seem to react identically to tension whether intrinsic or extrinsic in origin, quasi-static or cyclic, in vitro or in vivo (table 1). Tension results in wider, more fibrous sutures abutted by thinner but elongated bones. The mechanical stimulus induces expression of markers of connective tissue and bone proliferation and differentiation through mechanisms that may initially involve calcium uptake and/or integrin binding.

Delivered cyclically (either naturally or artificially), compressive strain behaves generally like tensile strain, maintaining sutural width and bone elongation. Because sutures in vivo are constructed to convert compression into tension via the sutural ligament, there may be little functional difference between cyclic tension and compression. It is also possible that a suture released periodically from compression experiences the release as a tensile strain, and vice versa.

In contrast, compressive strain delivered quasi-statically narrows sutures, retards bone growth in length but promotes bone thickening (table 1). Although synostosis sometimes accompanies compressive loading regimes, compression itself does not cause fusion. Rather, compression contributes to an osteogenic environment. Stimuli that enhance osteogenesis (or incapacitate osteogenic inhibitors) are well known to be associated with suture fusion [75, 87–95]. The narrowing of the suture space, development of cartilage, and immobility that sometimes accompany compression also facilitate fusion, but these effects are all indirect.

The most remarkable finding from the studies reviewed is the absence of a difference between the responses of braincase versus facial sutures to mechanical loads, despite the presence of the dura mater, a potent source of growth factors, in the former but not the latter. Similarly, in vitro and in vivo studies have yielded very similar findings even though a vascular supply accompanied by pericytes is absent in vitro. Thus the sutural tissues themselves must have sufficient responding elements.

Acknowledgments

I thank NIDCR for support of my work cited herein through award DE 08513 and Dr. Michael Cunningham for continuing interesting discussions on these topics.

References

1 Weinmann JP, Sicher H: Bone and Bones; Fundamentals of Bone Biology. St Louis, Mosby, 1947.
2 Wang JH-C, Yang G, Li Z: Controlling cell responses to cyclic mechanical stretching. Ann Biomed Eng 2005;33:337–342.
3 Wang JH-C, Yang G, Li Z, Shen W: Fibroblast responses to cyclic mechanical stretching depend on cell orientation to the stretching direction. J Biomech 2004;37:573–576.
4 Ikegame M, Ishibashi O, Yoshizawa T, Shimomura J, Komori T, Ozawa H, Kawashima H: Tensile stress induces bone morphogenetic protein 4 in preosteoblastic and fibroblastic cells, which later differentiate into osteoblasts leading to osteogenesis in the mouse calvariae in organ culture. J Bone Miner Res 2001;16:24–32.
5 Chiquet M, Renedo AS, Huber F, Flück M: How do fibroblasts translate mechanical signals into changes in extracellular matrix production? Matrix Biol 2003;22:73–80.

6 Von den Hoff JW: Effects of mechanical tension on matrix degradation by human periodontal ligament cells cultured in collagen gels. J Periodontal Res 2003;38:449–457.
7 Redlich M, Roos HA, Reichenberg E, Zaks B, Mussig D, Baumert U, Golan I, Palmon A: Expression of tropoelastin in human periodontal ligament fibroblasts after stimulation of orthodontic force. Arch Oral Biol 2004;49:119–124.
8 Shimomura J, Ishibashi O, Ikegame M, Yoshizawa T, Ejiri S, Noda T, Kawashima H: Tensile stress induces α-adaptin C production in mouse calvariae in an organ culture: possible involvement of endocytosis in mechanical stress-stimulated osteoblast differentiation. J Cell Physiol 2003;195:488–496.
9 Mao JJ, Wang P, Kopher RA: Biomechanics of craniofacial sutures: orthopedic implications. Angle Orthod 2003;73:128–135.
10 Mao JJ: Mechanobiology of craniofacial sutures. J Dent Res 2002;81:810–816.
11 Mao JJ, Nah HD: Growth and development: hereditary and mechanical modulations. Am J Orthod Dentofacial Orthop 2004;125:676–689.
12 Warren SM, Greenwald JA, Spector JA, Bouletreau P, Mehrara BJ, Longaker MT: New developments in cranial suture research. Plast Reconstr Surg 2001;107:523–540.
13 Opperman LA: Cranial sutures as intramembranous bone growth sites. Dev Dyn 2000;219: 472–485.
14 Yu JC, Borke JL, Zhang G: Brief synopsis of cranial sutures: optimization by adaptation. Semin Pediatr Neurol 2004;11:249–255.
15 Huggare J, Rönning O: Growth of the cranial vault; in Dixon AD, Hoyte DAN, Rönning O (eds): Fundamentals of Craniofacial Growth. Boca Raton, CRC Press, 1997, pp 363–387.
16 Rice DPC, Rice R, Thesleff I: Molecular mechanisms in calvarial bone and suture development, and their relation to craniosynostosis. Eur J Orthod 2003;25:139–148.
17 Martin RB, Burr DB, Sharkey NA: Skeletal Tissue Mechanics. New York, Springer, 1998.
18 Carter DR, Beaupré GS: Skeletal Function and Form. Cambridge, Cambridge University Press, 2001.
19 Gussekloo SWS, Vosselman MG, Bout RG: Three-dimensional kinematics of skeletal elements in avian prokinetic and rhynchokinetic skulls determined by Roentgen stereophotogrammetry. J Exp Biol 2001;204:1735–1744.
20 Iordansky NN: Evolution of cranial kinesis in lower tetrapods. Neth J Zool 1990;40:32–54.
21 Herring SW, Teng S: Strain in the braincase and its sutures during function. Am J Phys Anthropol 2000;112:575–593.
22 Herring SW, Rafferty KL: Cranial and facial sutures: functional loading in relation to growth and morphology; in Davidovitch Z, Mah J (eds): Biological Mechanisms of Tooth Movement and Craniofacial Adaptation. Boston, Harvard Society for the Advancement of Orthodontics, 2000, pp 269–276.
23 Hubbard RP, Melvin JW, Barodawala IT: Flexure of cranial sutures. J Biomech 1971;4:491–496.
24 Jaslow CR: Mechanical properties of cranial sutures. J Biomech 1990;23:313–321.
25 Jaslow CR, Biewener AA: Strain patterns in the horncores, cranial bones and sutures of goats *(Capra hircus)* during impact loading. J Zool 1995;235:193–210.
26 Herring SW: Sutures and craniosynostosis: a comparative, functional, and evolutionary perspective; in Cohen MMJ, MacLean RE (eds): Craniosynostosis, ed 2. New York, Oxford University Press, 2000, pp 3–10.
27 Popowics TE, Herring SW: Load transmission in the nasofrontal suture of the pig, *Sus scrofa*. J Biomech 2007;40:837–844.
28 Woo SL-Y, Akeson WH: Response of tendons and ligaments to joint loading and movements; in Helminen HJ, Tammi M, Kiviranta I, Paukkonen K, Säämänen A-M, Jurvelin J (eds): Joint Loading. Bristol, Wright, 1987, pp 287–315.
29 Tanaka E, Miyawaki Y, del Pozo R, Tanne K: Changes in the biomechanical properties of the rat interparietal suture incident to continuous tensile force application. Arch Oral Biol 2000;45:1059–1064.
30 Radhakrishnan P, Mao JJ: Nanomechanical properties of facial sutures and sutural mineralization front. J Dent Res 2004;83:470–475.
31 Pritchard JJ, Scott JH, Girgis FG: The structure and development of cranial and facial sutures. J Anat 1956;90:73–87.

32 Persson M: Structure and growth of facial sutures. Odont Revy 1973;24(suppl 26):1–146.
33 Margulies SS, Thibault KL: Infant skull and suture properties: measurements and implications for mechanisms of pediatric brain injury. J Biomech Eng 2000;122:364–371.
34 Henderson JH, Chang LY, Song HM, Longaker MT, Carter DR: Age-dependent properties and quasi-static strain in the rat sagittal suture. J Biomech 2005;38:2294–2301.
35 Gefen A, Gefen N, Zhu Q, Raghupathi R, Margulies SS: Age-dependent changes in material properties of the brain and braincase of the rat. J Neurotrauma 2003;20:1163–1177.
36 McLaughlin E, Zhang Y, Pashley D, Borke J, Yu J: The load-displacement characteristics of neonatal rat cranial sutures. Cleft Palate Craniofac J 2000;37:590–595.
37 Oudhof HAJ, van Doorenmaalen WJ: Skull morphogenesis and growth: hemodynamic influence. Acta Anat 1983;117:181–186.
38 Rafferty KL, Herring SW, Marshall CD: The biomechanics of the rostrum and the role of facial sutures. J Morphol 2003;257:33–44.
39 Henderson JH, Longaker MT, Carter DR: Sutural bone deposition rate and strain magnitude during cranial development. Bone 2004;34:271–280.
40 Persson M, Roy W: Suture development and bony fusion in the fetal rabbit palate. Arch Oral Biol 1979;24:283–291.
41 Prahl-Andersen B: Sutural Growth; doctoral dissertation, University of Nijmegen, 1968.
42 Koskinen L: Adaptive sutures. Proc Finnish Dent Soc 1977;73(suppl 10):1–67.
43 Mooney MP, Siegel MI, Opperman LA: Animal models of craniosynostosis: experimental, congenital, and transgenic models; in Mooney MP, Siegel MI (eds): Understanding Craniofacial Anomalies: the Etiopathogenesis of Craniosynostoses and Facial Clefting. New York, Wiley-Liss, 2002, pp 209–249.
44 Herring SW: The ontogeny of mammalian mastication. Am Zool 1985;25:339–349.
45 Persson M: The role of movements in the development of sutural and diarthrodial joints tested by long-term paralysis of chick embryos. J Anat 1983;137:591–599.
46 Moss ML: Extrinsic determination of sutural area morphology in the rat calvaria. Acta Anat 1961;44:263–272.
47 Byron CD, Borke J, Yu J, Pashley D, Wingard CJ, Hamrick M: Effects of increased muscle mass on mouse sagittal suture morphology and mechanics. Anat Rec 2004;279A:676–684.
48 Engström C, Kiliaridis S, Thilander B: The relationship between masticatory function and craniofacial morphology. II. A histological study in the growing rat fed a soft diet. Eur J Orthod 1986;8:271–279.
49 Kaku M, Kawata T, Kawasoko S, Fujita T, Tokimasa C, Tanne K: Remodeling of the sagittal suture in osteopetrotic *(op/op)* mice associated with cranial flat bone growth. J Craniofac Genet Dev Biol 1999;19:109–112.
50 Kawata T, Tokimasa C, Fujita T, Kaku M, Kawasoko S, Sugiyama H, Ozawa S, Tanne K: Morphological change of the nasopremaxillary suture in growing 'toothless' osteopetrotic *(op/op)* mice. J Craniofac Genet Dev Biol 1999;19:48–55.
51 Herring SW, Ochareon P: Bone – special problems of the craniofacial region. Orthod Craniofac Res 2005;8:174–182.
52 Markey M, Main R, Marshall C: In vivo cranial suture function and suture morphology in extant fish: implications for inferring skull function in fossil taxa. J Vert Paleontol 2005;25(suppl): 88A–89A.
53 Herring SW, Mucci RJ: In vivo strain in cranial sutures: the zygomatic arch. J Morphol 1991;207:225–239.
54 Sun Z, Lee E, Herring SW: Cranial sutures and bones: growth and fusion in relation to masticatory strain. Anat Rec 2004;276A:150–161.
55 Rafferty KL, Herring SW: Craniofacial sutures: morphology, growth and in vivo masticatory strains. J Morphol 1999;242:167–179.
56 Jaslow CR: Sexual dimorphism of cranial suture complexity in wild sheep *(Ovis aries)*. Zool J Linn Soc 1989;95:273–284.
57 Miyawaki S, Forbes DP: The morphologic and biochemical effects of tensile force application to the interparietal suture of the Sprague-Dawley rat. Am J Orthod 1987;92:123–133.
58 Tanaka E, Miyawaki Y, Tanaka M, Watanabe M, Lee K, del Pozo R, Tanne K: Effects of tensile forces on the expression of type III collagen in rat interparietal suture. Arch Oral Biol 2000;45:1049–1057.

59 Morinobu M, Ishijima M, Rittling SR, Tsuji K, Yamamoto H, Nifuji A, Denhardt DT, Noda M: Osteopontin expression in osteoblasts and osteocytes during bone formation under mechanical stress in the calvarial suture in vivo. J Bone Miner Res 2003;18:1706–1715.
60 Parr JA, Garetto LP, Wohlford ME, Arbuckle GR, Roberts WE: Sutural expansion using rigidly integrated endosseous implants: an experimental study in rabbits. Angle Orthod 1997;67:283–290.
61 Takahashi I, Onodera K, Sasano Y, Mizoguchi I, Bae JW, Mitani H, Kagayama M: Effect of stretching on gene expression of beta1 integrin and focal adhesion kinase and on chondrogenesis through cell-extracellular matrix interactions. Eur J Cell Biol 2003;82:182–192.
62 Southard KA, Forbes DP: The effects of force magnitude on a sutural model: a quantitative approach. Am J Orthod Dentofacial Orthop 1988;93:460–466.
63 Cleall JF, Bayne DI, Posen JM, Subtelny JD: Expansion of the midpalatal suture in the monkey. Angle Orthod 1965;35:23–35.
64 Chang H-N, Garetto LP, Katona TR, Potter RH, Roberts WE: Angiogenic induction and cell migration in an orthopaedically expanded maxillary suture in the rat. Arch Oral Biol 1996;41: 985–994.
65 Chang H-N, Garetto LP, Potter RH, Katona TR, Lee C-H, Roberts WE: Angiogenesis and osteogenesis in an orthopedically expanded suture. Am J Orthod Dentofacial Orthop 1997;111:382–390.
66 Sasaki A, Sugiyama Y, Tanaka E, Sugiyama M: Effects of sutural distraction osteogenesis applied to rat maxillary complex on craniofacial growth. J Oral Maxillofac Surg 2002;60:667–675.
67 Jackson GW, Kokich VG, Shapiro PA: Experimental and postexperimental response to anteriorly directed extraoral force in young *Macaca nemestrina*. Am J Orthod 1979;75:318–333.
68 Elder JR, Tuenge RH: Cephalometric and histologic changes produced by extraoral high-pull traction to the maxilla in *Macaca mulatta*. Am J Orthod 1974;66:599–617.
69 Bradley JP, Shahinian H, Levine JP, Rowe NM, Longaker MT: Growth restriction of cranial sutures in the fetal lamb causes deformational changes, not craniosynostosis. Plast Reconstr Surg 2000;105:2416–2423.
70 Koskinen-Moffett L, Moffett BC: Sutures and intrauterine deformation; in Persing JA, Edgerton MT, Jane JA (eds): Scientific Foundations and Surgical Treatment of Craniosynostosis. Baltimore, Williams & Wilkins, 1989, pp 96–106.
71 Koskinen-Moffett LK, Moffett BC Jr, Graham JM Jr: Cranial synostosis and intra-uterine compression: a developmental study of human sutures. Prog Clin Biol Res 1982;101:365–378.
72 Lin KY, Nolen AA, Gampper TJ, Jane JA, Opperman LA, Ogle RC: Elevated levels of transforming growth factors beta 2 and beta 3 in lambdoid sutures from children with persistent plagiocephaly. Cleft Palate Craniofac J 1997;34:331–337.
73 Anton SC, Jaslow CR, Swartz SM: Sutural complexity in artificially deformed human *(Homo sapiens)* crania. J Morphol 1992;214:321–332.
74 Burrows AM, Caruso KA, Mooney MP, Smith TD, Losken HW, Siegel MI: Sutural bone frequency in synostotic rabbit crania. Am J Phys Anthropol 1997;102:555–563.
75 Opperman LA, Chhabra A, Cho RW, Ogle RC: Cranial suture obliteration is induced by removal of transforming growth factor (TGF)-β3 activity and prevented by removal of TGF-β2 activity from fetal rat calvaria in vitro. J Craniofac Genet Dev Biol 1999;19:164–173.
76 Al-Mubarak R, Da Silveira A, Mao JJ: Expression and mechanical modulation of matrix metalloproteinase-1 and -2 genes in facial and cranial sutures. Cell Tissue Res 2005;321:465–471.
77 Collins JM, Ramamoorthy K, Da Silveira A, Patston P, Mao JJ: Expression of matrix metalloproteinase genes in the rat intramembranous bone during postnatal growth and upon mechanical stresses. J Biomech 2005;38:485–492.
78 Kopher RA, Mao JJ: Suture growth modulated by the oscillatory component of micromechanical strain. J Bone Miner Res 2003;18:521–528.
79 Vij K, Mao JJ: Geometry and cell density of rat craniofacial sutures during early postnatal development and upon in vivo cyclic loading. Bone 2006;38:722–730.
80 Satoyoshi M, Kawata A, Koizumi T, Inoue K, Itohara S, Teranaka T, Mikuni-Takagaki Y: Matrix metalloproteinase-2 in dentin matrix mineralization. J Endod 2001;27:462–466.
81 Hirukawa K, Miyazawa K, Maeda H, Kameyama Y, Goto S, Togari A: Effect of tensile force on the expression of IGF-1 and IGF-1 receptor in the organ-cultured rat cranial suture. Arch Oral Biol 2005;50:367–372.

82 Yu JC, Lucas JH, Fryberg K, Borke JL: Extrinsic tension results in FGF-2 release, membrane permeability change, and intracellular Ca^{2+} increase in immature cranial sutures. J Craniofac Surg 2001;12:391–398.
83 Miao D, Bai X, Panda DK, Karaplis AC, Goltzman D, McKee MD: Cartilage abnormalities are associated with abnormal Phex expression and with altered matrix protein and MMP-9 localization in Hyp mice. Bone 2004;34:638–647.
84 Borke JL, Yu JC, Isales CM, Wagle N, Do NN, Chen JR, Bollag RJ: Tension-induced reduction in connexin 43 expression in cranial sutures is linked to transcriptional regulation by TBX2. Ann Plast Surg 2003;51:499–504.
85 Ogle RC, Tholpady SS, McGlynn KA, Ogle RA: Regulation of cranial suture morphogenesis. Cells Tissues Organs 2004;176:54–66.
86 Tarnowski CP, Ignelzi MA Jr, Wang W, Taboas JM, Goldstein SA, Morris MD: Earliest mineral and matrix changes in force-induced musculoskeletal disease as revealed by Raman microspectroscopic imaging. J Bone Miner Res 2004;19:64–71.
87 Yu P, Gosain AK, Khanna A: The role of transforming growth factor-beta in the modulation of mouse cranial suture fusion. Plast Reconstr Surg 2001;108:916–924.
88 Yoshida T, Phylactou LA, Uney JB, Ishikawa I, Eto K, Iseki S: Twist is required for establishment of the mouse coronal suture. J Anat 2005;206:437–444.
89 Warren SM, Brunet LJ, Harland RM, Economides AN, Longaker MT: The BMP antagonist noggin regulates cranial suture fusion. Nature 2003;422:625–629.
90 Dodig M, Tadic T, Kronenberg MS, Cacic S, Liu Y-H, Maxson R, Rowe DW, Lichtler AC: Ectopic *Msx2* overexpression inhibits and *Msx2* antisense stimulates calvarial osteoblast differentiation. Dev Biol 1999;209:298–307.
91 Greenwald JA, Mehrara BJ, Spector JA, Warren SM, Fagenholz PJ, Smith LP, Bouletreau PJ, Crisera FE, Ueno H, Longaker MT: In vivo modulation of FGF biological activity alters cranial suture fate. Am J Pathol 2001;158:441–452.
92 Liu Y-H, Tang Z, Kundu RK, Wu L, Luo W, Zhu D, Sangiorgi F, Snead ML, Maxson REJ: Msx2 gene dosage influences the number of proliferative osteogenic cells in growth centers of the developing murine skull: a possible mechanism for MSX2-mediated craniosynostosis in humans. Dev Biol 1999;205:260–274.
93 Opperman LA, Chhabra A, Nolen AA, Bao Y, Ogle RC: Dura mater maintains rat cranial sutures in vitro by regulating suture cell proliferation and collagen production. J Craniofac Genet Dev Biol 1998;18:150–158.
94 Yu H-MI, Jerchow B, Sheu T-J, Liu B, Costantini F, Puzas JE, Birchmeier W, Hsu W: The role of Axin2 in calvarial morphogenesis and craniosynostosis. Development 2005;132:1995–2005.
95 Nacamuli RP, Fong KD, Lenton KA, Song HM, Fang TD, Salim A, Longaker MT: Expression and possible mechanisms of regulation of BMP3 in rat cranial sutures. Plast Reconstr Surg 2005;116:1353–1362.

Susan W. Herring
Department of Orthodontics, University of Washington
Box 357446
Seattle, WA 98195-7446 (USA)
Tel. +1 206 543 3203, Fax +1 206 685 8163, E-Mail herring@u.washington.edu

Rice DP (ed): Craniofacial Sutures. Development, Disease and Treatment.
Front Oral Biol. Basel, Karger, 2008, vol 12, pp 57–78

Suture Neontology and Paleontology: The Bases for Where, When and How Boundaries between Bones Have Been Established and Have Evolved

Michael J. Depew, Claudia Compagnucci, John Griffin

Laboratory of Craniofacial Development and Evolution, Department of Craniofacial Development, King's College, London, UK

Abstract

Much of what has been written about sutures has either focused on the genetic and biologic etiologies of specific sutural development, maintenance, and pathogenesis or on the utilization of sutures as character states in vertebrate cladistic analyses. There is a much more modest literature explicitly concerned with the evolution of sutures. We provide a small bridge of these literatures by presenting a discussion of the evolutionary biologic bases for the patterns of where, when, and how sutural boundaries between skeletal and dental elements have been established and have evolved. As sutural boundaries do not exist in the absence of the nucleation events that initiate the generation of skeletal elements, we explore historic models seeking to identify the inductive events dictating the specific times and places where a cranial skeletal element forms, the elaboration of its sutural boundaries, and the mechanisms whereby subsequent phyletic changes may be manifested and recognized.

Where, When and How Boundaries between Skeletodontal Elements Have Been Established and Evolved: An Introduction

A review of the scientific literature on sutures reveals that much of what has been written has generally fallen into one of two broad categories: (1) the genetic and biologic etiology of specific sutural development, maintenance, and pathogenesis and (2) the utilization of sutures as character states in the examination of vertebrate cladistic analyses. The former class of manuscripts and texts would include, for instance, anthropologic studies of cranial deformation, the biomechanical bases of suture morphologic elaboration, and the genetic, molecular, and cellular basis of both normal and craniosynostotic sutures. The latter class includes the vast neontologic and paleontologic literature in which sutures are almost passive, secondary character states of the bones that are the primary objects of description and comparison. A much more modest literature concerned primarily with the development and evolution of sutures in their own right exists, and it is the purpose of the present chapter to provide a small bridge of these literatures by presenting a discussion of the evolutionary biologic bases for the patterns of where, when, what and how boundaries (as we presently will, in an evolutionary context, define sutures) between skeletal (herein to include both bone and cartilage) and dental elements have been established and have evolved.

Sutures: Of Homology, Boundaries, and Typology

To discuss the evolution of sutures we must place them in both neontologic and paleontologic contexts by establishing a working definition to identify them and a means of recognizing how and when they change. The development of the gnathostome (jawed vertebrate) skull is characterized both by a developmental adherence to a basic seminal structural bauplan and by the manifestation of varied ontogenetic elaborations of this bauplan into the wide diversity of sizes, shapes, and articulations of skeletodontal elements and overall forms observed [1–27]. To reach these conclusions, neontologists and paleontologists have applied the concept of homology to their investigations of these traits. Originally defined by Richard Owen as 'the same organ in different animals under every variation of form and function', homology as a concept underlies all of comparative biology [28], including that of the evolution of sutures. For a concept that is so central to biology, many attempts have been made to re-define or re-nuance notions of homology and of the related idea of homoplasy (the occurrence of similarity in structure not due to common decent). Hall [29], for instance, defines homology, as the 'continuous occurrence of the same feature (gene, structure or behavior) in two organisms whose common ancestor also possessed the feature'.

A 'feature' or 'character state' is any trait of the phenotype, and thus one's recognition of a 'feature' dictates in large part the invocation of homology. A major component of the invocation of homology between two elements is their shared topologic relations to other structures. Thus, one can reduce the character state of a skeletodontal element to (1) that which is the boundary of the element and (2) that which lies within the boundary. Primacy can thus be placed on the boundary. From an evolutionary biology vantage, by their nature, and regardless of their unique histological or ontogenetic constitutions, sutures form identifiable boundaries between elements. Hence, with regard to the skull elements, if the suture defines the boundary then the suture becomes a prime unit in the identification of homology between elements. Historically, any particular suture may have been considered a character state of an associated skeletal element, but the emphasis has generally been in the characterization of the element rather than in the particular make up of its boundaries: more rarely have such particulars as the cellular, molecular, histological, and functional characteristics of a suture been the focus of comparison. While the exact morphologies of two structures may have diverged over time, they may be deemed homologous if they maintain their relative boundary (topographic) relationships with other structures. Recognition of the boundary is therefore key, and at it simplest may follow from detection of articulations, or junctures of tissue and cellular discontinuities, during the ontogeny of skull development. (Clearly, however, not all tissue and cellular discontinuities are sutural boundaries.)

The boundaries between bones form articulations (or junctures) of many types, and they are often classified by the nature of the juncture between the bones [20]. Emphasis has typically been either on (1) the form of, and relationship between, the osseous components of the juncture twixt the bones, (2) on the type and nature of the tissue in the space between the osseous components, or (3) its topographical relationship to the involved bones (e.g., 'sagittal' sutures between parietal bones). Thus, multiple classifications may apply to any particular suture.

Phenotypic alterations due to change in developmental processes have traditionally been attributed to *heterochronic* (change in the timing of an event) or *heterotopic* (change in the topology of an event) shifts, though change due to *heterofacience* (change in the active capacitance, or the elaboration of capacity, of a developmental event) is also recognized. Unfortunately, little is known about the comparative molecular and cellular neontology of sutures; slightly more is known regarding the patterns of structural changes of sutures within evolutionary clades. Thus, to investigate the evolution of sutures one applies the notion of homology (the central comparative concept in biology) to sutural boundaries as central character states. The traits of this central character state are what then are compared and may include any aspect of the phenotype that can be described – e.g., topography, morphology, histocytochemistry, or gene expression. Comparisons of the phenotype can then be filtered through analyses of heterotopy, heterochrony or heterofacience if mechanistic etiologies are desired for any observed changes.

Overview of the Skeletal Systems Involved in Generating Sutural Boundaries

Relative position, morphology, histocytochemistry, and gene expression are all aspects of the phenotypes of sutural boundaries. They are described in reference to the parts of the skull capable of establishing boundaries – that is the bones, cartilages and teeth of the skull. The gnathostome skull is a complex, composite, modular assemblage of skeletal and dental elements with diverse developmental origins that encases the brain, its associated primary sensory organs, and the oral and respiratory openings [1–26]. The initial, embryonic cranial skeletal structures to appear are the chondrocranial elements whose development is highly conserved and reflects the initial bauplan of the gnathostome skull. The chondrocranium is composed of those structures that initially develop as cartilaginous units. These units have numerous possible fates: quiescence, endochondral ossification, direct investment by dermal bone, degeneration, transdifferentiation, or synchondroses with other chondrocranial units. That there are multiple, genetically regulated, fates to the chondrocranial elements is of obvious significance with regard to sutures and skeletal boundaries.

The perinatal skull arises with the advent of the nascent dentition and the dermatocranium, the ossified elements of the skull that develop around the chondrocranium. These bones are typically classified topologically. Osteichthyans are characterized by large numbers of dermal bones while tetrapods are characterized by large-scale reductions in number, known as 'Williston's law' [30], and chondrychthyans do not possess any as such. The skull of the adult develops with the refined modeling and remodeling of the cranial elements. In basal gnathostome taxa, the brain is more or less fully protected by the chondrocranial neurocranium; in higher taxa, the calvarial dermatocranium provides the roofing protection for the dorsal brain, and develops in apposition to the dural mesenchyme covering the brain. This mesenchyme thus provides potential influences on the sutural patterns of the calvarium that other dermal bones of the head will not encounter. Overall, great phylogenetic differences between taxa occur in the number and articulations of the dermatocranial elements.

Adaptations of tooth attachment have played significant roles in vertebrate evolution, and the association of the evolution of dental units and dermal skeletal units (see below) makes the sutures of the teeth and the skull notable with regard to skeletodontal boundaries. In conjunction with modifications of the dentition, jaws, skull, and facial musculature it has facilitated the development of highly specialized feeding mechanisms and the expansion of vertebrates into a vast array of ecological niches [2, 3, 7, 9, 11, 19, 20, 24, 34, 35, 62, 70–95].

This is reflected in the variety of tooth attachment modes observed in both extant and extinct organisms, ranging from relatively primitive rigid attachments to the complex gomphosis of mammals. Despite the considerable evident gnathostome dental specializations, there are but three basic modes of sutural connectivity: ankylosis, direct fibrous attachment and pedicellate (indirect) fibrous attachment.

Sutures thus form in the context of the boundaries generated by the developing and maturing cartilaginous, osseous, and dentigerous elements of the skull. To study and compare the development and evolution of sutures the ontogeny of the elements giving rise to the suture neontology and paleontology must be considered as well as the morphology, topography, and histocytochemistry.

Sutures, Cranial Kinesis, and the Interplay of Form and Function

Discussion of sutural neontology and paleontology has often centered around form-function analyses of intracranial mechanics or cranial kinesis [7, 10, 17, 20, 24, 31–69]. Cranial kinesis involves the relative movements of the neurocranium, dermatocranium and splanchnocranium (fig. 1). With metakinesis there is a relative movement of the neurocranium and the dermatocranium, which generally involves the specialization of five neurocranial-dermatocranial contact points: (1) the supraoccipital and parietal along the midline, (2) the bilateral paroccipital processes and their associated dermatocranial side walls, and (3) the basipterygoid process of either side of the basal plate and the pterygoids (i.e., the palate). According to Frazetta [31], metakinesis may have evolved to help shield the brain from stresses and then subsequently aided in head positioning and gape width. Streptostyly involves the movement of the quadrate relative to the dermatocranium. To accommodate movement, both dorsal and ventral joints are often modified. Dorsally, a special joint surface between the quadrate and squamosal (along with a slender supratemporal and paroccipital process) forms. Ventrally, the quadrate must be freed from the palate, usually by loss of its articulation with the pterygoid or by linking it with the pterygoid but freeing both of them. Both metakinesis and streptostyly involve synovial joints, often neomorphic, derived from the branchial arches [43]. Mesokinesis differs as it involves the acquisition of syndesmotic joints between dermatocranial elements, mainly between the frontals and parietals, and within the palate (forming hypokinetic joints) and an accommodation point either within the postorbital bar or between this bar and the temporal region. Mesokinesis is apparently not seen outside of the squamae.

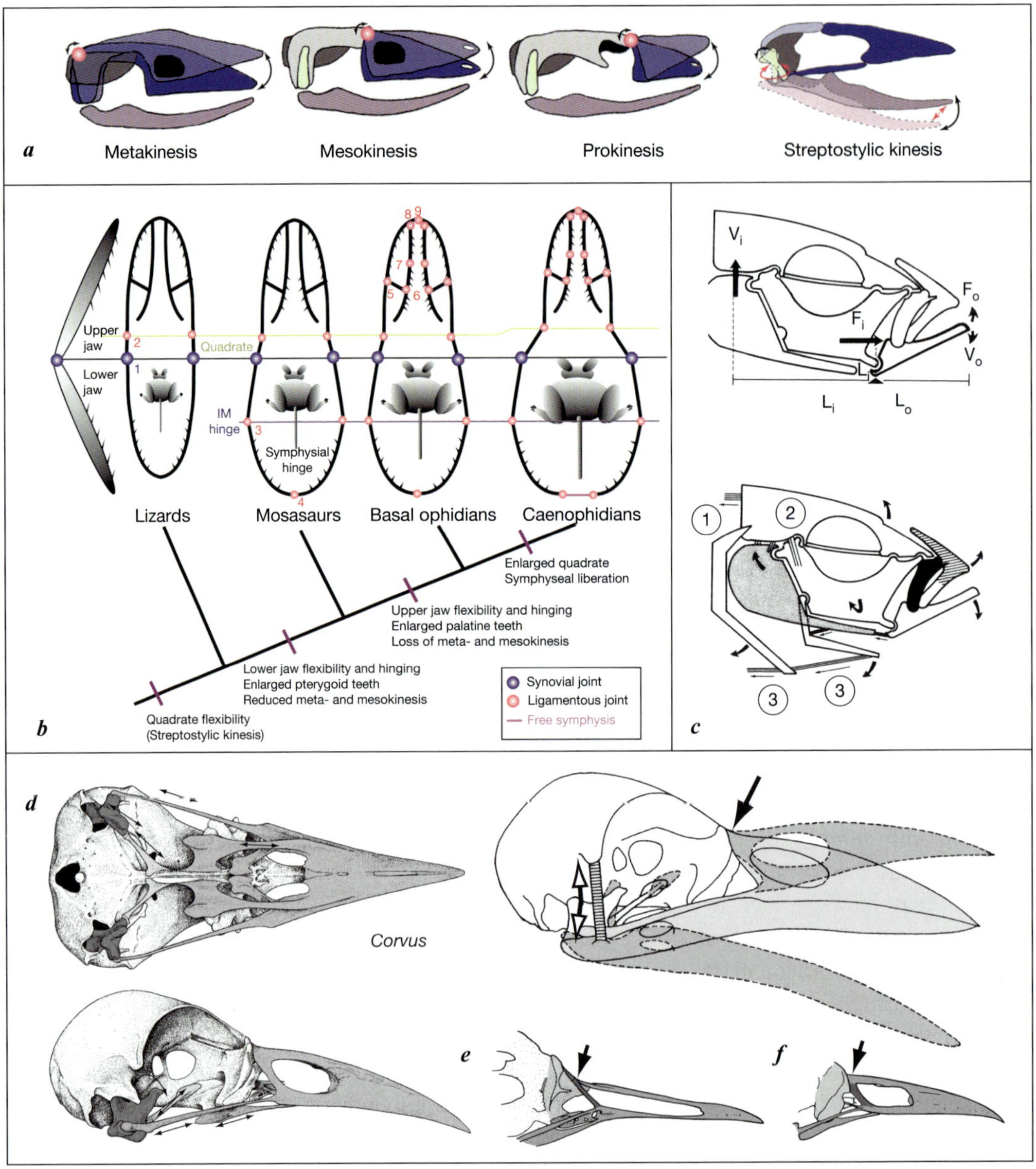

Fig. 1. Cranial kinesis. ***a*** Schemas of four major modes of cranial kinesis. Red circles indicate main axes of movement, including metakinesis, mesokinesis, prokinesis and streptostylic kinesis. Dark blue structures indicate mobile neurocranial units at rest, steel blue indicates a kinetic movement of the neurocranium, while light blue indicates static neurocranium. Yellow indicates a quadrate complex, while lavender indicates the lower jaw. ***b*** Diagram indicating the evolutionary trends in the elaboration of neomorphic kinetic sutural boundaries

Historic Evolutionary Perspectives on Basic Skeletodontal Units and Their Establishment

The remains of the earliest vertebrates consist of fragments of composites of mineralized tissues such as dentine, enameloid and bone (or, rather, an acellular, matrix-rich mineralized tissue known as *aspidin*), generally in the forms of either conodont oral 'teeth' or the more extensive dermal bony armor plates belonging to a group of agnathan (jawless) vertebrates collectively known as ostracoderms [2, 9, 10, 14, 15, 19, 95, 99, 102, 109, 112–117]. These three tissue types (dentine, enameloid and bone) apparently form an ancient coupling [6, 9, 10, 15, 20, 62, 95–99, 102–104, 109–117].

The classification of ostracoderms is based in large part on the pattern and number of the ossified dermal plates forming the carapace over their heads and trunks [9, 22, 95, 114]. These plates ranged in number from 2 to 4 large plates to many small polygonal elemental plates known as tesserae (fig. 2). Which state – few or many – is more primitive? Were the few subdivided into the many, or were the many used to form the few? This presents an ongoing question. One argument has suggested that the greater number meant more flexibility – and flexibility was thought to be under positive selective pressure – and hence was more advanced. This does not seem to follow with the sequence in which the various ostracodems appear in the fossil record, however.

Sutural boundaries do not exist in the absence of nucleation events generating skeletodontal elements [95–113], and the question of the few versus the many serves to highlight a number of issues regarding the evolution of individual skeletal elements – and their boundaries. Among these are the following: (1) Is there a basic skeletal unit, or building block, whose variously regulated development may explain the establishment of larger bones, and, if so, what is the nature of this unit? (2) What mechanisms exist for establishing the position of the nucleating event during bone and dental development, and are they universal? (3) Is there a developmental relationship between disparate structures such as neurogeneic placodes and the bones of the head? (4) What establishes a relationship between units – how do they come together and how do they establish boundaries?

in the ophidian (snake) lineage. IM = Intramandibular joint. Numbers indicate joints [modified after 56]. ***c*** Basic kinetic diagram of the teleostean jaws [modified after 22]. ***d*** Depiction of prokinesis in a crow (*Corvus*). Skulls on the left are differentially shaded to indicate mobile units (neurocranium, quadrate complex, pterygoid, and upper jaw plus palate) formed by the selective synostosis of cranial sutures. Double-headed arrows indicate direction of movement, while arrow indicates the craniofacial hinge [after 37]. Depictions of the nares in schizorhinal (***e***) and holorhinal (***f***) birds [after 132].

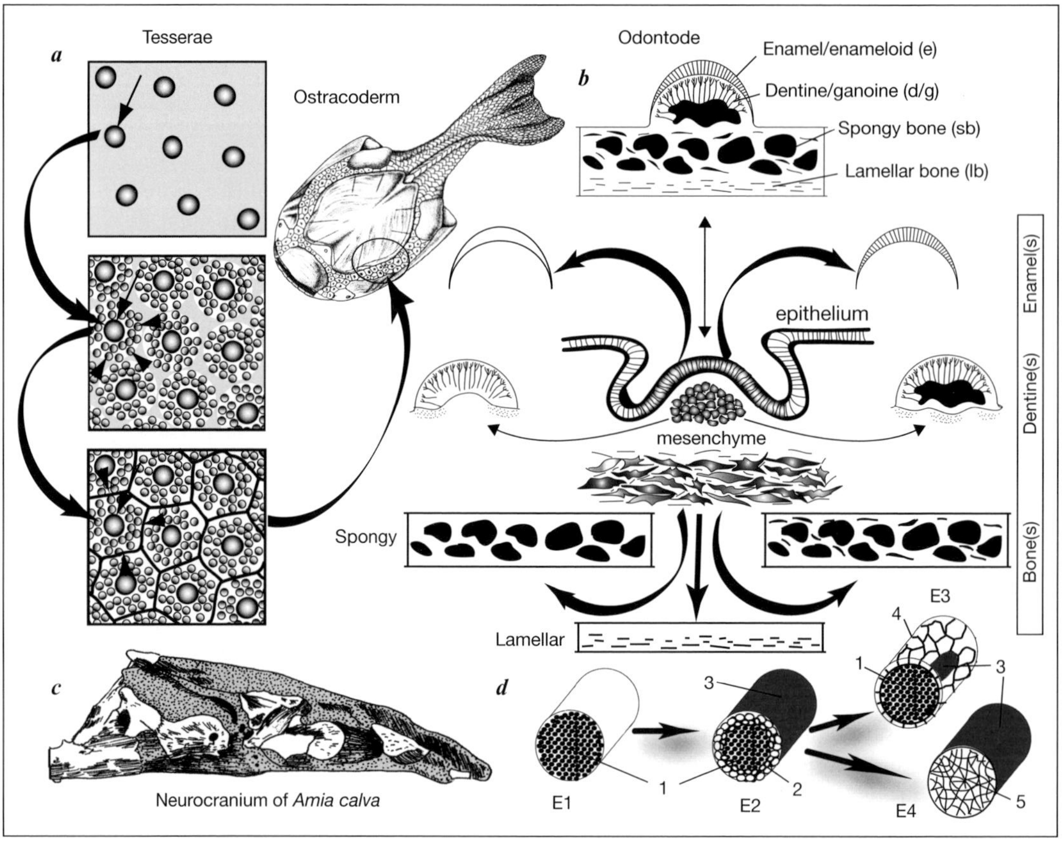

Fig. 2. Element nucleation I. ***a*** Diagram using the heterostracan *Drepanaspis* to depict the presence of many tiny plates referred to as tesserae. Tesserae are small dermal modules. In small individuals, a tiny tubercle may be nucleated (arrow) under some patterning systems. During ontogeny, growth occurs by the subsequent addition of much smaller tubercles (arrowheads) around the initial nucleating tubercle until a suture, or boundary (black lines), with another growing tesserae develops. ***b*** Depiction of tesserae as an 'odontode' indicating the conserved coupling of a developmental module for the manifestation of dermal bones, scales and teeth. Histological examination of the tesserae plates has demonstrated that they consist of units formed of a number of layers in a pattern which has been taken as plesiomorphic for primitive vertebrates. This unit is hypothesized to form from the interactions of competent epithelia and mesenchyme and to yield an outer epithelial enamel (or mesenchymal enameloid) layer, a dentine or ganoine layer, an ostensibly vascularized spongy bone layer and a deep layer of lamellar bone. ***c*** Depiction of the neurocranium of *A. calva* highlighting the idea that the ossified, suture-forming skull also includes a significant chondrocranial component, one for which there is scant theoretical literature expounding a developmental module for its formation. The ossified portions of the neurocranium are depicted in white, while the cartilaginous portion is in grey stippling. ***d*** Schema, modified from Janvier [10], indicating the evolution in the nature of the cartilaginous portion of the vertebrate skull.

In a backdrop of utility in phylogenetic reconstruction, investigators of the first of these questions have often used teeth and scales as one set of basic units of cranial hard tissue construction and evolution. Donoghue [113] cites, among others, the early work of Williamson, Klaatsch, Hertwig, Goodrich, and the more recent work of Stensio, Orvig and Reif, in suggesting that the dermal and oral skeleton is the product of an elaboration of skeletodontal developmental modules (units). Such modules have variously been given the names 'lepidomoria' (Stensio and Orvig) or 'odontodes' (Orvig and Reif), and two main means of transforming individual modules into larger structures have been presented: (1) by concrescence whereby a coalescence of modules forms a higher order pattern or (2) higher order pattern is the result of differentiation due to increased morphological specialization and/or subdivision of modules (fig. 3).

In the lepidomorial theory of Stensio and Orvig, a theoretical model was generated to explain the patterning of the dermal skeleton, and it was to be used for phylogenetic resolution twixt taxa. In essence, the model is just a generalized description of how a 'placoid scale' from a shark develops. Placoid scales were utilized as the conceptual bases for these models because: (1) shark scales were traditionally thought to be reflective of the primitive condition in dermal skeletons, (2) sharks themselves were thought to be primitive, and (3) the placoid scale was structurally simple. The basic tenet of the lepidomoria theory was that the dermal and oral skeleton is, at the most basic level, the product of developmental modules termed lepidomoria: each lepidomorium was recognized by its enamel-coated crown of dentin and an ossified basal plate situated in the deep vascular inner layer of the skin (corium/dermis). Each lepidomorium arose ontogenetically from a simple 'papilla' formed around a single vascular loop that ascended in a superficial direction from the subepidermal vascular plexus of the dermis. Subsequent development occurs as with a placoid scale – i.e., enameloid from an enamel organ makes a rigid mold in which the dentine begins to form – thus, the scale attains size and shape at once. As interpreted by Donoghue [113], this suggested that the basic unit was actually even simpler, consisting of a single vascular capillary loop entering the pulp cavity from below (placoid scales actually have supernumerary loops). Moreover, while placoid scales do not seem to coalesce, the notion was that the lepidomoria – that is, a basic skeletal unit – had done so prior to mineralization. Thus, higher order morphology was due to coalescence rather than differentiation (as was thought by many to be the case during dental development and evolution). The odontode theory of Orvig offered

E1 = Normal cartilage (1); E2 = globular calcified cartilage (2), as seen in certain ostracoderms, placoderms and acanthodians; E3 = prismatic calcified cartilage (4) with remnants of perichondral bone (3) as seen in some chondrichtyans; E4 = perichondral and endochondral bone (5) as seen in osteichthyans such as in ***c***.

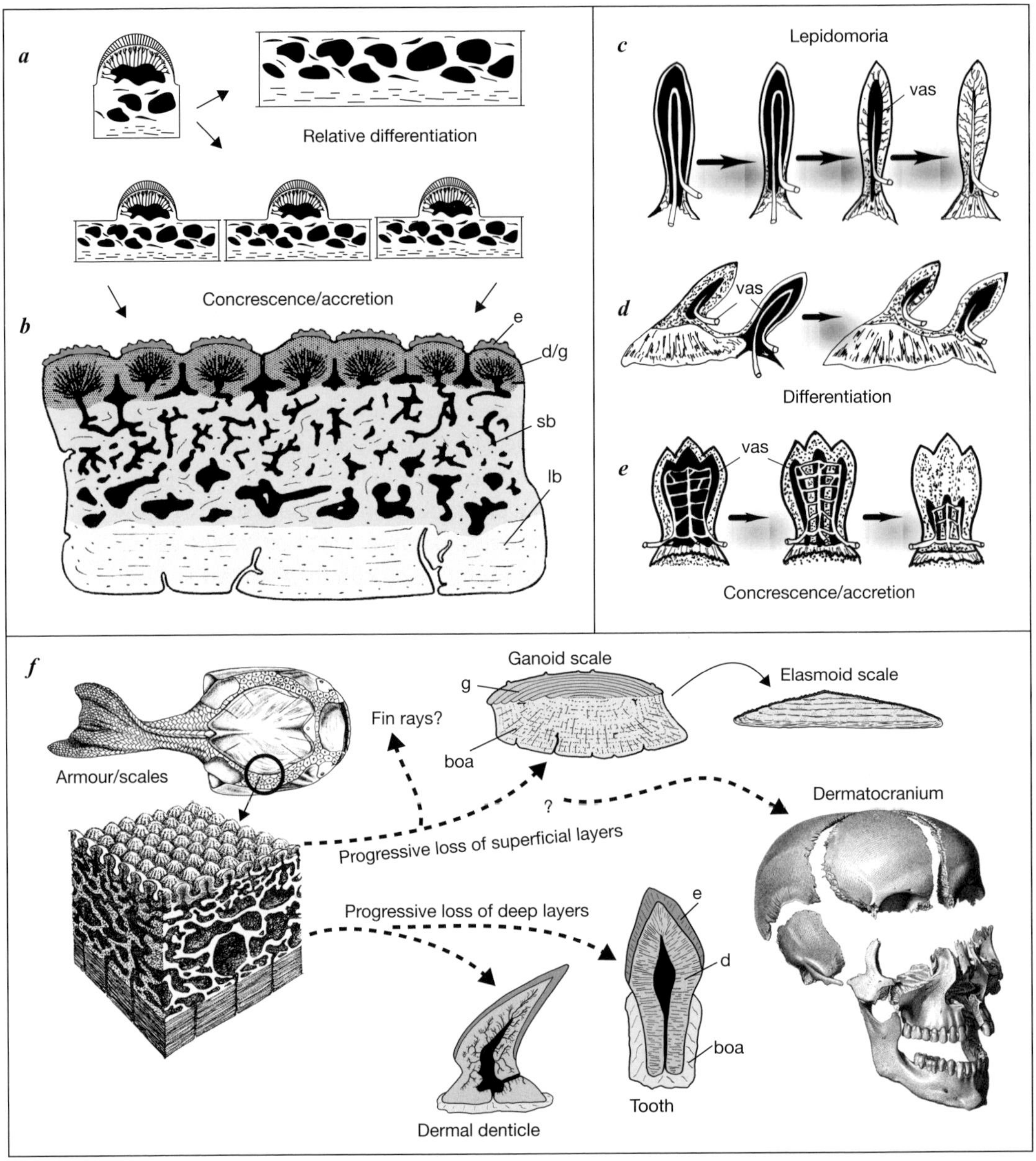

Fig. 3. Element nucleation II. Elaboration. ***a***, ***b*** Taking the odontode as a developmental module, elaboration of larger order bones. ***a*** Hypothesized to occur either through the relative differentiation of one or more portions of the module unit (here depicted as the spongy and lamellar bone forming a large dermal ossification) or through the concrescence, or accretion, of many units (***b***). e = Enamel; d/g = dentine/ganoid; sb = spongy bone; lb = lamellar bone. ***c*** Schemas depicting the ontogenetic formation of lepidomoria, hypothetical developmental

little operationally different from lepidomoria in terms of delineating tractable fundamental skeletal units.

As an alternative, Reif [117] offered the odontode regulation theory, making odontodes into morphogenetic entities to encompass a theory of morphogenesis. Like others before him, Reif saw the placoid scale as reflecting the basic morphogenetic unit within the vertebrate dermal skeleton. Reif looked at placoid scales but found, however, no evidence of a differentiation of dental papilla into a series of distinct 'lepidomoria'. Reif, therefore, modified Orvig's odontode concept into a transformational theory by suggesting that morphological changes take place through differentiation: thus large or complex teeth and scales arise through the changes in morphogenesis of individual primordia rather than through concrescence of primordia.

It bears reiterating that these reductionist, theoretical models were: (1) proposed in the context of explaining patterns of dermal elements (or subsections thereof) that were found in the head shields of ostracoderms, (2) proposed with an evolutionary context with sharks, and hence their placoid scales, in mind, and (3) explanations of mechanisms of dermal bone morphogenesis. These were not models, however, to explain the mechanisms underlying the inductive events dictating the specific times and specific places where a placoid scale, odontode, lepidomoria, or an entire dermal bone was established. If, as it has been supposed, the early vertebrate head was covered by tesserae of micromeric elements made of odontodes or odontode analogues (i.e., were covered by 'microsquamose' scutes or scales) then it is reasonable to seek a mechanism whereby subsequent phyletic changes (in at least some taxonomic groups) of subpopulations of these micromeric elements resulted in the emergence of relatively large, definitive bones.

While such explanations are even today largely tenuous, more than a century ago Allis [118, 119] proffered a causal explanation of the position of the dermal bones in the skull of the fish, *Amia calva*. The patterns of dermal bones of the skull – and thus their sutures – form the basis of comparing the vast majority of vertebrates; Allis suggested that the lateral line system, consisting of mechanoreceptive neuromasts and electroreceptive ampullary organs housed within canals coursing along cranial dermal bones of basal gnathostomes, dictated where the dermal bones began to form and thus might be used to homologize skeletal elements between fish (fig. 4) [2, 3, 7, 14, 15, 18–20, 100, 101, 105–107, 118–121].

units, as centered around a vascular loop (vas). ***d*** Relative differentiation as seen in a lepidomoria. ***e*** Concrescence or accretion as seen in a lepidomoria. ***f*** Schematic representation of the transition from the tesserae – odontode – lepidomoria developmental unit associated with primitive vertebrates to extant skeletal structures that they are hypothesized to have given rise to. e = Enamel; d = dentine; boa = bone of attachment.

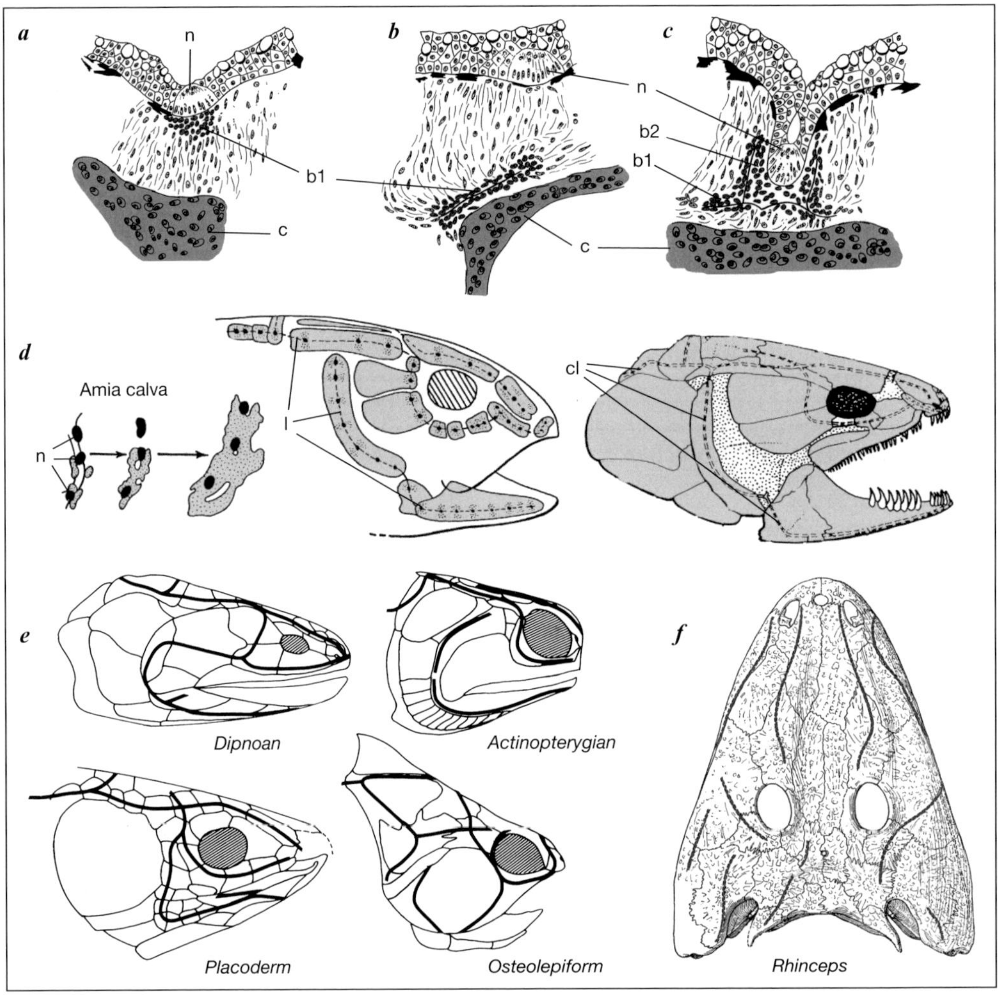

Fig. 4. Element nucleation III. Lateral line. Neuromast induction of dermal ossification. ***a–c*** Histological schemas suggesting the developmental relationship of forming neuromasts and the associated condensations of skeletogenic mesenchyme. b1, b2 = Dermal bone blastemata; c = cartilage; n = neuromast. ***d*** Diagram of the developmental association of the neuromasts (n) of the lateral lines and the nucleation event initiating osteogenesis (outlined in grey) in *A. calva* [modified from 10]. Note that multiple neuromasts may be associated with a single bone and that not all bones contain lateral line canals (cl) housing neuromasts. l = Lateral line. ***e*** Outlines of the lateral line canals in four taxa of fish [after 15]. ***f*** Lateral lines as evident in an early tetrapod, the labirynthodont, *Rhinceps* [after 133].

The primitive condition in basal gnathostomes appears to have been a system of lateral lines that developed from six pairs (subdivided as preotic or postotic) of cephalic lateral line placodes [122–124]. Following the initial formation of the placode (an epithelial thickening ostensibly coupled with an associated population of neural crest cells), ganglionic cells demarginate. Neurites from these ganglia enter the medulla while also contacting the placode. Sequent to this, the mitotic activity of the placode cells increases and the cephalic placodes elongate (placodes forming the trunk lateral lines migrate onto the trunk). Variably through cell division or migration, placodes elaborate an orientation forming a sensory ridge. From these ridges, initially within the central zone of the ridge, neuromasts (receptor primordia) form. (Elctroreceptive primoria are distinct and form at the periphery.) The neuromast primoria erupt to the surface and are spaced in a pattern suggestive of a mechanism involving lateral inhibition [125]. While in extant amphibians these neuromasts remain relatively superficial, in other basal gnathostomes ectodermal ridges form around the lateral line ridges of neuromasts, fused above them and so enclose them within an epithelial canal. Twixt each such enclosed neuromast, an opening to the surface remains patent. The epithelial canals encapsulating the neuromasts are themselves subsequently encapsulated by cartilage or bone. What Allis initially described in *Amia* was the process of the sinking of the neuromasts into the dermis, the formation of patent canals via the union of separate forming sections, and the opening to the surface of the pores between neuromasts; this association has been confirmed and reconfirmed in numerous basal gnathostomes (fig. 4).

Thus the question has been: is the close association of dermal bones of the head and the neuromasts housed in their laterosensory canals a causal one whereby the neuromast induces the osteogenesis or are they only secondarily topographically coincident? [15, 100, 101, 105, 120–123]. Evidence for the former includes: (1) the temporospatial coincidence of the sinking of the neuromasts into the dermis in *Amia* and the initiation of osteogenesis in the immediate vicinity, (2) the course of the canals actually passes through what is the center of radiation of bone growth of the implicated dermal bones, (3) neuromasts could act as centers of aggregation of osteogenic mesenchyme [126, 127], and (4) neurogenic placodes, including the otic, olfactory, and dental placodes, have skeletogenic-inducing properties. Evidence for the latter has included: (1) the basal gnathostome skull consists of numerous bones, known as 'anamestic' bones, that seemed to develop just to fill in space, lacking lateral-line canals passing through them; (2) Moy-Thomas [128] removed the lateral-line primordia from the frontal region of a trout embryo prior to the onset of ossification and found that in this region bones without canals still formed – albeit it was developmentally delayed; (3) the course of lateral lines in some lineages shifted without change in the fundamental pattern of the homologous

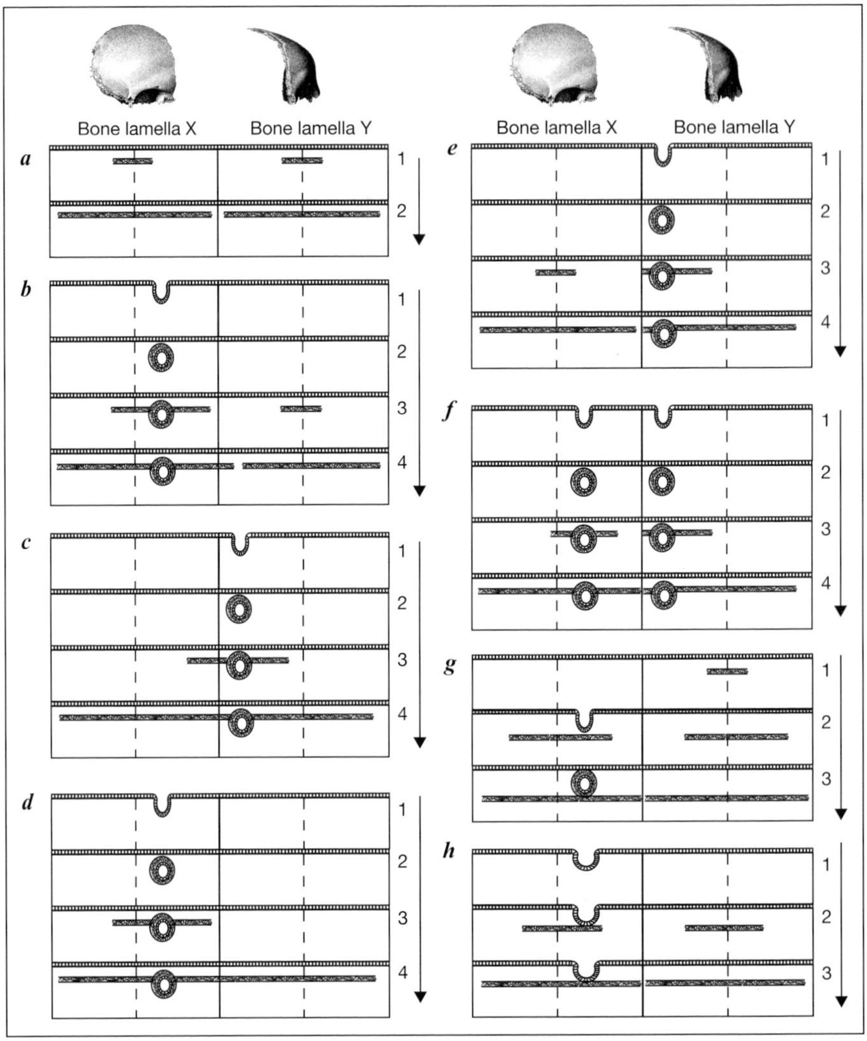

Fig. 5. Element nucleation III. Theoretical association of anamestic and neuromast-induced bones formed during dermagenesis and membranogenesis as proposed by Graham-Smith [100, 101]. Arrow and numbers indicate ontogenetic progression of the potential bone lamella X (left of each column) and bone lamella Y (right). The top of each numbered progression depicts the epithelial layer from which the inductive event is initiated. Neuromasts are taken as invaginated epithelia. Dark lines represent the horizontal, lamellar ossification while tubular, laterosensory ossifications are depicted as dark lamellar lines encapsulating neuromast epithelia that have sunk into the dermis. ***a*** The default state in which a nonneuromast induction event has generated lamellae in bones X and Y. ***b*** Dermogenesis, in which the sunk neuromast has nucleated, or induced, an encapsulating ossification in X. This ossification grows by lateral extension while a nonlaterosensory induction initiates ossification of bone Y. As the initiation

bone; (4) the size and number of the postorbital and intraorbital canal bones in *Amia* varied from one specimen to another, and (5) higher gnathostomes have no apparent lateral line systems.

Resolution of the above question is incomplete; however, attempts have been made to incorporate both data sets (fig. 5) into a coherent mechanism of dermal bone initiation and development in basal gnathostomes [15, 100, 101]. It has been suggested, based on experimental evidence from the varieties of ossification sequences seen in numerous fish, that canal-containing bones consist of two fundamental components: a 'tubular', laterosensory ossification formed via a process termed 'dermogenesis' and a basal, 'lamellar' ossification formed via a process termed 'membranogenesis' [1, 100, 101, 126]. In dermogenesis, the neuromasts sink, become encapsuled, and initiate the ossification. Growth of the tubular bone occurs by the lateral extension, in the form of horizontal lamina, of the initial ossification. In cases of membranogenesis, however, the initial focus of ossification could occur at some distance from a neuromast if the neuromast remained close to the surface. Ossification would progress by lateral extensions. A neuromast and its focal ossification could either stay superficial or subsequently sink and join the deeper membranous bone lamella. Alternatively, no neuromast could also be associated with the forming deeper membranous bone lamella, a situation subsequently considered to be the default state with regard to the dermal elements of the gnathostome skull [100, 101]. Thus, the skeletal patterns of both canal and anamestic bones can be explained by the relative elaboration of dermogenesis and membranogenesis (fig. 5).

For our current purposes, this two-component system (tubulogenesis and dermogenesis) still leaves a number of issues. The first issue concerns the proximate developmental mechanisms that initiate the establishment of the

of ossification occurred earlier in X, it may invade the territory of bone Y. ***c*** Depiction of the event in which the induction of the neuromast itself has topographically shifted to a region where nucleation has previously been unrelated to laterosensory induction. In this case, dermogenesis in the region of Y acts as a nucleator for both bones X and Y, which are thereafter a single bone. ***d*** Where the territory of Y loses its own nucleation event, or the bone is initiated but then resorbs, the laterosensory-initiated ossification in X can grow laterally to encompass territory formerly occupied by Y. ***e*** Depicts the case where bone X loses its dermogenetic induction and reverts back to the default state while a heterotopic neuromast initiates ossification in Y. ***f*** Two adjacent neuromasts share timing of ossification nucleation and grow laterally to form a single bone. ***g*** A sinking, but superficial, neuromast initiates lamellar ossification in X followed ontogenetically by tubulogenesis. Co-ossification may then occur, but with the canal bone relatively superficial. ***h*** A sinking, but superficial, neuromast initiates lamellar ossification in X, but this is not followed ontogenetically by tubulogenesis.

particular time and place where either 'dermogenetic' or 'membranogenetic' foci form. If, for example, the lateral line system is proximate to the ossification, and keeping in mind that both neuromasts and the associated mesenchyme migrate to their eventual positions, then what patterns the placement of the neuromasts? While studies of the genetic, molecular, and cellular underpinnings of placodogenesis (both neurogenic and odontogenic) have progressed significantly in the past 20 years [124], we are still significantly far from full understanding of lateral line placodogenesis and elaboration. We are, moreover, still unclear whether, in fact, both 'dermogenetic' or 'membranogenetic' foci are elaborated by the same, or related, patterning systems or if the one leads the other (i.e., the causal relationship of the lateral lines to canal bones may, in fact, be spurious).

The second issue concerns the establishment and elaboration of sutural boundaries. A salient question becomes: What mechanism(s) direct the decision to coalesce specific ossification centers to form a unified element? The relative rate of growth of an ossification center, once initiated, that of the dermis in which it grows, and its relative competence to manifest and maintain its own boundaries, not to mention the capacity to direct the functionally appropriate histogenesis within the sutural boundary, are each factors that undoubtedly interrelate to the establishment and regulation of the positions where the bones meet and where sutures form (and are the purview of other chapters within this volume).

Some paleontologists have considered that an ossification spreads from its center until it meets another thereby establishing a sutural line: this is, perhaps, too simplistic a notion, however. The position of a mature bone is only partially determined by the foci of its initial ossification. It has been demonstrated repeatedly that an individual skeletal element (as determined by the boundaries formed of its sutures) may have been formed by multiple ossification centers. Westoll [100] proposed the term 'anmestic' to refer to bones that develop to fill in space, and in those regions where, in fish, the dermal bones are tightly associated with the subjacent neurocranium, and where they do not transmit a unique set of mechanical forces (e.g., snout), a mosaic pattern (i.e., each specimen displays a distinct pattern) of bones often is to be found. Alternatively, formation of extra bones has also been attributed to the increase in mechanical forces. Patent, unossified fontanelles between dermal bones are moreover found in adult gnathostomes, such as with the calvaria of the King Charles Spanial [129] or in the snout of *Acanthostega* [130]. In fact, it has also been demonstrated that an ossification center may be initiated, but then be resorbed – rather than fused to another element – before its topographic position subsequently taken by the growth of another bone (e.g., the parietal of the actinopterygian fish *Polypterus* [131]).

Conclusions

A common trend in the cranial evolution of most groups is toward the reduction in the total number of bones, expressed in 'Williston's law', and is usually accounted for by loss or fusion [30]. Can the patterns of gnathostome dermal bones observed be explained by ad hoc hypotheses of changes in relative growth, subdivision, loss and replacement? Do the major intertaxa differences in pattern, as seen for example with those between placoderms and osteichthyeans, represent obfuscation of a shared common bone pattern control system plesiomorphic to gnathostomes? Or, rather, do they represent distinct, disparate control mechanisms? What of patterns of ossification within the developing chondrocranium? All are unresolved questions. Lastly, we must ask: what mechanisms are responsible for positioning the points of initiation of the molecular cascades known to initiate ossification centers in cartilaginous primordia? How are sutures within the endocranium established?

To address this one must address at least two processes. The first is the mechanism that establishes the conserved pattern of development of the elements of the chondrocranium. The second is the mechanism that establishes the idiosyncratic fates (e.g. quiescence, endochondral ossification, direct investment by dermal bone, degeneration, transdifferentiation, or synchondroses with other chondrocranial units) of these chondrocranial elements.

Acknowledgments

The authors would like to thank Per Ahlberg, Jenny Clack, Susan Evans and Tom Kemp for their considered opinions. Funding was through the Royal Society (MJD) and EU Marie Curie Fellowships (CC and JG).

References

1 de Beer GR: The Development of the Vertebrate Skull. Chicago, University of Chicago Press, 1985.
2 Goodrich ES: Studies on the Structure and Development of Vertebrates. New York, Dover Publications, 1958.
3 Romer AS: The Osteology of the Reptilia. Chicago, University of Chicago Press, 1956.
4 Schmalhausen II: The Origin of Terrestrial Vertebrates. New York, Academic Press, 1968.
5 Barghusen HR, Hopson A: The endoskeleton: the comparative anatomy of the skull and visceral skeleton; in Wake M (ed): Hyman's Comparative Anatomy. Chicago, University of Chicago Press, 1979, pp 265–326.
6 Holmgren N: Studies on the head of fishes, embryological, morphological, and phylogenetical researches. I. Development of the skull in sharks and rays. Acta Zool 1940;21:267–561.
7 Gregory WK: Fish skulls. A study of the evolution of natural mechanisms. Trans Am Phil Soc 1933;23:i–vii, 75–481.

8 Reynolds SH: The Vertebrate Skeleton. Cambridge, Cambridge University Press, 1913.
9 Carroll RL: Vertebrate Paleontology and Evolution. New York, Freeman, 1988.
10 Janvier P: Early Vertebrates. Oxford, Clarendon Press, 1996.
11 Moore WJ: The Mammalian Skull. Cambridge, Cambridge University Press, 1981.
12 Trueb L: Patterns of cranial diversity among the lissamphibia; in Haken J, Hall BK (eds): The Skull. Chicago, University of Chicago Press, 1993, vol 2: Patterns of Structural and Systematic Diversity, pp 255–343.
13 Novacek M: Patterns of diversity in the mammalian skull; in Haken J, Hall BK (eds): The Skull. Chicago, University of Chicago Press, 1993, vol 2: Patterns of Structural and Systematic Diversity, pp 438–545.
14 Schultze HP: Patterns of diversity in the skulls of jawed fishes; in Haken J, Hall BK (eds): The Skull. Chicago, University of Chicago Press, 1993, vol 2: Patterns of Structural and Systematic Diversity, pp 189–254.
15 Thomson KS: Segmentation of the adult skull and the problem of homology; in Haken J, Hall BK (eds): The Skull. Chicago, University of Chicago Press, 1993, vol 2: Patterns of Structural and Systematic Diversity, pp 366–368.
16 Heilmann G: The Origin of Birds. London, Witherby, 1926.
17 Rieppel O: Patterns of diversity in the reptilian skull; in Haken J, Hall BK (eds): The Skull. Chicago, University of Chicago Press, 1993, vol 2: Patterns of Structural and Systematic Diversity, pp 344–390.
18 Jarvik E: Basic Structure and Evolution of Vertebrates. London, Academic Press, 1980.
19 Jollie M: Chordate Morphology. New York, Reinhold, 1926.
20 Hildebrand M: Analysis of Vertebrate Structure. New York, Wiley, 1988.
21 Kingsley JS: The Vertebrate Skeleton from the Developmental Standpoint. Philadelphia, Blakiston's Sons, 1925.
22 Radinsky LB: The Evolution of Vertebrate Design. Chicago, University of Chicago Press, 1987.
23 Romanoff AL: The Avian Embryo: Structural and Functional Development. New York, MacMillan, 1960.
24 Peyer B: Comparative Odontology. Chicago, University of Chicago Press, 1968.
25 Kemp TS: The Origin and Evolution of Mammals. Oxford, Oxford University Press, 2005.
26 Depew MJ, Tucker A, Sharpe P: Craniofacial development; in Rossant J, Tam PPL (eds): Mouse Development: Patterning, Morphogenesis, and Organogenesis. London, Academic Press, 2002, pp 421–498.
27 Depew MJ, Simpson CA: 21st century neontology and the comparative development of the vertebrate skull. Dev Dyn 2006;235:1256–1291.
28 Hall BK: Homology: the Hierarchical Basis of Comparative Biology. San Diego, Academic Press, 1994.
29 Hall BK: Descent with modification: the unity underlying homology and homoplasy as seen through an analysis of development and evolution. Biol Rev Camb Philos Soc 2003;78:409–433.
30 Gregory WK: 'Williston's law' relating to the evolution of skull bones in the vertebrates. Am J Phys Anthropol 1935;20:123–152.
31 Frazetta TH: A functional consideration of cranial kinesis in lizards. J Morphol 1962;111:287–319.
32 Albright RG, Nelson EM: Cranial kinetics of the generalized colubrid snake *Elaphe obsoleta quadrivittata*. J Morphol 1959;105:193–291.
33 Beecher RM: Adaptations for food-gathering in the American blackbirds. Auk 1979;68:411–439.
34 Bemis WE: Feeding Systems of Living Dipnoi: Anatomy and Function. J Morphol Suppl 1986;1: 249–275.
35 Bemis WE, Lauder GV: Morphology and function of the feeding apparatus of the lungfish, *Lepidosiren paradoxa* (Dipnoi). J Morphol 1986;187:81–108.
36 Bock WJ: Secondary articulation of the avian mandible. Auk 1960;77:19–55.
37 Bock WJ: Kinetics of the avian skull. J Morphol 1964;114:1–42.
38 Bock WJ, Morioka H: Morphology and evolution of the ectethmoid-mandibular articulation in the Meliphagidae (Aves). J Morphol 1971;135:13–50.
39 Bout RG, Zweers GA: The role of cranial kinesis in birds. Comp Biochem Physiol A Mol Integr Physiol 2001;131:197–205.

40 Buhler P, Martin LD, Witmer LM: Cranial kinesis in the late cretaceous birds Hesperornis and Parahesperornis. Auk 1988;105:111–122.
41 DeMar R, Barghusen HR: Mechanism and the evolution of synapsid jaw. Evolution 1972;26: 622–637.
42 Eaton TH: Evolution of the upper jaw mechanism in teleost fishes. J Morphol 1935;58:157–172.
43 Evans SE: At the feet of the dinosaurs: the early history and radiation of lizards. Biol Rev 2003;78:513–551.
44 Frazzetta TH: Adaptation and function of cranial kinesis in reptiles: a time motion analysis of feeding in alligator lizards; in Rhodin A, Miyata K (eds): Advances in Herpetology and Evolutionary Biology. Cambridge, Harvard University, 1983, pp 222–224.
45 Frazzetta TH: Adaptations and significance of the cranial feeding apparatus of the sunbeam snake *(Xenopeltis unicolor)*. I. Anatomy of the skull. J Morphol 1999;239:27–43.
46 Gans C: The feeding mechanism of snakes and its possible evolution. Am Zool 1961;1:217–227.
47 Gregory JT: Convergent evolution: the jaws of Hesperornis and the Masasaurs. Evolution 1951;5:345–354.
48 Gregory JT: The jaws of the Cretaceous toothed birds, Ichthyornis and Hesperornis. Condor 1952;54:73–88.
49 Gussekloo SWS, Vosselman MG, Bout RG: Three-dimensional kinematics of skeletal elements in avian prokinetic and rhynchokinetic skulls determined by roentgen stereophotogrammetry. J Exp Biol 2001;204:1735–1744.
50 Herrel A, Aerts P, De Vree F: Cranial kinesis in geckoes: functional implications. J Exp Biol 2000;203:1415–1423.
51 Herrel A, De Vree F, Delheusy VV, Gans C: Cranial kinesis in gekkonid lizards. J Exp Biol 1999;202:3687–3698.
52 Herring SW: Sutures and craniosynostosis: a comparative, functional and evolutionary perspective; in Cohen MM Jr, MacLean RE (eds): Craniosynostosis: Diagnosis, Evaluation, and Management. New York, Oxford University Press, 2000, pp 3–10.
53 Herring SW: Formation of the vertebrate face: epigenetic and functional influences. Am Zool 1993;33:472–483.
54 Herring SW: Sutures – a tool in functional cranial analysis. Acta Anat 1972;83:222–247.
55 Herring SW: A biometric study of suture fusion and skull growth in peccaries. Anat Embryol 1974;146:167–180.
56 Lee MSY, Bell GL Jr, Caldwell MW: The origin of snake feeding. Nature 1999;400:655–659.
57 Markey MJ, Main RP, Marshall CR: In vivo cranial suture function and suture morphology in the extant fish Polypterus: implications for inferring skull function in living and fossil fish. J Exp Biol 2006;209:2085–2102.
58 Markey MJ, Marshall CR: Linking form and function of the fibrous joints in the skull: a new quantification scheme for cranial sutures using the extant fish *Polypterus endlicherii*. J Morphol 2007;268:89–102.
59 Rieppel O: The evolution of the naso-frontal joint in snakes and its bearing on snake origins. Z Zool Syst Evolut Forsch 1978;16:14–27.
60 Rieppel O: The evolution of the Ophidian feeding system. Zool Jahrb Anat 1980;103:551–564.
61 Scapino R: Morphological investigation into functions of the jaw symphysis in carnivorans. J Morphol 1981;167:339–375.
62 Shellis RP: Comparative anatomy of tooth attachment; in Berkovitz BKB, Moxham BJ, Newman HN (eds): The Periodontal Ligament in Health and Disease. Oxford, Pergamon Press, 1982, pp 3–24.
63 Simonetta AM: On the mechanical implications of avian skull and their bearing on the evolution and classification of birds. Q Rev Biol 1960;35:206–220.
64 Tokita M: The skull development of parrots with special reference to the emergence of a morphologically unique cranio-facial hinge. Zoolog Sci 2003;20:749–758.
65 Westneat MW: A biomechanical model for analysis of muscle force, power output and lower jaw motion in fishes. J Theor Biol 2003;223:269–281.
66 Wilga CD: A functional analysis of jaw suspension in elasmobranches. Biol J Linn Soc 2002;71:165–185.

67 Wu EH: Kinematic analysis of jaw protrusion in orectolobiform sharks: a new mechanism for jaw protrusion in elasmobranchs. J Morphol 1994;222:175–190.
68 Zivanovic S: A note on the effect of asymmetry in suture closure in mature human skulls. Am J Phys Anthropol 1983;60:431–435.
69 Anton SC, Jaslow CR, Swartz SM: Sutural complexity in artificially deformed human *(Homo sapiens)* crania. J Morphol 1992;214:321–332.
70 Tomes CS: A Manual of Dental Anatomy – Human and Comparative. London, Churchill, 1923.
71 Bemis WE: Morphology and growth of lepidosirenid lungfish tooth plates (Pisces: Dipnoi). J Morphol 1984;179:73–93.
72 Fink WJ: Ontogeny and phylogeny of tooth attachment modes in actinopterygian fishes. J Morphol 1981;167:167–184.
73 Bemis WE, Giuliano A, McGuire B: Structure, attachment, replacement and growth of teeth in bluefish, *Pomatomus saltatrix* (Linnaeus, 1776), a teleost with deeply socketed teeth. Zoology 2005;108:317–327.
74 Bhatti HK: The integument and dermal skeleton of Siluroidea. Trans Zool Soc Lond 1938;24:1–79.
75 Kerr T: Development and structure of some actinopterygian and urodele teeth. Proc Zool Soc Lond 1960;133:401–422.
76 Parsons T, Williams EE: The teeth of amphibia and their relation to amphibian phylogeny. J Morphol 1962;110:375–389.
77 Gillette R: The dynamics of continuous succession of teeth in the frog *(Rana pipiens)*. Am J Anat 1955;96:1–36.
78 Katow H: Structure and formation of ankylosis in *Xenopus laevis*. J Morphol 1979;162:327–342.
79 Oltmanns E: Zur Morphologie der Zähne rezenter Amphibien. Anat Anz 1952;98:369–389.
80 Hertwig O: Über das Zahnsystem der Amphibien und seine Bedeutung für die Genese des Skeletts der Mundhöhle. Eine vergleichend anatomische, entwicklungsgeschichtliche Untersuchung. Arch Mikr Anat 1874;11(suppl):208.
81 Krause R: Mikroskopische Anatomie der Wirbeltiere in Einzeldarstellungen. III. Amphibien. Berlin, de Gruyter, 1923.
82 Jarvik E: On the structure of the snout of crossopterygians and lower gnathostomes in general. Zool Bidrag 1942;21:235–675.
83 Cooper JS, Poole DFG: The dentition and dental tissues of the agamid lizard, Uromastix. J Zool 1973;169:192–201.
84 Taub AM: Comparative histological studies on Duvernoy's gland of colubrid snakes. Bull Am Mus Nat Hist 1967;138:1–50.
85 Edmund AG: Dentition; in Gans C, Bellairs Ad'A, Parsons TS (eds): Biology of the Reptilia. London, Academic Press, 1969, pp 115–200.
86 Savitzky AH: Hinged teeth in snakes: an adaptation for swallowing hard-bodied prey. Science 1981;212:346–349.
87 Patchell FC, Shine R: Hinged teeth for hard-bodied prey: a case of convergent evolution between snakes and legless lizards. J Zool 1986;208:269–275.
88 Modesto SP: The cranial skeleton of the early permian aquatic reptile *Mesosaurus tenuidens*: implications for relationships and paleobiology. Zool J Linn Soc 2006;146:345–368.
89 McIntosh JE, Anderton X, Flores-de-Jacoby L, Carlson DS, Shuler CF, Diekwisch TG: Caiman periodontium as an intermediate between basal vertebrate ankylosis-type attachment and mammalian 'true' periodontium. Microsc Res Tech 2002;59:449–459.
90 Ferguson MW: Palate development. Development 1988;103(suppl):41–60.
91 Thomas HF, Kollar EJ: Differentiation of odontoblasts in grafted recombinants of murine epithelial root sheath and dental mesenchyme. Arch Oral Biol 1989;34:27–35.
92 Hopson JA: Tooth replacement in cynodont, dicynodont and therocephalian reptiles. Proc Zool Soc Lond 1964;142:235–675.
93 Osborn JW: From reptile to mammal: evolutionary considerations of the dentition with emphasis on tooth attachment. Symp Zool Soc Lond 1984;52:549–574.
94 Crompton AW, Parker P: Evolution of the mammalian masticatory apparatus. Am Sci 1978;66:192–201.
95 Halstead LB: The Pattern of Vertebrate Evolution. San Francisco, Freeman, 1968.

96 Halstead LB: Calcified tissues in the earliest vetebrates. Calcif Tissue Res 1969;3:107–124.
97 Halstead LB: The vertebrate invasion of fresh water. Phil Trans R Soc Lond 1985;309:243–258.
98 Beresford WA: Cranial skeletal tissue: diversity and evolutionary trends; in Haken J, Hall BK (eds): The Skull. Chicago, University of Chicago Press, 1993, vol 2: Patterns of Structural and Systematic Diversity, pp 69–130.
99 Donoghue PC, Sansom IJ, Downs JP: Early evolution of vertebrate skeletal tissues and cellular interactions, and the canalization of skeletal development. J Exp Zoolog B Mol Dev Evol 2006;306:278–294.
100 Graham-Smith W: On some variations in the latero-sensory lines of the placoderm fish Bothriolepis. Phil Trans R Soc Lond 1978;282:1–39.
101 Graham-Smith W: On the lateral lines and dermal bones in the parietal region of some crossopterygian and dipnoan fishes. Phil Trans R Soc Lond 1978;282:41–105.
102 Janvier P, Arsenault M: Palaeobiology: calcification of early vertebrate cartilage. Nature 2002;417:609.
103 Johanson Z, Smith MM: Placoderm fishes, pharyngeal denticles, and the vertebrate dentition. J Morphol 2003;257:289–307.
104 Johanson Z, Smith MM: Origin and evolution of gnathostome dentitions: a question of teeth and pharyngeal denticles in placoderms. Biol Rev 2005;80:303–345.
105 Moodie RL: The influence of the lateral-line system on the peripheral osseous elements of fishes and amphibia. J Comp Neurol 1922;34:319–335.
106 Patterson C: Cartilage bones, dermal bones and membrane bones, or the exoskeleton versus the endoskeleton; in Mahala Andrews S, Miles RS, Walker AD (eds): Problems in Vertebrate Evolution. London, Linnean Society of London by Academy Press, 1977, pp 77–121.
107 Pehrson T: Some points in the cranial development of teleostomian fishes. Acta Zool 1922;3:1–63.
108 Sansom IJ, Donoghue PCJ, Albanesi G: Histology and affinity of the earliest armoured vertebrate. Biol Lett 2005;1:446–449.
109 Sire JY: Teeth outside the mouth in teleost fishes: how to benefit from a developmental accident. Evol Dev 2001;3:104–108.
110 Sire JY, Akimenko MA: Scale development in fish: a review, with description of sonic hedgehog (shh) expression in the zebrafish *(Danio rerio)*. Int J Dev Biol 2004;48:233–247.
111 Sire JY, Huysseune A: Formation of dermal skeletal and dental tissues in fish: a comparative and evolutionary approach. Biol Rev Camb Philos Soc 2003;78:219–249.
112 Smith MM, Hall BK: Development and evolutionary origins of vertebrate skeletogenic and odontogenic tissue. Biol Rev 1990;65:277–373.
113 Donoghue PC: Evolution of the development of the vertebrate dermal and oral skeletons: unraveling concepts, regulatory theories, and homologies. Paleobiology 2002;28:474–597.
114 Janvier P: Patterns of diversity in the skull of jawless fishes; in Haken J, Hall BK (eds): The Skull. Chicago, University of Chicago Press, 1993, vol 2: Patterns of Structural and Systematic Diversity, pp 131–188.
115 Janvier P: Major events in early vertebrate evolution. Trends Ecol Evol 1999;14:298–299.
116 Smith MM: Vertebrate dentitions at the origin of jaws: when and how patterns evolved. Evol Dev 2003;5:394–413.
117 Reif W: Evolution of dermal skeleton and dentition in vertebrates: the odontode regulation theory. Evol Biol 1982;15:287–368.
118 Allis EP: The anatomy and development of the lateral line system in *Amia calva*. J Morphol 1889;2:463–566.
119 Allis EP: On morphology of certain of the bones of the cheek and snout of *Amia calva*. J Morphol 1898;14:423–466.
120 Hanken J, Hall BK: Introduction; in de Beer G (ed): The Development of the Vertebrate Skull. Chicago, University of Chicago Press, 1985.
121 Meinke DK: Morphology and evolution of the dermal skeleton in lungfishes. J Morphol 1986;1:133–149.
122 Northcutt RG: Evolution of gnathostome lateral line ontogenies. Brain Behav Evol 1997;50:25–37.
123 Northcutt RG: Development of the lateral line system in the channel catfish; in Browman HI, Skiftesvik AB (eds): The Fish Big Bang. Proceedings of the 26th Annual Larval Fish Conference, Helsinki, 2003, pp 137–159.

124 Baker CV, Bronner-Fraser M: Vertebrate cranial placodes. I. Embryonic induction. Dev Biol 2001;232:1–61.
125 Gompel N, Cubedo N, Thisse C, Thisse B, Dambly-Chaudiere C, Ghysen A: Pattern formation in the lateral line of zebrafish. Mech Dev 2001;105:69–77.
126 Devillers C: Recherches sur la crâne dermique des téléostéens. Ann Paleont 1947;33:1–94.
127 Devillers C: The role of morphogenesis in the origin of higher levels of organization. Syst Zool 1965;14:259–271.
128 Moy-Thomas JA: Development of the frontal bones of the rainbow trout. Nature 1941;147: 681–682.
129 Weidenreich F: The brain and its role in the phylogenetic transformation of the human skull. Trans Am Phil Soc 1941;31:320–442.
130 Clack JA: A revised reconstruction of the dermal skull roof of *Acanthostega gunnari*, an early tetrapod from the Late Devonian. Trans R Soc Edinb Earth Sci 2003;93:163–165.
131 Pehrson T: The ontogeny of the lateral line system in the head of dipnoans. Acta Zool Stockh 1949;30:153–182.
132 Zusi RL: Patterns of diversity in the avian skull; in Haken J, Hall BK (eds): The Skull. Chicago, University of Chicago Press, 1993, vol 2: Patterns of Structural and Systematic Diversity, pp 391–437.
133 Watson DMS: The evolution of the labrynthodonts. Phil Trans R Soc Lond 1954;245:219–265.

Michael J. Depew
Laboratory of Craniofacial Development and Evolution
Department of Craniofacial Development, King's College London
Floor 27, Guy's Hospital
London Bridge
London SE1 9RT (UK)
E-Mail michael.depew@kcl.ac.uk

Rice DP (ed): Craniofacial Sutures. Development, Disease and Treatment.
Front Oral Biol. Basel, Karger, 2008, vol 12, pp 79–90

Single Suture Craniosynostosis: Diagnosis and Imaging

Jyri Hukki[a], *Pia Saarinen*[a], *Marko Kangasniemi*[b]

[a]Department of Plastic Surgery, Cleft Palate and Craniofacial Centre and
[b]Department of Radiology, Helsinki University Hospital, Helsinki, Finland

Abstract

Craniosynostosis, premature suture fusion, is one of the most common craniofacial anomalies affecting approximately 1 in 2,500 live births. Craniosynostosis is most commonly an isolated (nonsyndromic) condition with the sagittal suture being the most commonly affected suture. In this review we describe the range of isolated synostoses and show how these can lead to a variety of different morphological and functional abnormalities.

Introduction

Together with cleft lip and/or palate and branchial arch syndromes such as hemifacial microsomia, craniosynostosis belongs to the group of the most common congenital malformations of the head and face. Craniosynostosis refers to premature ossification of one or several sutures of the skull. This condition may lead to an abnormal skull shape depending on the suture affected. The characteristic features can be identified in the neonate with relative ease. Routine radiological examinations for identifying a synostotic suture are neither necessary nor recommended. Radiological imaging, however, is reserved for patients with a high suspicion of craniosynostosis or related conditions. In these patients, three-dimensional computerized tomography (3D-CT) imaging is performed to identify not only the cranial sutures but the bony structures of the head as a whole. Modern imaging techniques have revealed numerous details of clinical importance not visible in a plain X-ray.

Treatment of craniosynostosis is surgical intervention aimed to correct the shape of the head and, importantly, to give space for the brain to grow in a normal fashion. Neuropsychological development disorders have been associated with the premature fusion of only one suture; therefore, monitoring these children during the period of growth is indicated. Further research is needed regarding the connection between craniosynostosis and disturbances of brain function.

Craniosynostosis refers to the premature ossification of one or several sutures of the skull. This condition may lead to abnormal skull shape or retarded skull growth. Brain volume increases 3-fold during the first year of life. During the first 2 years, the volume increases 4-fold compared to the moment of birth [1]. It is important that the skull expands adequately to accommodate the growing brain. If a single suture has ossified and prevents normal skull growth in that region, the growth of the brain leads to compensatory changes in other parts of the skull. This gives rise to morphological deformity typical for synostosis of each individual suture. The condition can usually be identified on the basis of the appearance of the skull.

Craniosynostosis can be primary, in which case one or several sutures have ossified either completely or in part during the fetal period due to a developmental disorder affecting the suture itself. Ossification disturbances of one suture (simple craniosynostosis) represent the most common type, and the etiology of these disturbances often remains unexplained. Multiple suture synostoses are often associated with syndromes of genetic origin (e.g. Apert syndrome, Crouzon syndrome, Pfeiffer syndrome and Saethre-Chotzen syndrome). Syndromes are usually suspected on the basis of other associated developmental disorders, such as anomalies affecting the extremities.

Secondary craniosynostosis is associated with developmental disorders of the central nervous system, metabolic diseases or hematological diseases. The reason for an abnormal skull shape may also be an unconventional fetal position in the uterus during the late stages of pregnancy, in which case mechanical pressure leads to premature closure of the suture [2]. Secondary craniosynostosis may also develop after birth, for example as a complication of shunt therapy of the cerebrospinal fluid circulation.

Estimates of the incidence of craniosynostoses vary. The best estimates come from Atlanta, Ga., USA: 34.3/100,000 live births, and from France: 47.6/100,000. Craniosynostosis syndromes are rare; their incidence is about 1.5/100,000 [1].

Scaphocephaly

Scaphocephaly or boat skull (scaphos = boat, cephalos = head) is the most common form of cranial deformity in craniosynostosis. This deformity is the result of premature closure of the sagittal suture and therefore it is also called sagittal synostosis. The head form varies considerably depending on the

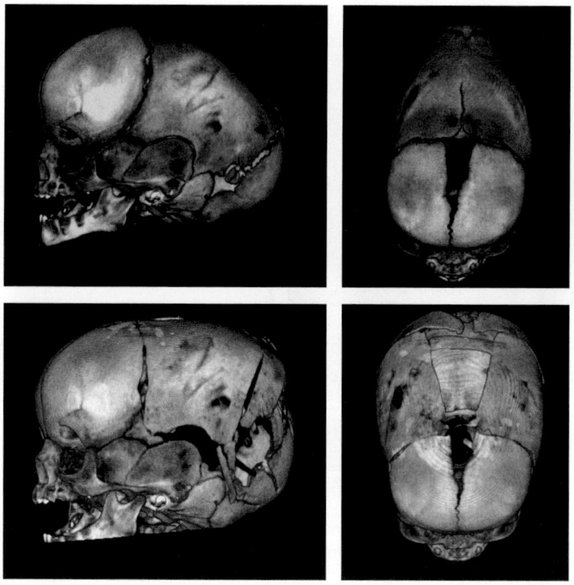

a b c d

Fig. 1. Scaphocephaly. Boy, 4 months of age. ***a*** Side view with posteriorly elongated skull. ***b*** View from above shows posterior synostosis in the sagittal suture. ***c*** Side view postoperatively. ***d*** Postoperative view from above shows expansion of the posterior skull.

localization and length of the synostotic site. The typical boat form is not necessarily seen except in patients where the synostosis is situated anteriorly or affects the whole length of the sagittal suture including the anterior fontanelle. In contrast, with posterior synostosis of the sagittal suture, the skull is typically narrow in the occipital area and the whole forehead is broad and high. The synostotic site can usually be palpated easily as a longitudinal prominent ridge. One of the most typical features of the head form in addition to extra length, a palpable ridge and narrow skull is the side profile. In most cases, the highest part of the skull is the area of the anterior fontanelle and the head is sloping downwards towards the neck (figs 1, 2).

3D-CT images reveal the site and length of the synostosis which can vary from a few millimeters (fig. 2) to the whole length of the suture. Other typical features seen are erosions of the calvarial bone which are localized posterior to the coronal sutures in the skull. They are seldom seen in the forehead in spite of the often considerable bulging of the anterior skull. These erosions can be severe enough to produce multiple perforations in the bone. More often however, the outer surface of the calvarial bone as seen during surgery seems intact and the erosions have made the bone paper-thin from the inside.

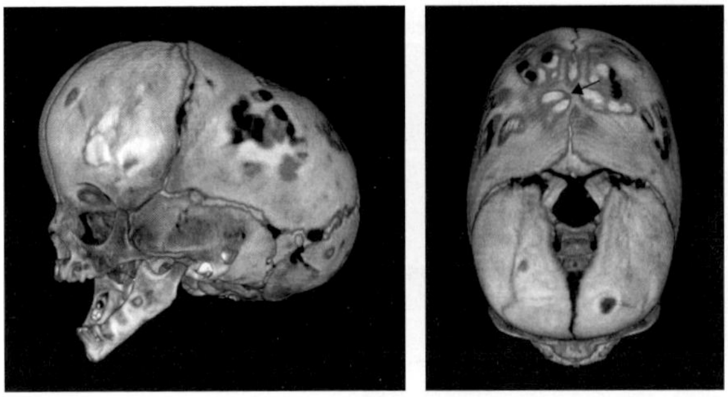

a *b*

Fig. 2. Scaphocephaly. Girl, 5 months of age. ***a*** Side view shows a bulging forehead and elongated downslanting cranium posteriorly from coronal sutures. ***b*** View from above shows a 1-cm-long synostosis in the middle of the sagittal suture (arrow). The length of the synostosis does not necessarily correlate with the severity of the deformity.

Taking these erosions into account, the commonly held belief that sagittal synostosis rarely if ever has an adverse effect on the child's neurological development should be overthrown as nonscientific. Although increased intracranial pressure does not seem to be present in more than 25% of cases [3], behavioral studies from numerous authors suggest mild to severe cognitive and behavioral disturbances in up to 50% of children with sagittal synostosis, operated or unoperated [4, 5]. Whereas patients with increased intracranial pressure can be assumed to have disturbances in brain function it may be relevant to assume that brain dysfunctions can be present with normal intracranial pressure especially when the brain is compressed mechanically as in craniosynostosis.

Metopic Synostosis and Trigonocephaly

Depending on the timing and extent of premature suture fusion, a synostosis in the metopic suture may present as a spectrum of manifestations ranging from a vertical frontal ridge (metopic ridge, fig. 3) to a triangular head shape (trigonos = triangular) with a keel-shaped forehead, narrow bitemporal width and hypotelorism. Usually there is widening and an increase in height in the parietal area as a result of compensatory growth of the brain and cranial bone posteriorly. Typical features revealed by 3D-CT include narrow anterior cranial vault width, retruded lateral orbital rims, and a narrowed bitemporal width. The orbits are slanting upwards and medially and the forehead may present as a keel of various angles (fig. 4). In addition to these findings, a distribution of digital impressions inside the calvarium is often seen. The forehead appears smooth in

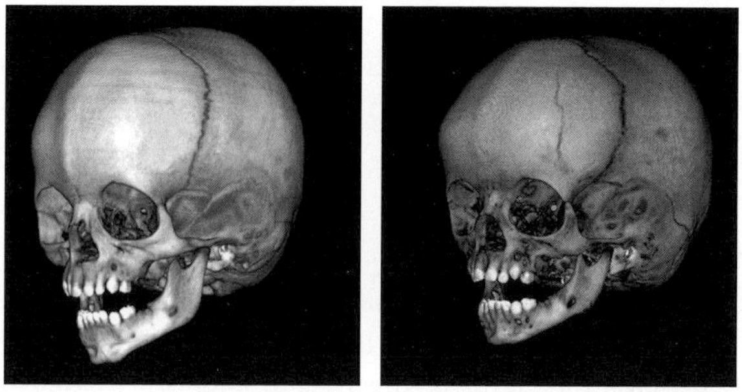

a b

Fig. 3. Metopic ridge. ***a*** The ridge extends from the site of anterior fontanelle to the radix of the nose. ***b*** The ridge is visualized only in upper part of the forehead. Both represent minimal alterations caused by metopic closure. Sometimes the metopic ridge is formed after birth. No treatment is required.

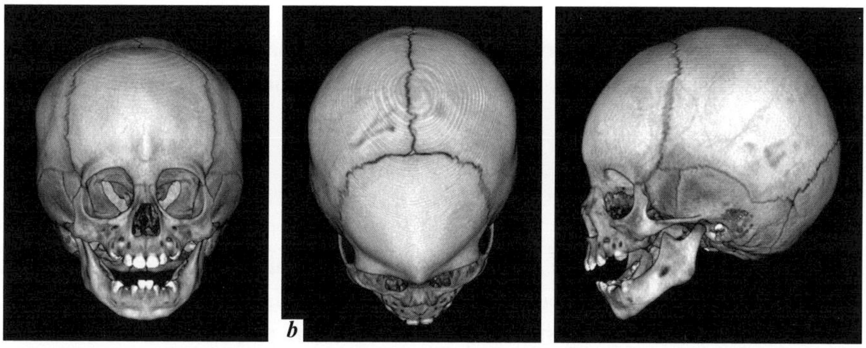

a b c

Fig. 4. Metopic synostosis, trigonocephaly. Boy, 10 months of age. ***a*** Frontal view shows hypotelorism as well as upwards and medially slanting orbits. ***b*** View from above with keel-shaped forehead. Note that the narrowing of the skull begins behind the patent coronal sutures. ***c*** Side view.

this respect in spite of the alleged compression of cranial bone due to synostosis, whereas the parieto-occipital area often shows numerous digital markings.

Plagiocephaly

Plagiocephaly (plagios = oblique) is a descriptive term used for describing asymmetric flattening of the calvarium. If the flattening is situated on either side of the frontal area the term anterior plagiocephaly can be used.

Correspondingly, posterior plagiocephaly refers to unilateral flattening in the occipitoparietal area. Both conditions can result either from external forces (positional molding or deformational plagiocephaly) either in utero or postpartum or from malformation (synostosis).

Anterior Plagiocephaly: Unilateral Coronal Synostosis

In anterior synostotic plagiocephaly, the coronal suture is partly or completely fused prematurely. The synostosis results in compensatory widening of the ipsilateral palpebral fissure together with posterior and superior displacement of the ipsilateral supraorbital rim, eyebrow and forehead and often the anterior position of the ear on that side. The deviation of the nasal root is toward the flattened side. In 3D-CT scan, the coronal suture is involved either partially or in whole length. Nearby joints in the skull base may also be affected. In addition, there is also deviation of the lambdoid sutures on the ipsilateral side which is shifted towards the synostotic coronal suture. Thus, there is a deviation of midlines both on anterior and posterior cranial bases and the whole hemisphere on the affected side is smaller (fig. 5). On the contralateral side of the forehead there is often compensatory bulging and the superior orbital rim is depressed due to pressure of the brain in the anterior fossa.

Anterior Plagiocephaly without Synostosis

At first glance, it may be possible to confuse the nonsynostotic form of anterior plagiocephaly with the synostotic type. When assessing a child with deformational frontal plagiocephaly several clearly distinctive features separate it from a synostotic type. Ipsilateral narrowing of the palpebral fissure and lowering of the ipsilateral eyebrow are seen. There is no angulation of the nasal root, and a ridge indicating synostosis over the coronal suture cannot be palpated. The ipsilateral ear is shifted away from the flattened forehead. When viewed from above, the compression of the forehead results in bulging of the ipsilateral occipitoparietal region. Thus, the overall clinical features are quite opposite from those of the synostotic type. In 3D-CT, all of the typical features of unilateral coronal synostosis are absent except diminished space in the anterior fossa on the affected side (fig. 6).

Posterior Plagiocephaly

The diagnosis and treatment of infants with posterior plagiocephaly is one of the most controversial aspects in craniofacial surgery. The great majority of babies with posterior flatness of the skull represent deformational posterior plagiocephaly, which is considered to be due to positional molding of the skull postpartum. The incidence of deformational plagiocephaly increased considerably

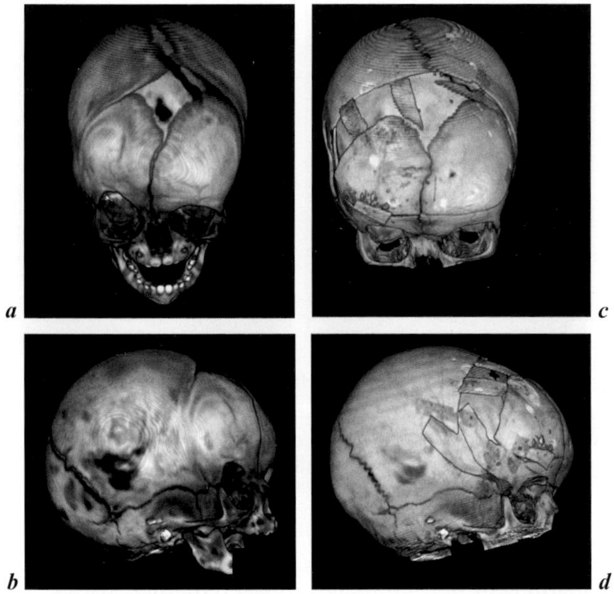

Fig. 5. Right coronal synostosis. Girl, 4 months of age. ***a*** Upper frontal view. Typical features of coronal synostosis are seen: there is posterior and superior displacement of the ipsilateral supraorbital rim and forehead. The deviation of the nasal root is towards the flattened side. The posterior skull is deviated towards the synostotic side. ***b*** Side view reveals almost complete coronal synostosis on the right side. ***c*** 1 week after bilateral fronto-orbital correction. Age 7 months. Upper frontal view. ***d*** Side view. The technique of fronto-orbital advancement is clearly visualized.

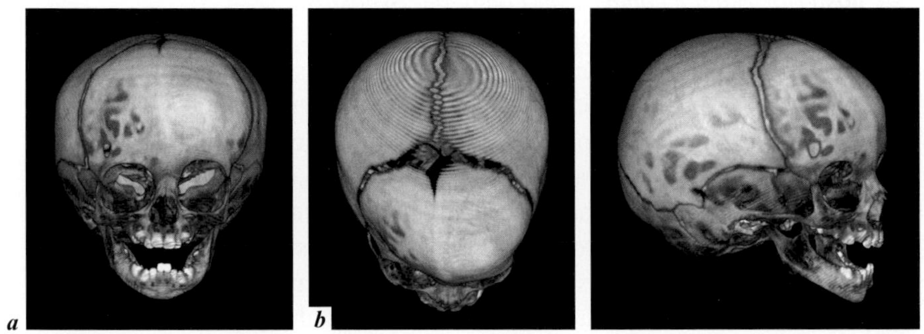

Fig. 6. Deformational anterior (frontal) plagiocephaly. ***a*** Flattening of the forehead on the affected side has caused inferior displacement of the orbit. ***b*** There is no deviation in the nasal root or in the sagittal suture (compare fig. 5). ***c*** Note that bony erosions and perforations occur mainly in the forehead (compare fig. 5).

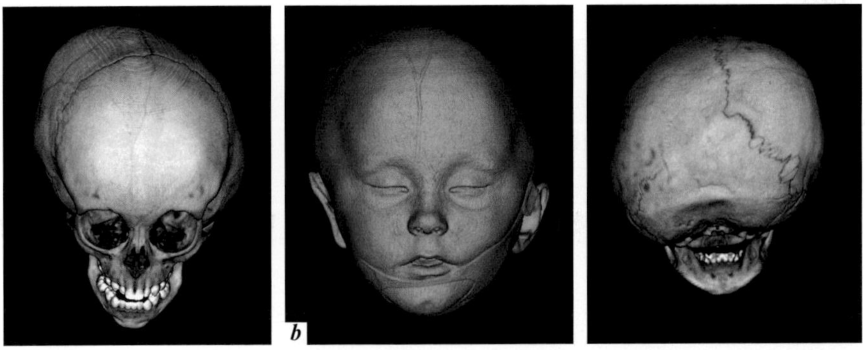

a b c

Fig. 7. Posterior plagiocephaly with synostosis of the left lambdoid suture. Boy, 1 year 10 months. ***a*** Upper frontal view shows cranioscoliosis towards the right. ***b*** The left ear is typically displaced inferiorly. ***c*** Posterior view reveals closure of the left lambdoid suture. Ipsilateral occipitomastoid bulge and inferior tilt of the skull base are typical features.

after 1998 when recommendations of putting babies to sleep on their backs in order to avoid sudden infant death syndrome were made worldwide. However, only a relatively small number of newborn infants develop posterior flatness while in the rest of the babies, the head shape remains completely normal in spite of a similar sleeping position. While the previous hypothesis may be relevant with respect to some of the babies it can be speculated that the deformity may have already developed in utero. The head molding during delivery may have temporarily disguised the existing deformity which will return a few weeks after birth. So far, the etiology remains unknown.

Posterior Plagiocephaly with Lambdoid Synostosis

Synostosis of the lambdoid suture is rare. Huang et al. [6] reported 4 cases of true lambdoid synostoses in a series of 102 babies assessed for posterior plagiocephaly. As in other synostoses it can affect the suture either partially or in its entirety. True lambdoid synostosis causes a dramatic effect in the calvarium. The affected occipitoparietal area is flattened whereas on the contralateral side there is considerable compensatory bossing parietally and sometimes frontally. There is an ipsilateral occipitomastoid bulge and the skull base has an ipsilateral inferior tilt (fig. 7). The external ear on the ipsilateral side is displaced inferiorly. This feature separates the true lambdoid synostosis from the deformational posterior plagiocephaly where the characteristics are opposite no matter how severe the deformity is. In deformational plagiocephaly, the ipsilateral ear is shifted forwards along with the flattened side and the compensatory bossing in the forehead is always on the ipsilateral side.

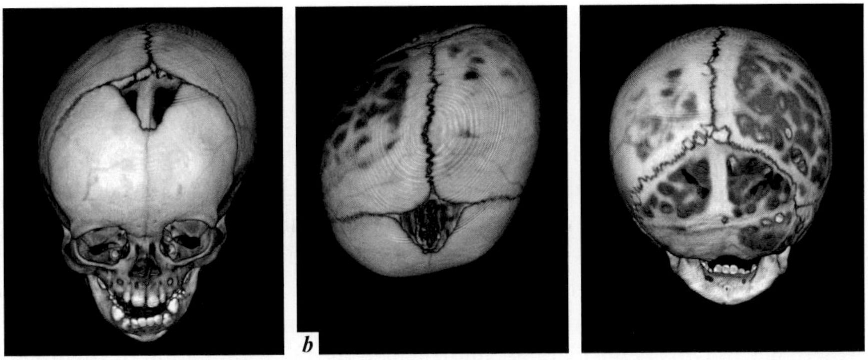

a b c

Fig. 8. Deformational posterior plagiocephaly. Boy, 11 months. Upper frontal (***a***) and parietal (***b***) views show patent sutures and typical rhomboid head shape. ***c*** Posterior view. The sutures are open. There is no occipitomastoid bulge on the affected (right) side and the posterior skull base is horizontal. The right occipitoparietal area is filled with intracranial erosions. Nearly ten holes of 5–10 mm in diameter can be seen.

Deformational Posterior Plagiocephaly

Patients who are assessed to have posterior plagiocephaly due to positional molding are usually managed conservatively or with helmet therapy. The latter method seems to be popular in the United States whereas in Europe and especially in Scandinavian countries it is less often used. In most of the babies with deformational plagiocephaly, the shift toward a more normal head shape starts already before the age of 6 months and is accelerated between 6 months and 1–1.5 years. The reason is simply natural growth of the brain and the baby's ability to turn over onto his belly. However, in this group of babies there is a subgroup where severe unilateral posterior flatness does not normalize by 1.5 years, or where the deformity is progressive. This group forms a minority of less than 1 out of 10 babies assessed for posterior plagiocephaly. Radiological examination using 3D-CT can be justified in this subgroup. This examination often reveals severe unilateral erosion of the calvarial bone but also true perforations of the calvarium (fig. 8). The etiology is unknown, however, the term 'positional molding' is hardly justified in this subgroup. Surgery may be considered in selected patients.

3D-CT Imaging

Today, the most precise picture of cranial anatomy, cranial base anatomy and the structure of sutures and bones is achieved by means of 3D-CT. In young children the examination can often be carried out by means of 'feeding bottle anesthesia'. The child is kept awake for a few extra hours and fed to satiety just before the examination, in which case the infant usually falls asleep. Older children need general anesthesia up to about the age of 5. The examination causes radiation load, and therefore unnecessary imaging examinations should be avoided. Imaging examinations should not be carried out just to check whether the sutures are open or not as the diagnosis can usually be established by means of a clinical examination. Imaging is only indicated when treatment plans are being formulated, at which point imaging not only verifies the diagnosis but also provides valuable information about the anatomy of cranial bones. In our experience, this has considerable significance for the formulation of treatment plans and for the documentation of results. It should be noted that craniosynostoses are often associated with changes not only in the calvarium but also in the cranial base, mandibular joints and other structures. For this reason, including the entire head in the imaging examinations is justified.

The Department of Radiology at our hospital is equipped with optimized imaging technology and postprocessing of images. This enables optimum benefit to be derived from CT imaging as regards diagnostics and treatment plans. The imaging examination is conducted by means of a CT device with four detector rows using helical technique. The examination starts from the lower jaw and covers the entire face and skull area. Three protocols are used depending on the patient's age: there are separate settings for patients under 2 years of age, patients aged 2–8 years, and patients over 8 years of age.

When the equipment at our hospital is used for the examination (GE Lightspeed QX/i; GE Medical Systems, Milwaukee, Wisc., USA), the radiation dose received by the patient is about 5% of the dose that Hall et al. [7] suspect may have an impact on cognitive development. For example, at the imaging settings we have used 140 kV and 70 mA; the radiation dose received by the patient is about 13 mGy. Minimum requirement for documentation in craniofacial surgery is 3D-CT examination preoperatively and 1 year postoperatively. Native scans of the skull should be abandoned in diagnostics and follow-up.

Craniosynostoses and Brain Function

Craniosynostosis affecting a single suture has traditionally been considered an esthetic inconvenience, perhaps causing a problem when selecting hats and sports helmets. Ossification of a single suture does not necessarily cause clinical symptoms in a young child even if the shape of the skull is clearly abnormal. If the other sutures are open and functional, the situation will not usually require rapid intervention. However, intracranial pressure can be elevated in single-suture synostosis even if there are no clinical signs indicating intracranial hypertension. Elevated intracranial pressure seems to occur in about 25% of patients with sagittal synostosis, in which case the disturbances of brain function can be assumed to be associated with elevated intracranial pressure [3, 8].

Several neuropsychological studies have demonstrated disturbances in cognitive development and behavior in up to 50% of children with single suture synostosis [4, 5]. However, isolated study materials are small, and the studies are associated with many methodological problems. There have been variations in the children's age at the time of diagnosis, and they have been treated at different ages by means of different surgical methods, which have not been clarified. Control groups have not always been used, and unspecified tests may have been employed [4]. The significance of the findings has remained unclear. It is not known for certain whether the neuropsychological abnormalities are due to craniosynostosis as such or whether there is a more extensive developmental disorder in the background of which craniosynostosis is just one part. The significance of surgical methods or the timing of surgery has not been investigated so far. This being the case, debating the possible superiority of some surgical methods over others is unnecessary. We need a greater number of controlled studies with higher patient numbers and better documentation. We also need more direct research of brain function in order to establish the etiology and significance of published neurological findings. Disturbances in brain function could be demonstrated in nearly 50% of the asymptomatic children who were referred for examination due to their abnormal skull shape [9]. Disturbances also occurred in patients with unilateral occipital flattening without synostosis. It can probably be assumed that disturbances of brain function may occur if the brain is compressed, even if the patient has no synostosis and the intracranial pressure remains within the normal range. Symptoms may develop as late as school age.

Conclusion

If craniosynostosis is suspected in an outpatient setting, the child should be referred to specialized healthcare at a clinic with appropriate experience of the condition in order to establish the diagnosis and formulate a treatment plan. According to current views, not only multiple-suture synostoses but also single-suture synostoses should be surgically corrected during the first year of life in order to give the brain enough space to grow. Removal of the suture area is not a sufficient procedure alone [10]. Taking into account the frequency of neuropsychological symptoms, these children should also be monitored during the period of growth in order to enable rapid intervention if developmental disorders should occur. As synostosis may recur, performing a control CT scan at the age of 5–7 years has also been suggested [1]. At the craniofacial outpatient clinic of Töölö Hospital, Helsinki, Finland follow-up of patients undergoing surgery for scaphocephaly and occipital problems is carried out regularly until the age of 8 years and until the age of 15 years if the synostosis has affected the front of the skull. Computerized scans are only used in selected cases.

References

1 Cohen MJ, Maclean R: Craniosynostosis, Diagnosis, Evaluation, and Management, ed 2. Oxford, Oxford University Press, 2000.

2 Marion R: Syndromes, genetics and the craniofacial complex; in Goodrich J, Hall Y (eds): Craniofacial Anomalies: Growth and Development from a Surgical Perspective. New York, Thieme Medical, 1995.

3 Renier D, Sainte-Rose C, Marchac D, Hirsch JF: Intracranial pressure in craniostenosis. J Neurosurg 1982;57:370–377.

4 Speltz ML, Kapp-Simon KA, Cunningham M, Marsh J, Dawson G: Single-suture craniosynostosis: a review of neurobehavioral research and theory. J Pediatr Psychol 2004;29:651–668.

5 Becker DB, Petersen JD, Kane AA, Cradock MM, Pilgram TK, Marsh JL: Speech, cognitive, and behavioral outcomes in nonsyndromic craniosynostosis. Plast Reconstr Surg 2005;116:400–407.

6 Huang MH, Gruss JS, Clarren SK, Mouradian WE, Cunningham ML, Roberts TS, Loeser JD, Cornell CJ: The differential diagnosis of posterior plagiocephaly: true lambdoid synostosis versus positional molding. Plast Reconstr Surg 1996;98:765–776.

7 Hall P, Adami HO, Trichopoulos D, Pedersen NL, Lagiou P, Ekbom A, Ingvar M, Lundell M, Granath F: Effect of low doses of ionising radiation in infancy on cognitive function in adulthood: Swedish population based cohort study. BMJ 2004;328:19.

8 Thompson DN, Malcolm GP, Jones BM, Harkness WJ, Hayward RD: Intracranial pressure in single-suture craniosynostosis. Pediatr Neurosurg 1995;22:235–240.

9 Balan P, Kushnerenko E, Sahlin P, Huotilainen M, Naatanen R, Hukki J: Auditory ERPs reveal brain dysfunction in infants with plagiocephaly. J Craniofac Surg 2002;13:520–526.

10 Posnick J: Craniofacial and Maxillofacial Surgery in Children and Young Adults. Philadelphia, Saunders, 2000, vol 1.

Dr. Jyri Hukki
Associate Professor of Plastic Surgery
Cleft Palate and Craniofacial Centre, Department of Plastic Surgery
Helsinki University Hospital, PO Box 266
FIN–00290 Helsinki (Finland)
Tel. +358 40 7254600, Fax +358 9 47187650, E-Mail jyri.hukki@hus.fi

Rice DP (ed): Craniofacial Sutures. Development, Disease and Treatment.
Front Oral Biol. Basel, Karger, 2008, vol 12, pp 91–106

Clinical Features of Syndromic Craniosynostosis

David P. Rice

Departments of Orthodontics and Craniofacial Development, King's College London, London, UK; Department of Orthodontics, University of Helsinki, Helsinki, Finland

Abstract
Disruption of normal suture development and function can result in premature suture fusion, craniosynostosis. This review focuses on syndromic forms of craniosynostosis. More than 100 syndromes in which craniosynostosis is a feature have been documented and here the most common conditions including Apert and Crouzon syndromes are described as well as other conditions with a particularly interesting molecular etiology, such as Saethre-Chotzen and craniofrontonasal syndrome.

Introduction

Craniosynostosis is the process of premature cranial suture fusion, although the term is commonly used to describe the result, for which the term craniostenosis may also be used [1]. Synostosis can also affect the facial skeleton with the sphenofrontal, frontoethmoidal and frontonasal sutures being most frequently affected. Craniosynostosis occurs in approximately 1 in 2,500 live births [2]. It is a heterogeneous condition which may be the result of a number of different causes all leading to the same final pathological condition. It may be an isolated finding (nonsyndromic) or be part of a collection of abnormalities (syndromic) such as Apert, Carpenter or Crouzon syndromes.

Craniosynostosis may also be secondary to another disorder. An example of this is seen in patients who have hydrocephalus which is treated by draining the cerebral spinal fluid with a shunt. Although intracranial pressures may be normalized the developing brain may grow inwards to occupy the ventricles which are expanded due to the previous raised intracranial pressure, instead of growing outwards and placing pressure on the sutures. This lack of pressure on the calvaria and sutures causes the bones to thicken and the sutures to fuse [3]. Fetal head constraint which physically limits the expansion of one or more sutures has been suggested as a major cause of nonsyndromic craniosynostosis [4]. Also, metabolic conditions such as hyperthyroidism or rickets, and hematological disorders such as thalassemia or sickle cell anemia are associated with craniosynostosis.

Over 100 craniosynostotic syndromes have been described, many of which are inherited in a dominant fashion, such as Apert, Crouzon, Pfeiffer and Saethre-Chotzen syndromes. Others, such as Carpenter and Antley-Bixler syndromes, exhibit recessive inheritance [5]. The salient clinical features of some syndromal craniosynostoses are summarized in this chapter. A comprehensive overview of the human genetics of craniosynostosis is given by Passos-Bueno et al. [pp. 107–143].

Although the genetic basis of many patients with craniosynostosis as part of a syndrome is known, there is still a significant proportion of patients with unknown mutations. Therefore in this chapter conditions are classified by the name of their syndrome rather than on their genetic basis. The key sources of reference in this field are the Online Mendelian Inheritance in Man database (www.ncbi.nlm.nih.gov/entrez) and the book *Craniosynostosis, Diagnosis, Evaluation, and Management* by Cohen and MacLean [1].

Apert Syndrome (OMIM 101200)

Apert syndrome is characterized by craniosynostosis especially affecting the coronal sutures, brachysphenocephalic acrocephaly, midface malformations and symmetrical syndactyly of the limbs. Apert syndrome, together with Crouzon syndrome, is the most common syndrome with craniosynostosis. It has a prevalence of 1 in 64,500 live births [6]. It is inherited in an autosomal dominant manner and caused by mutations in *fibroblast growth factor receptor 2 (FGFR2)* with most mutations arising spontaneously [7, 8]. As in Crouzon, Pfeiffer and Muenke syndromes new mutations causing Apert syndrome are of paternal origin and their risk of occurrence increases with increasing paternal age [9]. Craniosynostosis of the coronal suture usually occurs before birth. In contrast, cranial base abnormalities occur late in childhood.

Craniofacial Features

Patients with Apert syndrome have a large cranial volume, the rostral caudal head length is short and the head height is increased. The brain is large (megalencephaly) and abnormalities in the central nervous system are not

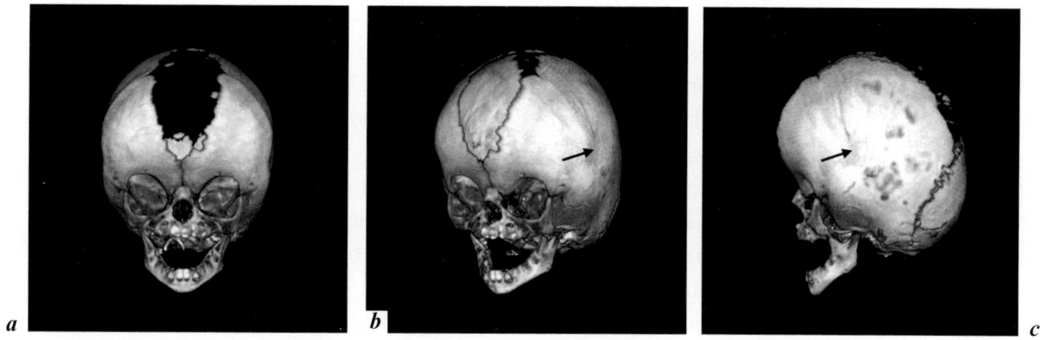

Fig. 1. Apert syndrome. 3D CT scan showing typical features in 6-month-old individual. ***a–c*** Wide defect in the midline of the calvaria stretching from the anterior section of the frontal bone to the occipital bone. Misshaped orbits, coronal suture synostosis (arrows), maxillary hypoplasia and the skull shape hyperacrobrachycephalic. The forehead is steep and wide. (Images courtesy of Jyri Hukki and Pia Saarinen.)

uncommon [1]. Anomalies of the septum pellucidum are associated with lower IQ [10]. The coronal sutures are typically closed at birth; however all other sutures and fontanelles are open and often expanded (fig. 1). The metopic and sagittal sutures are typically widened to form a broad midline defect in which bony islands form and then later coalesce to close the area [11]. In Apert patients the coronal suture initially fuses at an inferior location and this fusion progresses in a superior direction. Interestingly, fusion of the lambdoidal sutures has also been observed during the operation of Apert syndrome patients. However, in these lambdoidal sutures synostosis was not detected radiographically prior to surgery [11, 12].

The synchondroses are cartilaginous joints in the cranial base that act as growth sites. They control growth of the cranial base, the cranial fossae and indirectly growth of the midfacial region. Premature fusion of the spheno-occipital and petro-occipital synchondroses can occur in patients with Apert syndrome. If it does occur this will happen relatively late in childhood and not in infancy. This is in contrast to the cranial base in patients with Crouzon syndrome where very early fusion of the synchondroses is not uncommon [13].

Apert syndrome patients exhibit ocular proptosis which may be asymmetric. The proptosis is due to shallow orbits which are reduced in volume because of protrusion of the greater wing of the sphenoid, generalized maxillary hypoplasia, retrusion of the orbital rims, particularly the upper rim, and premature fusion of the sphenoparietal and sphenofrontal sutures which results in shortening of the orbital plate of the frontal bone [1, 14].

Oral features are dominated by maxillary abnormalities [15]. Seventy-six percent of patients have a cleft of the soft palate or uvula. Clefting of the hard palate, alveolus or lip is however relatively rare. The palate has a distinctive U shape. The palatal mucosa is often swollen, particularly in the tuberosity region and these swellings increase with age.

The dental development in Apert syndrome patients is delayed on average by 1 year and this delay gets more pronounced the older the individual becomes [16]. There is nearly always dental crowding in both the maxilla and mandible and tooth eruption is often delayed and ectopic. Apert syndrome patients usually exhibit a malocclusion between the upper and lower teeth. Most common malocclusions are posterior cross-bites, class III incisor and molar relationships (mandibular teeth occluding in an advanced horizontal position with the maxillary teeth), and anterior open bites (space in the vertical dimension between the anterior teeth) [15]. These malocclusions are largely the result of midface hypoplasia combined with a relatively normal mandible [14].

Other Features

Symmetric limb abnormalities are seen in all patients with Apert syndrome. These range from syndactyly of all five digits to fusion of only digits two, three and four. As well as bony fusions, abnormalities of the skin, muscles, tendons, aponeuroses, vessels and nerves of the hands and feet have all been documented in detail [1].

Approximately two thirds of Apert syndrome patients have cervical spine fusions. These occur most commonly between C5 and C6 and between C3 and C4. Fusions may occur between the vertebral bodies, articular facets, the neural arches or transverse processes. There is some evidence that fusions occur most commonly between vertebrae previously separated by a narrow intervertebral disc. This indicates that the condition is progressive and not due to developmental defects in somite segmentation [17, 18].

The trachea is normally made up of individual cartilaginous rings separated by fibromuscular membrane. In Apert syndrome patients the trachea may be a solid cartilaginous tube. This abnormality as well as other defects in the nasopharyngeal and oropharyngeal spaces can result in airway problems and respiratory distress [1].

Crouzon Syndrome (OMIM 123500)

Crouzon syndrome is typified by craniosynostosis, usually affecting the coronal suture in combination with craniosynostosis of the sagittal and/or lambdoid sutures, and midface malformations notably ocular proptosis [1]. In contrast

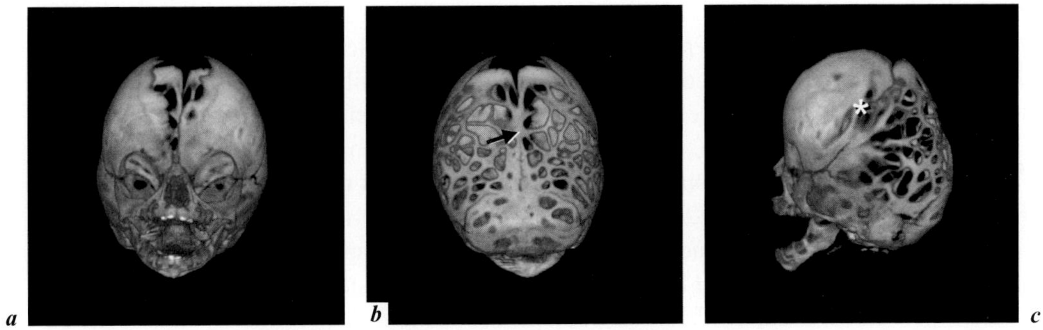

Fig. 2. Crouzon syndrome. 3D CT scan showing typical features in 2-month-old individual. ***a–c*** Coronal (asterisk) and sagittal (arrow) suture synostosis and maxillary hypoplasia. (Images courtesy of Jyri Hukki and Pia Saarinen.)

to Apert syndrome, the limbs of patients with Crouzon syndrome are normal. Together with Apert syndrome, Crouzon syndrome is the most common syndrome with craniosynostosis. It has a prevalence of 1 in 64,500 live births [6]. It is inherited in an autosomal dominant manner and caused by mutations in *FGFR2* [19, 20]. Similar to Apert, Pfeiffer and Muenke syndromes, new mutations causing Crouzon syndrome are of paternal origin and their risk of occurrence increases with increasing paternal age [9]. Craniosynostosis may be present at birth but usually develops during the first year of life.

Craniofacial Features

Nearly all cases of Crouzon syndrome have craniosynostosis of the coronal suture and this is usually in combination with craniosynostosis of the sagittal and lambdoid sutures. The shape of the head may be scaphocephalic (narrow, elongated from posterior to anterior), trigonocephalic (triangular shape with pointed forehead) or cloverleaf (trilobed) (fig. 2). The shape of the head is largely predictable and dependent on the time and order of fusion of the different sutures and synchondroses and the subsequent compensatory growth. The calvarial bones are thin and pronounced digital marking or fingerprint impressions are often seen on radiographs, which increases with age [21].

Premature fusion of the spheno-occipital and petro-occipital synchondroses in the cranial base is common in Crouzon syndrome and usually occurs in the late prenatal or in the early postnatal period [13]. The anterior, middle and posterior cranial fossae are all short and deformity is usually symmetrical.

Patients with Crouzon syndrome exhibit symmetric ocular proptosis and this is a result of small orbits. The maxilla is hypoplastic and this together with the retrusion of the lower orbital rim worsens the proptosis. The palate is narrow, high vaulted and in 50% of cases exhibits lateral swellings, but it is rarely cleft. The maxillary hypoplasia contributes to both dental crowding and malocclusion. The most common malocclusions are unilateral and bilateral posterior cross-bites, and class III incisor and molar relationships (mandibular teeth occluding in an advanced horizontal position with the maxillary teeth). Interestingly, ectopic eruption of first permanent molar teeth has been observed in 47% of cases [21]. The upper first permanent molar normally erupts behind the second deciduous molar and in front of the upper second permanent molar. Impaction against both of these teeth has been noted.

Conductive hearing problems are found in approximately half of patients with Crouzon syndrome and atresia (closure or absence) of the external auditory meatus is found in 13% [21].

Other Features

Abnormalities of the central nervous system are common. These include Chiari malformation, progressive hydrocephalus, headaches and seizures in order of decreasing prevalence [21]. Chiari malformation is the herniation of the cerebral tonsils and hindbrain through the foramen magnum. In Crouzon syndrome patients it has been proposed that premature fusion of both the lambdoid sutures and the synchondroses reduces the size of the posterior cranial fossae during the first 2 years after birth. The reduction in size of the posterior cranial base coincides with a stage of particularly active growth of the cerebella and is thought to contribute to the high incidence of Chiari malformation [22]. Stenosis of the jugular foramen and associated obstruction of the jugular vein has been observed in 60% of cases. This can result in the raised intracranial pressure and hydrocephalus.

Fusions of the cervical vertebrae occur in 22% of cases [21, 23]. These occur most commonly between C2 and C3 and also commonly between C5 and C6. Fusions of the vertebral bodies and posterior elements are seen as abnormal butterfly-shaped vertebrae caused by persistence of the notochord in the vertebral body, which results in an opening and in a characteristic appearance on radiograph.

In common with Apert syndrome tracheal abnormalities may occur in patients with Crouzon syndrome. The malformation may present as isolated fusion of the tracheal rings or the whole trachea may present as a solid cartilaginous tube. The abnormality may extend into the bronchi [24].

Crouzonodermoskeletal Syndrome (Crouzon Syndrome with Acanthosis Nigricans) (OMIM 134934.0011)

Crouzonodermoskeletal syndrome is characterized by craniosynostosis and skin thickening and hyperpigmentation especially at the flexures. The acanthosis nigricans in this condition is unusual as it has an early onset before puberty and it has a distinctive pattern of distribution. This distribution includes the abdomen, chest, axillae, neck, perioral region, perialar region, periorbital region and the nasolabial folds. Also reported in individuals with this condition is atresia of the choanae (opening between the nasal cavity and the nasopharynx), hydrocephalus, high-arched and cleft palate, supernumerary teeth, periapical cemental dysplasia in the jaws, and vertebral abnormalities that include shortening of the vertebral bodies, and a progressive narrowing of the interpediculate distances from the upper lumbar spine caudally [25, 26].

Crouzonodermoskeletal syndrome/Crouzon syndrome with acanthosis nigricans is distinct from Crouzon syndrome [1]. The condition has a phenotype distinct from Crouzon syndrome and it is caused by a specific mutation in the gene encoding FGFR3 [27]. The missense mutation results in an alanine 391 to glutamic acid substitution (Ala391Glu) in the transmembrane domain of the receptor.

Pfeiffer Syndrome (OMIM 101600)

Typical features of Pfeiffer syndrome are craniosynostosis, midface malformations including maxillary hypoplasia and ocular proptosis, widening of the thumbs and great toes, syndactyly and brachydactyly [1]. Mutations in *FGFR1* or *FGFR2* are known to cause Pfeiffer syndrome which can be inherited in an autosomal dominant manner [28]. New mutations are of paternal origin and their risk of occurrence increases with increasing paternal age [9]. As Pfeiffer syndrome is so rare its prevalence is hard to calculate and is at present unknown.

Three clinical types based on the presentation of the abnormalities and prognoses have been described [29]. All three types have craniosynostosis, broad thumbs and great toes, and brachydactyly. Type 1 is described as the classic or mild type. Type 1 Pfeiffer syndrome is characterized by craniosynostosis, usually involving the coronal suture and possibly the sagittal suture and usually resulting in brachycephaly (short, broad cranial vault). Patients with type 1 Pfeiffer syndrome are usually of normal or near normal intelligence and have a long life span. Type 2 Pfeiffer syndrome is more severe and characterized by craniosynostosis in multiple sutures resulting in a cloverleaf skull. Cloverleaf skull (trilobed shape) can be of varying severity and can result from a combination of different suture synostoses. In general cloverleaf-shaped skull involves premature fusion of the coronal, lambdoid and metopic sutures with the brain bulging through the sagittal and squamosal sutures resulting in a trilobed shape. Cloverleaf skull may also result from craniosynostosis of all the calvarial sutures with bulging through the fontanelles [1]. Type 2 Pfeiffer syndrome is also characterized by severe ocular proptosis, subnormal intellectual development, radiohumeral synostosis and ankylosis of the elbow joint, and a short life span. Type 3 Pfeiffer syndrome is similar to type 2 except patients do not exhibit a cloverleaf skull but more simple craniosynostoses, and the patients have a very short anterior cranial base.

Craniofacial Features

Pfeiffer syndrome patients have midface hypoplasia which compounds the dental crowding, cross-bite and class 3 malocclusion (mandible occluding in advance of the maxilla). The presence of multiple natal teeth has been reported in type 3 Pfeiffer syndrome [30]. The primary dentition normally starts to erupt into the mouth after 6 months. Although natal teeth are seen in the normal population, the presence of multiple teeth at birth is very rare. Pfeiffer syndrome patients may have low-set ears and ear tags.

Limb Features

Synostosis of the elbow is a feature of type 2 and type 3 Pfeiffer syndrome. Other features characteristic of Pfeiffer syndrome are mild soft tissue syndactyly (webbing) and brachydactyly (shortening of the digits). Shortening of the middle phalanges, brachymesophalangy, has been observed in both the hands and feet [1].

Other Features

Multiple other anomalies have been recorded in association with Pfeiffer syndrome. These include fusions of the cervical vertebrae, fusions of the cartilaginous tracheal rings and various cardiovascular, gastrointestinal and urogenital abnormalities.

Saethre-Chotzen Syndrome (OMIM 101400)

The craniofacial features of Saethre-Chotzen syndrome include craniosynostosis, ptosis or drooping of the eyelids, and a high forehead with low frontal hairline. Limb features include brachydactyly and soft tissue syndactyly [1, 31, 32]. Saethre-Chotzen syndrome is inherited in an autosomal dominant manner with high penetrance and is caused by mutations in the basic helix-loop-helix transcription factor *TWIST* [28]. Also reported is one patient with Saethre-Chotzen syndrome caused by a mutation in *FGFR2*, and there are some overlapping features between Saethre-Chotzen syndrome and Muenke syndrome which is caused by mutations in *FGFR3* [28].

Craniofacial Features

Craniosynostosis is present in most but not in all cases of Saethre-Chotzen syndrome. The coronal suture is most commonly affected resulting in a brachycephalic (short) or acrocephalic (pointed) skull. Other sutures involved include the lambdoid and metopic sutures. The craniosynostosis is often asymmetric which results in plagiocephaly and facial asymmetry. Late closing fontanelles are also a feature, as can be enlarged parietal foramina and other ossification defects. It has been reported that the length of the posterior cranial base can be short and the sella turcica enlarged and in a low position [33]. Saethre-Chotzen syndrome patients often have a broad depressed nasal base and a deviated nasal septum, the nose can be long, thin, pointed and beaked [34].

The maxilla is frequently hypoplastic which together with a high flat forehead can give a flattened facial appearance. The palate is often narrow, high vaulted or cleft. Dental anomalies associated with Saethre-Chotzen syndrome include hyperdontia (supernumerary teeth), enamel hypoplasia and dentine abnormalities resulting in thin, narrow roots and stones in the pulp chambers of the posterior teeth [35].

Limb Features

Saethre-Chotzen syndrome patients often exhibit partial soft tissue syndactyly. This most commonly occurs between the second and third fingers and may also occur between the toes. Brachydactyly, clinodactyly and bifurcation of the distal phalanges can also be observed [36].

Antley-Bixler Syndrome (OMIM 207410) and P450 Oxidoreductase Deficiency (POR) (OMIM 201750)

Antley-Bixler syndrome is characterized by craniosynostosis, midface hypoplasia, dysplastic ears, radiohumeral synostosis, and femoral bone bowing and fractures. It is thought to be inherited in an autosomal recessive manner. It is a rare condition with approximately 25 cases having been reported in the literature [37, 38]. The molecular basis of Antley-Bixler syndrome is a contentious issue with most of the controversies stemming from difficulties in the clinical diagnosis [39]. It has been reported that Antley-Bixler syndrome is caused by mutations in *FGFR2* [40]. Also, one case of Antley-Bixler syndrome has been reported with a mutation in *FGFR1* [41]. Interestingly, this case did not have radiohumeral synostosis but radioulnar synostosis. In common with cytochrome P450 oxidoreductase (POR) deficiency the patient had ambiguous genitalia. POR deficiency is a separate condition caused by mutations in the gene-encoding POR. Patients have a phenotype similar to individuals with Antley-Bixler syndrome but also have abnormal steroid metabolism, adrenal insufficiency and ambiguous genitalia [42].

Typical craniofacial features of Antley-Bixler syndrome include craniosynostosis especially of the coronal and lambdoid sutures, which leads to a brachycephalic shape skull with parietal and frontal bossing. Other features include an enlarged anterior fontanelle, ocular proptosis, severe midfacial hypoplasia, dysplastic nasal bridge, atresia or stenosis of the choanae (opening between the nasal cavity and the nasopharynx), and low-set protruding ears [37, 43].

Carpenter Syndrome (OMIM 201000)

The typical features of Carpenter syndrome are craniosynostosis and preaxial polydactyly of the feet. However, it has been suggested that polydactyly of the feet is not an absolute prerequisite for Carpenter syndrome, and that this allows the inclusion of Summitt and Goodman syndromes within the clinical spectrum of the disorder [44, 45]. Other syndromic features include soft tissue syndactyly, short or missing middle phalanges of the hands and feet, clinodactyly, short stature, obesity, congenital heart disease and mental retardation. The inheritance of Carpenter syndrome is autosomal recessive and until 2001 only 40 cases had been reported.

Craniofacial Features

Carpenter syndrome patients have craniosynostosis usually affecting the coronal, sagittal and lambdoid sutures with the coronal sutures being the last to fuse. The head shape is variable but may be cloverleaf-shaped and may be asymmetric. There is often midface hypoplasia, low-set ears and downward sloping palpebral fissures. Delayed eruption of the teeth is seen in Carpenter syndrome and there is some debate whether hypodontia, which has been recorded in several cases, is also associated with the syndrome [46].

Craniofrontonasal Syndrome (OMIM 304110)

Craniofrontonasal syndrome is caused by heterozygous loss-of-function mutations in the gene encoding ephrin-B1 [28]. It is an X-linked condition with the classical features exhibited in females. Craniofrontonasal syndrome is characterized by frontonasal dysplasia, craniosynostosis, ocular hypertelorism, a broad nasal tip, a central nasal groove and an anterior open bite [47, 48]. Craniofrontonasal syndrome was identified in a subpopulation of patients with craniofrontonasal dysplasia [49, 50]. The phenotype seen in males is less severe than that seen in females with males usually exhibiting ocular hypertelorism only. Despite this moderate phenotype, the number of male carriers is relatively small when compared to female carriers. This is due to a bias toward new mutations in the paternal germ line which result in increased numbers of affected female offspring. Other factors may include the possible increase in male prenatal death and reduced reproductive fitness in affected females [51, 52].

Craniofacial Features

Craniosynostosis of the coronal suture resulting in brachycephaly (short, broad cranial vault) is found in most female patients. Other diagnostic craniofacial features include ocular hypertelorism, and a bifid and broad nasal tip. The frontal region is frequently bossed, the faces asymmetric and the palate high-arched or cleft. Unilateral cleft lip has been recorded as has the rare abnormality of a median cleft lip. Most patients have a dental malocclusion. In females this is an anterior open bite, where the teeth at the front of the mouth do not overlap when the individual bites together. In males posterior open bites are seen as well as cross-bites, with the upper teeth occluding inside the lower teeth [48].

Other Features

Abnormalities in tissues of ectodermal origin are also seen in patients with craniofrontonasal syndrome including longitudinal grooving in nails and thick wiry hair. Other relatively common features include clinodactyly of the fifth finger, polydactyly, partial soft tissue syndactyly and asymmetry of the lower limbs.

Muenke Craniosynostosis (FGFR3-Associated Coronal Synostosis Syndrome, Nonsyndromic) (OMIM 602849)

Muenke syndrome is caused specifically by a heterozygous mutation in the gene encoding *FGFR3* which results in the proline 250 to arginine amino acid substitution (749C > G) [53]. Similar to Apert, Pfeiffer and Crouzon syndromes, new mutations causing Muenke craniosynostosis are of paternal origin and their risk of occurrence increases with increasing paternal age [9]. The condition is transmitted in an autosomal dominant manner with patients exhibiting variable expressivity. An example of this variability in phenotype is the finding

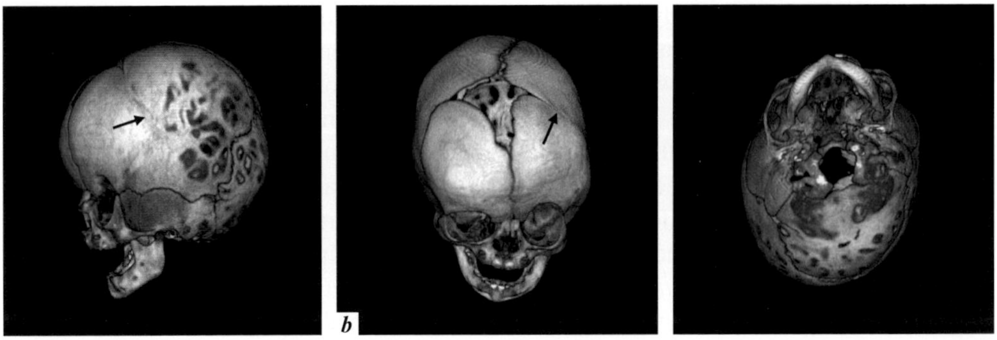

Fig. 3. Muenke craniosynostosis. 3D CT scan showing typical features in 5-month-old individual. ***a–c*** Left coronal suture synostosis (arrows), plagiocephaly, and maxillary hypoplasia. (Images courtesy of Jyri Hukki and Pia Saarinen.)

that coronal suture synostosis, a key feature of the condition, is not obligatory, indeed some individuals with the Pro250Arg mutation exhibit an extremely mild or even no phenotype [54]. The Pro250Arg mutation may account for a significant percentage of apparently nonsyndromic cases of coronal craniosynostosis [55]. Also, the Pro250Arg mutation increases the risk of re-operation in cases of apparently isolated coronal craniosynostosis [56].

In addition to either uni- or bilateral coronal suture synostosis, other craniofacial features include midfacial hypoplasia, downward slanting palpebral fissures, ptosis of the eyelids and a high-arched palate (fig. 3).

Limb abnormalities include brachydactyly, thimble-like, absent or fused middle phalanges, and tarsal and carpal joint fusions. Thirty percent of patients have mental retardation, developmental delay or borderline intelligence [53].

Thanatophoric Dysplasia Types I and II (OMIM 187600 and 187601)

Thanatophoric dysplasia is a lethal skeletal dysplasia with a birth prevalence of between 1 in 25,000 and 1 in 42,000 [1]. Individuals with thanatophoric dysplasia have severe growth disturbance. They have very short limbs, ribs and vertebral bodies, a narrow thorax, a disproportionately large head and usually die in the first few hours after birth. Type I thanatophoric dysplasia is characterized by curved femur bones and type II by straight femurs.

Types I and II thanatophoric dysplasia are caused by mutations in the gene encoding *FGFR3* [28].

Craniofacial Features

Typical features of type I thanatophoric dysplasia include macrocephaly, frontal bossing, cranial base dysplasia, relatively small face and a low nasal bridge. Craniosynostosis occurs in 28% of type I cases notably those encoding a Tyr373Cys amino acid substitution which causes a particularly severe phenotype [57].

Type II thanatophoric dysplasia is characterized by craniosynostosis; this often affects coronal, sagittal and lambdoid sutures resulting in a cloverleaf-shaped skull. Type II thanatophoric dysplasia is associated with *FGFR3* mutations that result in Lys650Glu substitution [57]. Individuals with type II thanatophoric dysplasia also have cranial base abnormalities including an enlarged middle cranial fossa and a hypoplastic posterior fossa with a small foramen magnum.

Acknowledgments

I thank Dr. Jyri Hukki and Dr. Pia Saarinen for permission to use the images in this chapter, and Dr. Ritva Rice and Eva Lana-Elola for help with the manuscript.

References

1 Cohen MJ, Maclean R: Craniosynostosis, Diagnosis, Evaluation, and Management, ed 2. Oxford, Oxford University Press, 2001.
2 Lammer EJ, Cordero JF, Wilson MJ, Oimette D, Ferguson S: Investigation of a suspected increased prevalence of craniosynostosis – Colorado 1978–1982. Proc Greenwood Genet Center 1987;6:126–127.
3 Kaufman B, Weiss MH, Young HF, Nulsen FE: Effects of prolonged cerebrospinal fluid shunting on the skull and brain. J Neurosurg 1973;38:288–297.
4 Graham JM Jr, Badura RJ, Smith DW: Coronal craniostenosis: fetal head constraint as one possible cause. Pediatrics 1980;65:995–999.
5 OMIM: Online Mendelian Inheritance in Man, John Hopkins University.
6 Cohen MM Jr, Kreiborg S: New indirect method for estimating the birth prevalence of the Apert syndrome. Int J Oral Maxillofac Surg 1992;21:107–109.
7 Wilkie AO, Slaney SF, Oldridge M, Poole MD, Ashworth GJ, Hockley AD, Hayward RD, David DJ, Pulleyn LJ, Rutland P, et al: Apert syndrome results from localized mutations of FGFR2 and is allelic with Crouzon syndrome. Nat Genet 1995;9:165–172.
8 Park WJ, Theda C, Maestri NE, Meyers GA, Fryburg JS, Dufresne C, Cohen MM Jr, Jabs EW: Analysis of phenotypic features and FGFR2 mutations in Apert syndrome. Am J Hum Genet 1995;57:321–328.
9 Wilkie AO: Bad bones, absent smell, selfish testes: the pleiotropic consequences of human FGF receptor mutations. Cytokine Growth Factor Rev 2005;16:187–203.
10 Renier D, Arnaud E, Cinalli G, Sebag G, Zerah M, Marchac D: Prognosis for mental function in Apert's syndrome. J Neurosurg 1996;85:66–72.

11 Cohen MM Jr, Kreiborg S: Suture formation, premature sutural fusion, and suture default zones in Apert syndrome. Am J Med Genet 1996;62:339–444.
12 Moore MH, Bourne AJ: Cranial suture disease in the Apert's syndrome infant. J Craniofac Surg 1996;7:271–274.
13 Kreiborg S, Marsh JL, Cohen MM Jr, Liversage M: Pedersen H, Skovby F, Borgesen SE, Vannier MW: Comparative three-dimensional analysis of CT-scans of the calvaria and cranial base in Apert and Crouzon syndromes. J Craniomaxillofac Surg 1993;21:181–188.
14 Kreiborg S, Aduss H, Cohen MM Jr: Cephalometric study of the Apert syndrome in adolescence and adulthood. J Craniofac Genet Dev Biol 1999;19:1–11.
15 Kreiborg S, Cohen MM Jr: The oral manifestations of Apert syndrome. J Craniofac Genet Dev Biol 1992;12:41–48.
16 Kaloust S, Ishii K, Vargervik K: Dental development in Apert syndrome. Cleft Palate Craniofac J 1997;34:117–121.
17 Thompson DN, Slaney SF, Hall CM, Shaw D, Jones BM, Hayward RD: Congenital cervical spinal fusion: a study in Apert syndrome. Pediatr Neurosurg 1996;25:20–27.
18 Kreiborg S, Barr M Jr, Cohen MM Jr: Cervical spine in the Apert syndrome. Am J Med Genet 1992;43:704–708.
19 Reardon W, Winter RM, Rutland P, Pulleyn LJ, Jones BM, Malcolm S: Mutations in the fibroblast growth factor receptor 2 gene cause Crouzon syndrome. Nat Genet 1994;8:98–103.
20 Jabs EW, Li X, Scott AF, Meyers G, Chen W, Eccles M, Mao JI, Charnas LR, Jackson CE, Jaye M: Jackson-Weiss and Crouzon syndromes are allelic with mutations in fibroblast growth factor receptor 2. Nat Genet 1994;8:275–279.
21 Kreiborg S: Crouzon syndrome. A clinical and roentgencephalometric study. Scand J Plast Reconstr Surg Suppl 1981;18:1–198.
22 Cinalli G, Spennato P, Sainte-Rose C, Arnaud E, Aliberti F, Brunelle F, Cianciulli E, Renier D: Chiari malformation in craniosynostosis. Childs Nerv Syst 2005;21:889–901.
23 Anderson PJ, Hall C, Evans RD, Harkness WJ, Hayward RD, Jones BM: The cervical spine in Crouzon syndrome. Spine 1997;22:402–405.
24 Devine P, Bhan I, Feingold M, Leonidas JC, Wolpert SM: Completely cartilaginous trachea in a child with Crouzon syndrome. Am J Dis Child 1984;138:40–43.
25 Schweitzer DN, Graham JM Jr, Lachman RS, Jabs EW, Okajima K, Przylepa KA, Shanske A, Chen K, Neidich JA, Wilcox WR: Subtle radiographic findings of achondroplasia in patients with Crouzon syndrome with acanthosis nigricans due to an Ala391Glu substitution in FGFR3. Am J Med Genet 2001;98:75–91.
26 Suslak L, Glista B, Gertzman GB, Lieberman L, Schwartz RA, Desposito F: Crouzon syndrome with periapical cemental dysplasia and acanthosis nigricans: the pleiotropic effect of a single gene? Birth Defects Orig Artic Ser 1985;21:127–134.
27 Meyers GA, Orlow SJ, Munro IR, Przylepa KA, Jabs EW: Fibroblast growth factor receptor 3 (FGFR3) transmembrane mutation in Crouzon syndrome with acanthosis nigricans. Nat Genet 1995;11:462–464.
28 Rice DP: Craniofacial anomalies: from development to molecular pathogenesis. Curr Mol Med 2005;5:699–722.
29 Cohen MM Jr: Pfeiffer syndrome update, clinical subtypes, and guidelines for differential diagnosis. Am J Med Genet 1993;45:300–307.
30 Alvarez MP, Crespi PV, Shanske AL: Natal molars in Pfeiffer syndrome type 3: a case report. J Clin Pediatr Dent 1993;18:21–24.
31 Pantke OA, Cohen MM Jr, Witkop CJ Jr, Feingold M, Schaumann B, Pantke HC, Gorlin RJ: The Saethre-Chotzen syndrome. Birth Defects Orig Artic Ser 1975;11:190–225.
32 Friedman JM, Hanson JW, Graham CB, Smith DW: Saethre-Chotzen syndrome: a broad and variable pattern of skeletal malformations. J Pediatr 1977;91:929–1023.
33 Evans CA, Christiansen RL: Cephalic malformations in Saethre-Chotzen syndrome. Acrocephalosyndactyly type III. Radiology 1976;121:399–403.
34 de Heer IM, de Klein A, van den Ouweland AM, Vermeij-Keers C, Wouters CH, Vaandrager JM, Hovius SE, Hoogeboom JM: Clinical and genetic analysis of patients with Saethre-Chotzen syndrome. Plast Reconstr Surg 2005;115:1894–1905.

35 Goho C: Dental findings in Saethre-Chotzen syndrome (acrocephalosyndactyly type III): report of case. ASDC J Dent Child 1998;65:136–137.
36 Kopysc Z, Stanska M, Ryzko J, Kulczyk B: The Saethre-Chotzen syndrome with partial bifid of the distal phalanges of the great toes. Observations of three cases in one family. Hum Genet 1980;56:195–204.
37 Hassell S, Butler MG: Antley-Bixler syndrome: report of a patient and review of literature. Clin Genet 1994;46:372–376.
38 Crisponi G, Porcu C, Piu ME: Antley-Bixler syndrome: case report and review of the literature. Clin Dysmorphol 1997;6:61–68.
39 Cohen MJ: FGFs/FGFRs and associated disorders; in Epstein C, Erickson R, Wynshaw-Boris A (eds): Inborn Errors of Development. Oxford, Oxford University Press, 2004, pp 380–400.
40 Chun K, Siegel-Bartelt J, Chitayat D, Phillips J, Ray PN: FGFR2 mutation associated with clinical manifestations consistent with Antley-Bixler syndrome. Am J Med Genet 1998;77: 219–224.
41 Hurley ME, White MJ, Green AJ, Kelleher J: Antley-Bixler syndrome with radioulnar synostosis. Pediatr Radiol 2004;34:148–151.
42 Fluck CE, Tajima T, Pandey AV, Arlt W, Okuhara K, Verge CF, Jabs EW, Mendonca BB, Fujieda K, Miller WL: Mutant P450 oxidoreductase causes disordered steroidogenesis with and without Antley-Bixler syndrome. Nat Genet 2004;36:228–230.
43 Antley R, Bixler D: Trapezoidocephaly, midfacial hypoplasia and cartilage abnormalities with multiple synostoses and skeletal fractures. Birth Defects Orig Artic Ser 1975;11:397–401.
44 Cohen DM, Green JG, Miller J, Gorlin RJ, Reed JA: Acrocephalopolysyndactyly type II – Carpenter syndrome: clinical spectrum and an attempt at unification with Goodman and Summit syndromes. Am J Med Genet 1987;28:311–324.
45 Gershoni-Baruch R: Carpenter syndrome: marked variability of expression to include the Summitt and Goodman syndromes. Am J Med Genet 1990;35:236–240.
46 Blankenstein R, Brook AH, Smith RN, Patrick D, Russell JM: Oral findings in Carpenter syndrome. Int J Paediatr Dent 2001;11:352–360.
47 Wieacker P, Wieland I: Clinical and genetic aspects of craniofrontonasal syndrome: towards resolving a genetic paradox. Mol Genet Metab 2005;86:110–116.
48 Saavedra D, Richieri-Costa A, Guion-Almeida ML, Cohen MM Jr: Craniofrontonasal syndrome: study of 41 patients. Am J Med Genet 1996;61:147–151.
49 Cohen MM Jr: Craniofrontonasal dysplasia. Birth Defects Orig Artic Ser 1979;15:85–89.
50 Reich E, Cox R, McCarthy J, Becker M, Genieser N, Converse J: A new inheritable syndrome with frontonasal dysplasia and associated extracranial anomalies; in Fifth International Conference on Birth Defects. Amsterdam, Excerpta Medica, 1977.
51 Twigg SR, Matsumoto K, Kidd AM, Goriely A, Taylor IB, Fisher RB, Hoogeboom AJ, Mathijssen IM, Lourenco MT, Morton JE, Sweeney E, Wilson LC, Brunner HG, Mulliken JB, Wall SA, Wilkie AO: The origin of EFNB1 mutations in craniofrontonasal syndrome: frequent somatic mosaicism and explanation of the paucity of carrier males. Am J Hum Genet 2006;78: 999–1010.
52 Twigg SR, Kan R, Babbs C, Bochukova EG, Robertson SP, Wall SA, Morriss-Kay GM, Wilkie AO: Mutations of ephrin-B1 (EFNB1), a marker of tissue boundary formation, cause craniofrontonasal syndrome. Proc Natl Acad Sci USA 2004;101:8652–8657.
53 Muenke M, Gripp KW, McDonald-McGinn DM, Gaudenz K, Whitaker LA, Bartlett SP, Markowitz RI, Robin NH, Nwokoro N, Mulvihill JJ, Losken HW, Mulliken JB, Guttmacher AE, Wilroy RS, Clarke LA, Hollway G, Ades LC, Haan EA, Mulley JC, Cohen MM Jr, Bellus GA, Francomano CA, Moloney DM, Wall SA, Wilkie AO, et al: A unique point mutation in the fibroblast growth factor receptor 3 gene (FGFR3) defines a new craniosynostosis syndrome. Am J Hum Genet 1997;60:555–564.
54 Robin NH, Scott JA, Cohen AR, Goldstein JA: Nonpenetrance in FGFR3-associated coronal synostosis syndrome. Am J Med Genet 1998;80:296–297.
55 Moloney DM, Wall SA, Ashworth GJ, Oldridge M, Glass IA, Francomano CA, Muenke M, Wilkie AO: Prevalence of Pro250Arg mutation of fibroblast growth factor receptor 3 in coronal craniosynostosis. Lancet 1997;349:1059–1062.

56 Thomas GP, Wilkie AO, Richards PG, Wall SA: FGFR3 P250R mutation increases the risk of reoperation in apparent 'nonsyndromic' coronal craniosynostosis. J Craniofac Surg 2005;16: 347–354.
57 Wilcox WR, Tavormina PL, Krakow D, Kitoh H, Lachman RS, Wasmuth JJ, Thompson LM, Rimoin DL: Molecular, radiologic, and histopathologic correlations in thanatophoric dysplasia. Am J Med Genet 1998;78:274–281.

Dr. David P. Rice
Professor of Orthodontics
Institute of Dentistry and Helsinki University Central Hospital
Box 41, University of Helsinki
FIN–00014 Helsinki (Finland)
E-Mail David.Rice@helsinki.fi

Rice DP (ed): Craniofacial Sutures. Development, Disease and Treatment.
Front Oral Biol. Basel, Karger, 2008, vol 12, pp 107–143

Genetics of Craniosynostosis: Genes, Syndromes, Mutations and Genotype-Phenotype Correlations

Maria Rita Passos-Bueno, Andréa L. Sertié, Fernanda S. Jehee, Roberto Fanganiello, Erika Yeh

Human Genome Center, Institute of Biosciences, University of São Paulo, São Paulo, Brazil

Abstract

Craniosynostosis is a very heterogeneous group of disorders, in the etiology of which genetics play an important role. Chromosomal alterations are important causative mechanisms of the syndromic forms of craniosynostosis accounting for at least 10% of the cases. Mutations in 7 genes are unequivocally associated with mendelian forms of syndromic craniosynostosis: *FGFR1, FGFR2, FGFR3, TWIST1, EFNB1, MSX2* and *RAB23*. Mutations in 4 other genes, *FBN1*, *POR*, *TGFBR1* and *TGFBR2*, are also associated with craniosynostosis, but not causing the major clinical feature of the phenotype or with an apparently low penetrance. The identification of these genes represented a great advance in the dissection of the genetics of craniosynostosis in the last 15 years, and today they explain the etiology of about 30% of the syndromic cases. The paucity in the identification of genes associated with this defect has partly been due to the rarity of familial cases. In contrast, very little is known about the molecular and cellular factors leading to nonsyndromic forms of craniosynostosis. Revealing the molecular pathology of craniosynostosis is also of great value for diagnosis, prognosis and genetic counseling. This chapter will review (1) the chromosomal regions associated with syndromic forms of the malformation, (2) the genes in which a large number of mutations have been reported by independent studies (*FGFR1, FGFR2, FGFR3, TWIST1* and *EFNB1*) and (3) the molecular mechanisms and genotype-phenotype correlations of such mutations.

Introduction

Cranial suture fusion occurs at specific periods during the lifetime of an individual, and therefore, abnormal activation of cell signaling triggered by genetic and/or environmental factors during embryogenesis or early childhood can alter the patency of the sutures. The two most common processes associated with cranial suture developmental defects are craniosynostosis, premature fusion of cranial sutures, and parietal foramina, delayed differentiation of the bones of the skull. Although common genes seem to be involved with these two cranial suture abnormalities, this chapter will focus on the genetics of craniosynostosis.

The prevalence of craniosynostosis is estimated to be 1 to 2,000–3,000 births [1]. The frequencies of different types of craniosynostosis vary according to ascertainment centers, but on average, of all craniosynostosis, sagittal synostosis is the most common (40–55%), followed by coronal (20–25%), metopic (5–15%), multiple suture synostosis (5–15%) and lambdoid (0–5%) [1].

Craniosynostosis has usually been classified as nonsyndromic (or isolated) and syndromic forms for genetic studies. Nonsyndromic craniosynostosis accounts for 70% of the cases [2–4], and occurs when cranial suture fusion is the only primary defect in the individual. Secondary symptoms, such as neurologic or ophthalmologic manifestations, can be present as a consequence of early sutural obliteration [1]. On the other hand, syndromic craniosynostosis occurs associated with other primary defects of morphogenesis. In practice, it is very hard to make this distinction and it is possible that some nonsyndromic forms actually represent the end of the spectrum of the clinical variability of syndromic forms.

Familial recurrence is reported for 14% in nonsyndromic coronal synostosis, 6% in sagittal synostosis, 3–9% in metopic synostosis and 22% in syndromic metopic synostosis [2–4, Jehee, unpubl. data]. Pedigrees from familial cases are compatible with autosomal dominant, autosomal recessive or X-linked inheritance [1–5]. Multifactorial inheritance also seems to play a role in the etiology of the nonsyndromic forms of craniosynostosis, although additional epidemiological studies should be performed.

The genetic etiology of the nonsyndromic craniosynostosis is still very poorly understood: to date, *EFNA4* is the only gene that when mutated causes only nonsyndromic craniosynostosis [6]. However, the understanding of the effect of mutations in this gene on the human phenotype still depends on the identification of a larger number of patients with *EFNA4* pathogenic changes. Conventional karyotype analysis is not recommended for nonsyndromic craniosynostosis.

Despite the lower proportion of syndromic forms, their genetic analysis has largely contributed to the elucidation of some important pathways for suture development and closure. There are at least 150 syndromes associated with craniosynostosis as a major clinical feature. Mendelian and chromosomal alterations are important causative mechanisms of this group of craniosynostosis. Linkage analysis in familial cases and molecular analysis of chromosomal alterations have led to the identification of six genes that when mutated are unequivocally associated with syndromic craniosynostosis: *FGFR1, FGFR2, FGFR3, TWIST1, EFNB1, MSX2* (table 1). More recently *RAB23* has been

Table 1. Genes and phenotypes associated with craniosynostosis

Gene	Gene symbol	Chromosome	Phenotypes	MIM	Penetrance craniosynostosis
Fibroblast growth factor receptor 1	*FGFR1*	8p11.2-p11.1	Pfeiffer	101600	high[a]
			osteoglophonic dysplasia	166250	apparently high
Fibroblast growth factor receptor 2	*FGFR2*	10q26	Crouzon	123500	high
			Crouzon with scaphocephaly		[b]
			Jackson-Weiss	123150	high
			Pfeiffer	101600	high
			Apert	101200	high
			SCS like	101400	high
			cutis gyrata syndrome of Beare-Stevenson	123790	high
			Antley-Bixley[c]	207410	apparently high
			nonclassifiable syndromes with craniosynostosis		[b]
			nonsyndromic coronal synostosis		[b]
Fibroblast growth factor receptor 3	*FGFR3*	4p16.3	Muenke syndrome	602849	high
			Crouzon with acanthosis nigricans	123500	high
			SCS like	101400	high
			thanatophoric dysplasia type I	187600	low (<30%)
			thanatophoric dysplasia type II	187601	high
Twist homolog Drosophila 1	*TWIST1*	7p21	SCS	101400	high
			nonsyndromic craniosynostosis	very few cases reported	
Ephrin-B1	*EFNB1*	Xq12	craniofrontonasal syndrome	304110	high
Ras-associated protein RAB23	*RAB23*	6p11	Carpenter syndrome	201000	high
Muscle segment homeobox homolog Drosophila 2	*MSX2*	5q34-35	craniosynostosis Boston type	604757	high

Table 1. (continued)

Gene	Gene symbol	Chromosome	Phenotypes	MIM	Penetrance craniosynostosis
Transforming growth factor-β receptor type I	*TGFBRI*	9q33-q34	Loeys-Dietz syndrome	609192	low (<30%)
Transforming growth factor-β receptor type II	*TGFBRII*	3p22	Loeys-Dietz syndrome		low (<30%)
Cytochrome P450 reductase gene	*POR*	7q11.2	Antley-Bixley	207410	apparently high
Fibrillin	*FBN1*	15q21	Shprintzen-Goldberg craniosynostosis syndrome	182212	very few cases reported

[a]High = Penetrance higher than 70%.
[b]Variability of the phenotype possibly related to the type of mutation.
[c]Under discussion.

included in this list [7]. Mutations in 4 other genes, *FBN1*, *POR*, *TGFBR1* and *TGFBR2* (table 1), are also associated with craniosynostosis, but not causing the major clinical feature of the phenotype and/or with an apparently low penetrance [8–10]. The identification of these genes represented a great advance in the dissection of the genetics of craniosynostosis in the last 15 years, even though they explain the etiology of about 30% of the syndromic cases. The paucity in the identification of genes associated with this defect has partly been due to the rarity of familial cases.

Revealing the molecular pathology of craniosynostosis has also been of great value for diagnosis, prognosis and genetic counseling. In this chapter we will deal with the genetics of the syndromic forms of craniosynostosis.

Chromosome Alterations in the Etiology of Craniosynostosis

All types of chromosomal abnormalities have already been described in patients with craniosynostosis, including deletions and duplications in almost all human chromosomes (fig. 1). The large number of chromosomal alterations and their ubiquitous location in the human genome indicate the vast genetic heterogeneity of this condition and reinforce the importance of performing karyotype analysis in patients with syndromic craniosynostosis that have been excluded for any of the known monogenic forms. It was estimated that approximately 16% of all cases of syndromic craniosynostosis are related to chromosomal abnormalities [11]. There is a high association of craniosynostosis with duplication 13q21-q34 and deletion 7p15-p21, 9p21-p24 and 11q23-q25 [50, 51]. Furthermore, an increasing number of craniosynostotic patients with deletion 22q11 and deletion and or duplication 1p36 have been reported [12, 33].

The mapping of important genes involved in suture closure based on chromosomal abnormalities has been limited. With the exception of 7p21, 9p21 and 11q23 deletions, the number of cases carrying each chromosomal alteration is not large enough to enable phenotype/genotype correlations. Furthermore, craniosynostosis is not present in all patients bearing the same chromosomal rearrangement; for instance, around 65–100% of patients with 9p21 deletions and only 50–70% of patients with deletions on 11q23 present metopic synostosis [52–55]. This suggests that other factors such as the environmental and genetic background of the individual could be important for the penetrance of craniosynostosis.

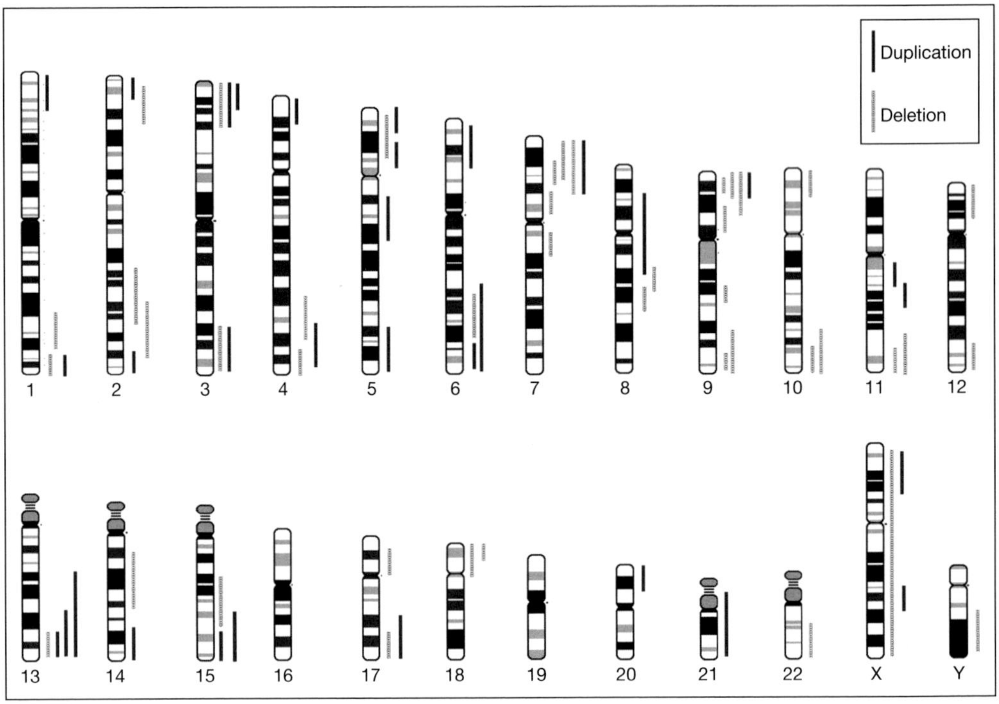

Fig. 1. Human chromosomal map depicting duplications and deletions associated with craniosynostosis [data based on 1, 12–49].

Mendelian Causes of Craniosynostosis

Herein we include a detailed description of the genes *FGFR1*, *FGFR2*, *FGFR3*, *TWIST1* and *EFNB1*, as several mutations in each of these genes have been associated with autosomal dominant forms of craniosynostosis, mostly syndromic forms as illustrated in figure 2.

Fibroblast Growth Factor Receptors (FGFRs)

FGFR Structure and Functions

The FGFR family consists of four closely related members of signal-transduction receptor tyrosine kinases (FGFR1–4). Each receptor is composed of three extracellular immunoglobulin-like domains (IgI, IgII and IgIII), a single-pass

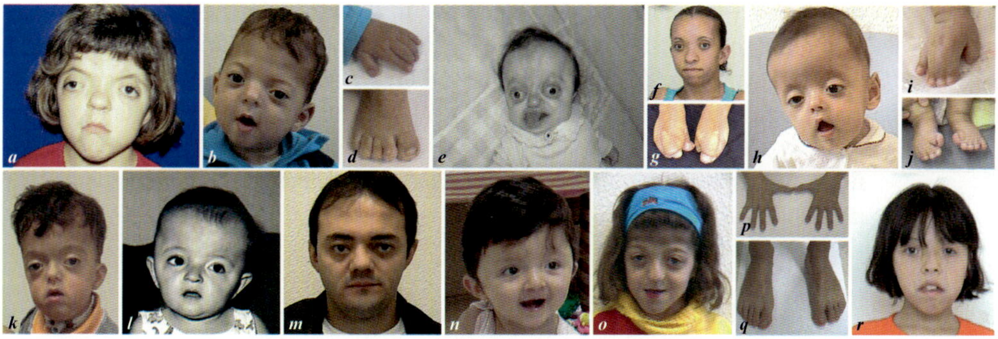

Fig. 2. Facial and limb appearance of patients with craniosynostosis. ***a*** Pfeiffer syndrome, FGFR1 p.Pro252Arg (courtesy of Dr. N. Alonso). ***b–d*** Pfeiffer syndrome, FGFR2 c.940-1G>C. ***e*** Pfeiffer syndrome, FGFR2 p.Trp290Cys. ***f, g*** Apert syndrome, FGFR2 p.Pro253Arg. ***h–j*** Apert syndrome, FGFR2 p.Ser252Trp. ***k*** Crouzon syndrome, FGFR2 p.Cys278Phe. ***l–n*** Three affected members of the same family, Muenke syndrome, FGFR3 p.Pro205Arg. ***o–q*** SCS, 46,XX, ins(7;9)(p21.2;p21.2p24.2). ***r*** SCS, TWIST1 c.385_405Ile135insAALRKII.

transmembrane domain (TM), and a split intracellular tyrosine kinase domain (TK1/TK2). The IgII and IgIII loops are critical for fibroblast growth factors (FGF) binding. The formation of a complex involving two FGFs, a FGFR dimer and cell surface heparan sulfate proteoglycans is required for autophosphorylation of various tyrosine residues in the TK domain [56]. Once phosphorylated, these tyrosines initiate signal transduction through a diverse array of signaling pathways, which may control phenomena such as cell proliferation, differentiation, migration and apoptosis according to the context [57, 58].

Complexity in FGFR signaling is enhanced by a wide array of alternative splicings. Most important is the alternative splicing of the exons encoding the C-terminal half of the third Ig loop of FGFR1–3. For these three receptors, the IgIII loop is encoded by two exons, an invariant exon termed IIIa and one of two exons, termed IIIb and IIIc, respectively, to which the IIIa exon is spliced. This generates two receptor isoforms with different ligand-binding specificities [59]. Best known are the variants of FGFR2: FGFR2b (encoded by the IIIb exon) is expressed mainly on the epithelia and is activated by ligands synthesized predominantly in the tissue mesenchyme; on the other hand, FGFR2c (encoded by the IIIc exon), the most abundant one, is located primarily in the mesenchyme and preferentially recognizes epithelial FGFs.

FGF-FGFR signaling plays a critical role in early embryonic development and in organogenesis and heterozygous mutations in the FGFR1–3 have been associated with a number of different dominant disorders, including craniosynostosis (gain-of-function mutations in FGFR1–3) [60–81], short-limbed bone dysplasias (gain-of-function mutations in FGFR3) [60, 82–85], Kallmann syndrome (haploinsufficiency for FGFR1) [86], lacrimo-auriculo-dento-digital (LADD) syndrome (dominant-negative FGFR2 and possibly FGFR3 mutations and happloinsufficiency for FGF10) [87] and camptodactyly, tall stature, scoliosis, and hearing loss (CATSHL) syndrome (dominant-negative FGFR3 mutation) [88]. In this section FGFR1–3 mutations associated with craniosynostosis are discussed.

Gain-of-Function FGFR Mutations Associated with Craniosynostosis: Overview

Heterozygous mutations in *FGFR1*, *FGFR2* and *FGFR3* genes account for the majority of cases of syndromic craniosynostosis. The FGFRs craniosynostotic syndromes share several craniofacial features including premature closure of coronal or other cranial sutures, but have distinct limb and dermatological features. In addition, some patients with nonclassifiable craniosynostotic syndromes or with nonsyndromic craniosynostosis have been shown to bear mutations in *FGFR2* and *FGFR3* genes (tables 1, 2).

The FGFR1–3 mutations associated with craniosynostosis identified so far are summarized in table 2 and illustrated in figure 3 [60–81]. All pathogenic FGFR1–3 mutations associated with craniosynostosis act dominantly and confer gain-of-function to the mutated receptor through different mechanisms, including (1) FGF-independent receptor dimerization and activation, (2) enhanced FGF-binding affinity, (3) loss of FGF-binding specificity and (4) ectopic splice form expression.

FGFR-related craniosynostoses are found both in familial and sporadic cases, and some mutations are highly recurrent. An exclusive paternal origin of de novo mutations has been described for several FGFRs mutations [89, 90].

Genotype-Phenotype Correlations

Analysis of FGFR1–3 mutations reveals a complex pattern of phenotype-genotype correlations. This is further complicated by the fact that the distinction between the craniosynostosis syndromes is not absolute and clinical overlapping is a common feature. There are several examples in which clinically different phenotypes can be caused by either the same mutation or by equivalent mutations on each of the FGFR1–3, while a given phenotype can be associated with many different mutations in the same or different FGFRs. In addition, low penetrance mutations have also been observed (table 2).

Table 2. *FGFR1–3* mutations associated with craniosynostosis

Gene	Nucleotide change[a]	Effects on protein or RNA[a]	Gene or protein region[b]	Phenotype	Reference No.[c]
FGFR 1	c.755C>G	p.Pro252Arg	IgII-IgIII linker	Pfeiffer syndrome; Jackson-Weiss syndrome	61
	c.929T>A	p.Asn330Ile	IgIIIc	osteoglophonic syndrome	62
	c.1115G>A	p.Tyr372Cys	IgIII-TM	osteoglophonic syndrome	62
	c.1135T>C	p.Cys379Arg	TM	osteoglophonic syndrome	62
FGFR 2	c.314A>G	p.Tyr105Cys	IgI	Crouzon syndrome	
	c.514-515GC>TT	p.Ala172Phe	IgII	Pfeiffer syndrome	
	c.755C>G	p.Ser252Trp	IgII-IgIII linker	Apert syndrome, Pfeiffer syndrome	
	c.755C>T	p.Ser252Leu[d]	IgII-IgIII linker	Crouzon syndrome	
	c.755 - 756 CG>TC	p.Ser252Phe	IgII-IgIII linker	Apert syndrome	
	c.755 - 757 CGC>TCT	p.Ser252Phe/Pro253Ser	IgII-IgIII linker	Pfeiffer syndrome	
	c.758C>G	p.Pro253Arg	IgII-IgIII linker	Apert syndrome	
	c.758C>T	p.Pro253Leu	IgII-IgIII linker	Crouzon syndrome	63
	c.760C>T	p.His254Tyr	IgII-IgIII linker	Crouzon syndrome	
	c.788C>T	p.Pro263Leu	IgII-IgIII linker	Crouzon syndrome	
	c.799T>C	p.Ser267Pro	IgII-IgIII linker	Crouzon syndrome, Pfeiffer syndrome	
	c.803insTGG	p.Thr268ThrGly	IgIIIa	Crouzon syndrome	
	c.804_809delGTGGTC	p.Val269_Val270del	IgIIIa	nonclassifiable disorder with craniosynostosis	
	c.818_820del	p.Asp273del	IgIIIa	Pfeiffer syndrome	64
	c.823_824ins12	p.Val274_Glu275ins4	IgIIIa	Crouzon syndrome	65
	c.826T>G	p.Phe276Val	IgIIIa	Crouzon syndrome, Pfeiffer syndrome	

Table 2. (continued)

Gene	Nucleotide change[a]	Effects on prctein or RNA[a]	Gene or protein region[b]	Phenotype	Reference No.[c]
	c.833G>A	p.Cys278Tyr [d]	IgIIIa	Crouzon syndrome; nonsyndromic sagittal/unilambdoid synostosis	66
	c.833G>T	p.Cys278Phe	IgIIIa	Crouzon syndrome, Pfeiffer syndrome, Jackson-Weiss syndrome	67
	c.842A>G	p.Tyr281Cys	IgIIIa	Crouzon syndrome	
	c.858_866delCCACATCCA	p.His287_Glndel	IgIIIa	Crouzon syndrome	
	c.863T>A	p.Ile288Asn	IgIIIa	Crouzon syndrome	68
	c.863T>G	p.Ile288Ser	IgIIIa	Crouzon syndrome	
	c.864_881del	p.Ile288Met; Gln289_Val294del	IgIIIa	Pfeiffer syndrome	
	c.866A>C	p.Gln289Pro	IgIIIa	Crouzon syndrome, Jackson-Weiss syndrome, SCS	69, 70
	c.868T>C	p.Trp290Arg	IgIIIa	Crouzon syndrome	
	c.868T>G	p.Trp290Gly	IgIIIa	Crouzon syndrome	
	c.870G>C	p.Trp290Cys	IgIIIa	Pfeiffer syndrome	
	c.870G>T	p.Trp290Cys	IgIIIa	Pfeiffer syndrome, nonclassifiable disorders with craniosynostosis	
	c.874A>G	p.Lys292Glu	IgIIIa	Crouzon syndrome	
	c.902A>G	p.Tyr301Cys	IgIIIa	Crouzon syndrome	
	c.923A>G	p.Tyr308Cys	IgIIIa	Crouzon syndrome	68
	c.940G>T	p.Ala314Ser	IgIIIa	Pfeiffer syndrome	
	c.940-1G>A	splicing	intron 9 – splice acceptor	Pfeiffer syndrome	
	c.940-1G>C	splicing	intron 9 – splice acceptor	Pfeiffer syndrome	
	c.940-2A>G[e]	splicing	intron 9 – splice acceptor	Pfeiffer syndrome; Apert syndrome	
	c.940-2A>T[e]	splicing	intron 9 – splice acceptor	Pfeiffer syndrome	

c.940-3T>G	splicing	intron 9 – splice acceptor	Pfeiffer syndrome	
c.940-3_-4insAlu[e]	splicing	intron 9	Apert syndrome	
c.940-3_946del10insACC	splicing	intron 9	Pfeiffer syndrome	
c.943G>T	p.Ala315Ser[d]	IgIIIc	nonsyndromic unicoronal synostosis	
c.958_959del AC[e]	p.Thr320GlyfsX5	IgIIIc	Jackson-Weiss syndrome	68
c.966A>C	p.Asp321Ala	IgIIIc	Pfeiffer syndrome	
c.983A>G	p.Tyr328Cys	IgIIIc	Crouzon syndrome	
c.992A>T	p.Asn331Ile	IgIIIc	Crouzon syndrome	
c.1009G>A	p.Ala337Thr[d]	IgIIIc	nonsyndromic unicoronal synostosis	71
c.1009G>C	p.Ala337Pro	IgIIIc	Crouzon syndrome	
c.1011-1012insGACGCT	p.AspAla377_378ins	IgIIIc	Crouzon syndrome	
c.1012G>C	p.Gly338Arg	IgIIIc	Crouzon syndrome	
c.1013G>A	p.Gly338Glu	IgIIIc	Crouzon syndrome	
c.1018T>C	p.Tyr340His	IgIIIc	Crouzon syndrome	
c.1019A>C	p.Tyr340Ser	IgIIIc	Crouzon syndrome	68
c.1019A>G	p.Tyr340Cys	IgIIIc	Pfeiffer syndrome	
c.1021A>C	p.Thr341Pro	IgIIIc	Pfeiffer syndrome	
c.1024T>A	p.Cys342Ser	IgIIIc	Crouzon syndrome, Jackson-Weiss syndrome, Pfeiffer syndrome	72
c.1024T>C	p.Cys342Arg	IgIIIc	Crouzon syndrome, Jackson-Weiss syndrome, Pfeiffer syndrome	73
c.1024T>G	p.Cys342Gly	IgIIIc	Pfeiffer syndrome	
c.1025G>A	p.Cys342Tyr	IgIIIc	Crouzon syndrome, Pfeiffer syndrome	
c.1025G>C	p.Cys342Ser	IgIIIc	Crouzon syndrome, Jackson-Weiss syndrome, Pfeiffer syndrome	74
c.1025G>T	p.Cys342Phe	IgIIIc	Crouzon syndrome, Jackson-Weiss syndrome	74
c.1025_1026GC>CT	p.Cys342Ser	IgIIIc	Pfeiffer syndrome	
c.1026C>G	p.Cys342Trp	IgIIIc	Crouzon syndrome, Pfeiffer syndrome	
c.1030G>C	p.Ala344Pro	IgIIIc	Pfeiffer syndrome	
c.1031C>G	p.Ala344Gly	IgIIIc	Jackson-Weiss syndrome, Crouzon syndrome	

Table 2. (continued)

Gene	Nucleotide change[a]	Effects on protein or RNA[a]	Gene or protein region[b]	Phenotype	Reference No.[c]
	c.1032G>A[f]	p.Ala344Ala (Splicing)[d]	IgIIIc	Crouzon syndrome; nonclassifiable disorders with craniosynostosis	
	c.1040C>G	p.Ser347Cys	IgIIIc	Crouzon syndrome	
	c.1041_1042insAlu[e]	splicing	IgIIIc	Apert syndrome	
	c.1052C>G	p.Ser351Cys	IgIIIc	Crouzon syndrome, Pfeiffer syndrome, unclassified craniosynostosis	75, 76
	c.1059C>A	p.Ser354Tyr	IgIIIc	Crouzon syndrome	66
	c.1061C>A	p.Ser354Tyr	IgIIIc	Crouzon syndrome	
	c.1061C>G	p.Ser354Cys	IgIIIc	Crouzon syndrome	
	c.1061C>T	p.Ser354Phe	IgIIIc	Crouzon syndrome	
	c.1066-1074delTGGTTGACA	p.Trp356_Thr358del	IgIIIc	Crouzon syndrome	
	c.1075G>T	p.Val359Phe	IgIIIc	Pfeiffer syndrome; Jackson-Weiss syndrome	74
	c.1084G>T	p.Ala362Ser[d]	IgIIIc	Crouzon syndrome	77
	c.1084+1G>T	splicing	intron 10 – splice donor	Pfeiffer syndrome	
	c.1084+3A>C	splicing	intron 10 – splice donor	Crouzon syndrome	66
	c.1084+3A>G	splicing	intron 10 – splice donor	Pfeiffer syndrome	
	c.1084_1085ins_TCAACA	p.Gly345_Pro361del	IgIIIc	Pfeiffer syndrome	
	c.1115C>G	p.Ser372Cys	IgIIIc-TM	Beare-Stevenson cutis gyrata syndrome	
	c.1124A>G	p.Tyr375Cys	IgIIIc-TM	Beare-Stevenson cutis gyrata syndrome; Pfeiffer syndrome	
	c.1150G>A	p.Gly384Arg	TM	unclassified craniosynostosis	
	c.1576A>G	p.Lys526Glu[d]	TK1	mild Crouzon syndrome, scaphocephaly	78, 79
	c.1645A>C	p.Asn549His	TK1	Crouzon syndrome	
	c.1646A>C	p.Asn549Thr	TK1	Pfeiffer syndrome	63

	c.1694A>C	p.Glu565Ala	TK1	Pfeiffer syndrome	80
	c.1694A>G	p.Glu565Gly	TK1	Pfeiffer syndrome	
	c.1922A>G	p.Lys641Arg	TK2	Pfeiffer syndrome	
	c.1977G>T	p.Lys659Asn	TK2	nonclassifiable syndrome with craniosynostosis	
	c.1988G>A	p.Gly663Glu	TK2	Pfeiffer syndrome	
	c.2032A>G	p.Arg678Gly	TK2	Crouzon syndrome	
FGFR 3	c.742C>T	p.Arg248Cys[g]	IgII-IgIII linker	thanatophoric dysplasia type I	
	c.749C>G	p.Pro250Arg[d]	IgII-IgIII linker	Muenke syndrome; Beare-Stevenson cutis gyrata syndrome	
	c.749C>T	p.Pro250Leu[d]	IgII-IgIII linker	nonsyndromic unicoronal craniosynostosis in child, macrocephaly in mother	81
	c.1118A>G	p.Tyr373Cys[g]	IgIII-TM linker	thanatophoric dysplasia type I	
	c.1172C>A	p.Ala391Glu	TM	Crouzonodermoskeletal syndrome[h]	
	c.1948A>G	p.Lys650Glu[i]	TK2	thanatophoric dysplasia type II	

[a]Nucleotide and amino acid residue numberings are in accordance with Cohen [1, 60] or the original reports. Mutation nomenclature is in accordance with the recommendations of the Human Genome Variation Society (http://www.hgvs.org/mutnomen/).
[b]Gene region or protein domain affected by the mutation.
[c]All the original reports of the mutations are cited here except for the ones included in Cohen [1, 60].
[d]Mutations either associated with reduced penetrance or with uncertain pathogenicity
[e]Mutations that lead to ectopic expression of the alternative FGFR2b splice form.
[f]Mutation that produces a cryptic donor splice site that causes a 17-amino acid deletion.
[g]Thanatophoric dysplasia type I mutations more frequently associated with craniosynostosis.
[h]Also referred to as Crouzon syndrome with acanthosis nigricans.
[i]Craniosynostosis is present in ~93% of thanatophoric dysplasia type II subjects with this mutation.

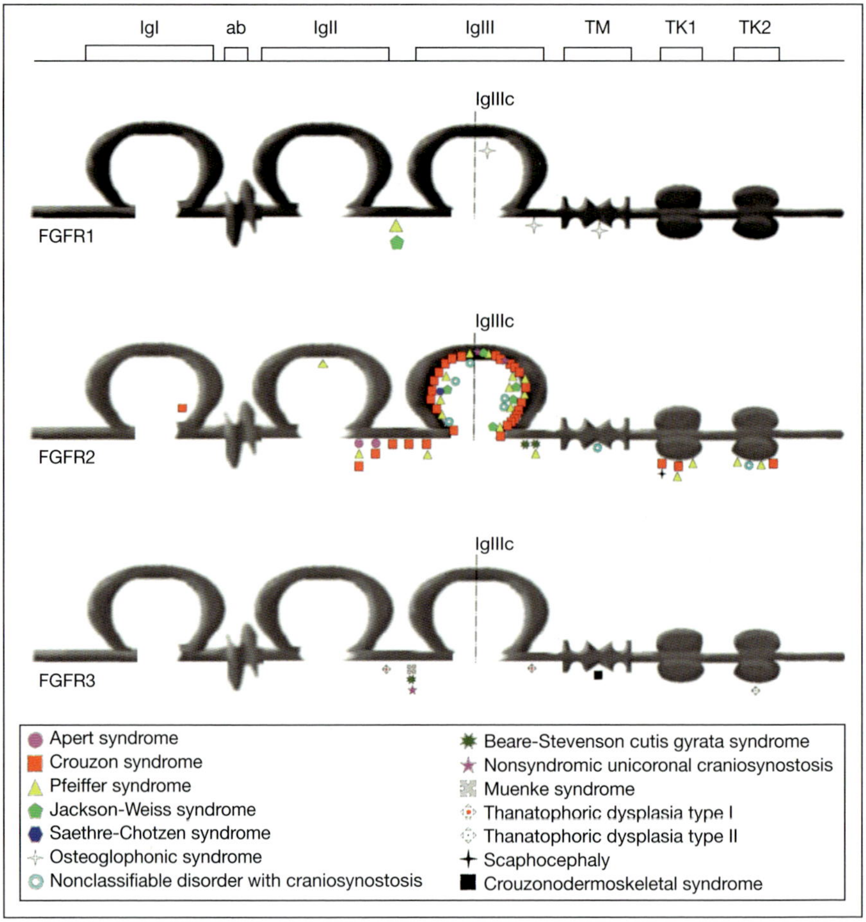

Fig. 3. Structure of FGFR proteins (types 1, 2 and 3) showing the approximate location of the mutations causing craniosynostosis. AB = Acid box; IgI, IgII, IgIII = immunoglobulin-like domains; IgIIIa = N-terminal portion of the IgIII loop (common to both FGFR1–3b and FGFR1–3c splice forms); IgIIIc = alternatively spliced form of the C-terminal portion of IgIII loop; TM = transmembrane domain; TK1 = first kinase domain; TK2 = second kinase domain.

FGFR1 Mutations

The most common FGFR1-activating mutation is the amino acid substitution p.Pro252Arg in the IgII-IgIII linker region. This heterozygous mutation has been found in a few cases of Pfeiffer syndrome (with a benign course) [60] and in a subject with Jackson-Weiss syndrome [61].

FGFR1 mutations were also found in patients with osteoglophonic dysplasia, a condition characterized by craniosynostosis, a prominent supraorbital ridge, depressed nasal bridge, rhizomelic dwarfism and nonossifying bone lesions [62]. This association reveals the critical role of FGFR1 in the modulation of bone elongation in humans.

Analogous mutations in FGFR2 or FGFR3 have been found for the four gain-of-function mutations in FGFR1 so far identified. Although there is phenotypic overlap among patients, these analogous mutations in different receptors are associated with different clinical entities. For example, FGFR1 p.Pro252Arg substitution is analogous to FGFR2 p.Pro253Arg and FGFR3 p.Pro250Arg that cause Apert and Muenke syndromes, respectively [60]. Another example is FGFR1 p.Asn330Ile mutation in the IgIIIc loop associated with osteoglophonic dysplasia [62], which is equivalent to FGFR2 p.Asn331Ile and FGFR3 p.Asn328Ile that cause Crouzon and hypochondroplasia syndromes, respectively [60].

FGFR2 Mutations

Mutations in FGFR2 account for approximately 90% of the syndromic craniosynostosis Apert, Crouzon, Pfeiffer, and Jackson-Weiss [60, 67, 68, 91] and for ~9% of all craniosynostosis [67, 71, 92]. No FGFR2 mutations have been found in any case of nonsyndromic sagittal or metopic synostosis [71].

In contrast to FGFR1 mutations, a broader spectrum of FGFR2 mutations has been associated with craniosynostosis. The majority of FGFR2 mutations are missense (to date about 65 amino acid substitutions reported) or splice-site type (about a dozen mutations reported) but small in-frame deletions and insertions have been also described. Several of the missense mutations (~20%) either create or destroy cysteine residues, resulting in unpaired cysteines that can produce intermolecular disulfide binding and ligand-independent constitutive receptor activation (table 2, fig. 3).

Mutations in the IgI and IgII Loops of FGFR2

Mutations within IgI and IgII domains have only been found in FGFR2 (table 2, fig. 3). The associated phenotypes resemble those with mutations in the hot spots of the *FGFR2* (exons IIIa and IIIc, or exons 8 and 10, respectively, encoding the IgIII domain) but with some unusual clinical features, such as Crouzon syndrome with scaphocephaly [60, 75] in one case and a Pfeiffer phenotype with severe limb abnormalities, including symphalangism [60, 93].

Mutations in the IgII-IgIII Linker Region of FGFR2

The two most frequent mutations in the linker region between IgII and IgIII of FGFR2 are p.Ser252Trp and p.Pro253Arg that cause 66 and 32.2% of

Apert syndrome cases, respectively. The p.Ser252Trp mutation is associated with a more severe craniofacial phenotype with cleft palate in some patients, while p.Pro253Arg mutation is associated with more severe syndactyly [60, 94]. Interestingly, one patient bearing the p.Ser252Trp mutation had such a mild syndactyly that the phenotype suggested Pfeiffer rather than Apert syndrome [60].

Few rare additional mutations in the IgII-IgIII linker region are also associated with Apert and Pfeiffer syndrome. The type of amino acid residue substitution has a specific clinical consequence, as illustrated by the observation of Crouzon-like phenotypes and nonpenetrance of the disease in cases with p.Ser252Leu or p.Pro253Leu substitutions.

Unlike mutations within other regions of FGFRs, the Apert syndrome p.Ser252Trp and p.Pro253Arg mutations are substitutions to bulky side-chain amino acids and are ligand dependent. It has been demonstrated that these substitutions define two gain-of-function mechanisms of FGFR2 mutations: enhanced FGF-binding affinity and loss of FGF-binding specificity [95–97]. Analogous mutations on FGFR1 and FGFR3 seem to behave similarly to the Apert FGFR2 mutations [98].

Mutations in the IgIII loop of FGFR2

The majority of FGFR2 mutations (~77%) are clustered in the IgIII loop of the receptor (table 2, fig. 3). Although several mutations have been associated with more than one syndrome, a genotype-phenotype correlation is observed in many cases. For example, Crouzon syndrome appears to be preferentially accounted for in the case of substitutions at residues p.Phe267, p.Cys278, p.Gln289, p.Gly338, p.Cys342, p.Ala344, p.Ser347 and p.Ser354; severe Pfeiffer syndrome cases, on the other hand, are more frequently associated with mutations at residues p.Trp290, p.Tyr340, p.Cys342 and p.Ser351 when they are substituted by a cysteine or if a cysteine residue is abolished. The residue that is substituted is also important for the phenotype, as exemplified by the conversion of the p.Trp290 and p.Tyr340 into other amino acid residues rather than cysteines (p.Trp290Arg/Gly, p.Tyr340His/Ser) that result in Crouzon syndrome [60, 68, 93].

One interesting category of FGFR2 mutations is the splicing mutations that are mostly associated with Pfeiffer syndrome (accounts for ~10% of mutations associated with this syndrome), and usually with a more severe limb phenotype [60, 93].

Another interesting class of mutations constitutes two de novo *Alu*-element insertions upstream or within exon IIIc (or exon 10) in 2 Apert syndrome patients. This type of mutation and a few other pathogenic changes affecting this domain lead to ectopic expression of the FGFR2b splice form in cells of mesenchyme origin [68, 99]. Therefore, these mutations define a new pathological class of FGFR2 mutations: ectopic splice form expression.

Mutations Either Near or within the Transmembrane Region of FGFR2

Two closely spaced mutations p.Ser372Cys and p.Tyr375Cys, in the linker region between IgIII and the transmembrane domain of FGFR2, have been associated with Beare-Stevenson cutis gyrata syndrome [60]. The latter was also recently found in a severe Pfeiffer phenotype, but in which cutis gyrata and acanthosis nigricans, clinical findings associated with Beare-Stevenson syndrome, were not observed [60, 91].

The only mutation within the transmembrane domain of FGFR2, p.Gly384Arg, has been associated with a nonclassifiable disorder with craniosynostosis [60].

Mutations in the Tyrosine Kinase Domain of FGFR2

A total of nine distinct mutations associated with syndromic craniosynostosis have been identified so far in the FGFR2 tyrosine kinase domain (table 2, fig. 3). There does not appear to be a set of clinical features that uniformly distinguishes patients with FGFR2 intracellular tyrosine kinase mutations from those with mutations in the extracellular region, except that patients tend to exhibit mild broadening of the thumbs and great toes [91, 93].

Some of these mutations occur at equivalent positions of FGFR3, but the associated phenotypes are different. For example, several FGFR2 mutations associated with Crouzon or Pfeiffer phenotypes occur at the position equivalent to constitutively activating mutations associated with short limb skeletal dysplasias [60].

FGFR3 Mutations

FGFR3 p.Pro250Arg mutation causes Muenke syndrome, the most common syndromic form of craniosynostosis [60]. Muenke syndrome expressivity is extremely variable and nonpenetrance has been reported in some families. It is estimated that about 30% of children with coronal synostosis and 6–8% of all craniosynostosis patients have this mutation [71, 92].

A recurrent mutation in the transmembrane region of FGFR3, p.Ala391Glu, accounts for a form of Crouzon syndrome that associates craniosynostosis and *acanthosis nigricans* also called crouzonodermoskeletal syndrome [60].

FGFR3 mutations are also associated with four forms of short-limbed bone dysplasias. Of these, only thanatophoric dysplasias (types I and II) and rarely hypochondroplasia are associated with craniosynostosis. It is interesting that the penetrance of craniosynostosis varies from approximately 28% in thanatophoric dysplasia type I cases, with the p.Arg248Cys and p.Tyr373Cys mutations, to 93% in thanatophoric dysplasias type II patients, carriers of the p.Lys650Glu mutation [60].

Twist Homolog Drosophila 1 (TWIST1)

Gene, Protein Structure and Functions

TWIST1 gene, which encodes a basic helix-loop-helix transcription factor (bHLH), has of a first exon with a translation start site (ATG) followed by an uninterrupted open reading frame of 606 nucleotides that encodes 202 amino acid residues (GenBank Accession No. U80998) and a second untranslated exon with two potential polyadenylation signals that are 65 and 415 bp away from the 5′ end of exon 2.

TWIST1 protein is characterized by two highly conserved regions: a DNA-binding domain, which consists mostly of basic amino acid residues and the bHLH motif, which consists of a short alpha helix (helix I) connected by a loop to a second, longer alpha helix (helix II). The loop region is essential for the protein tertiary structure and the correct functionality of the two alpha helices. The HLH region is necessary and sufficient for protein dimerization, and dimerization is needed prior to DNA binding [100]. The second HLH protein can be the same (creating a homodimer) or different (creating a heterodimer). The repertoire of proteins that dimerizes with TWIST1 is not fully known, but it seems that the type of heterodimer formed is critical for determining the specificity of downstream target genes [101].

TWIST1 protein contains additional functional motifs. One of these (amino acids 30–64 in humans) binds to histone acetyltransferase p300 and can be involved in *TWIST1* gene expression regulation through chromatin condensation [102]. Another motif is the 'Twist box' located at the C-terminal domain (amino acids 183–202 of the human protein), which interacts with the Runt-related factor DNA-binding domain, Runx2, and inhibits its function [103]. Nuclear localization sequences, other important functional domains, are located within and outside the HLH domain.

TWIST1 gene became a candidate for Saethre-Chotzen syndrome (SCS) after the gene was localized to chromosome 7p21, the region to which the SCS locus was previously mapped [104–107] and based on the observation that mice heterozygous for a *twist1*-null mutation exhibit subtle cranial and limb defects [108].

SCS, or acrocephalosyndactyly type III, is an autosomal dominantly inherited form of craniosynostosis. The classical clinical features are craniosynostosis, mainly involving the coronal sutures, low-set frontal hairline, facial asymmetry, ptosis of the eyelids, deviated nasal septum, brachydactily, partial soft tissue syndactly, especially of the second and third fingers, and various skeletal anomalies, such as defects of the cervical and lumbar spine or radioulnar synostosis among others. Short stature has been documented in some instances. Patients may have hearing loss, most commonly due to conductive hearing impairment as a consequence of abnormal configuration of the nasopharynx, cleft palate or both. Penetrance is high, but it is not complete. There is a wide spectrum of clinical variability, and mild cases can often be misdiagnosed. A better characterization of the clinical spectrum of variability is being established since the identification of *TWIST*1 as the causative gene.

TWIST1 Gene Mutations

Characterization and Distribution along the Gene

Although chromosomal structural alterations are not rare causative mechanisms of SCS, at least 97 different disease-causing mutations in the coding region of the *TWIST1* gene have been described among 153 patients worldwide mostly with SCS phenotype [109–115] (table 3). To date, no splice site and intronic mutations or changes within the promoter or in the second nontranslated exon have been reported. Among the mutations in the coding region of *TWIST1*, about 60% of are nucleotide substitutions leading to either missense (31%) or nonsense mutations (29%). The remaining 40% are deletions, duplications or insertions of less than 30 nucleotides, which will be referred to as small rearrangements (table 3). Two distinct mutations on the same allele have been reported in two unrelated patients.

The majority of the mutations (63/97; 65%) are located within the bHLH motif. The functional importance of the N- and C-terminal domains has also been shown by the identification of a few rare missense and in-frame mutations outside the bHLH motif [115]. Except for a few mutations, most of them are private with no apparent mutational hot spot. It is of note, however, that mutations involving the nucleotide at position c.309 (which encode the amino acid residue Tyr in the 5′ DNA-binding domain) account for 8% of all mutations or 13% of the nucleotide substitutions (table 3). There is also an apparent excess of duplications starting at nucleotides 416–420 (encoding for amino acid residues in the loop region) and unequal crossovers due to repeated sequences in this region have been suggested as the causative mechanism [115].

Large deletions including the *TWIST1* gene account for at least 10% of the SCS cases. These deletions were originally identified by fluorescence in situ hybridization or Southern blot analysis [115], and their detection has been greatly facilitated with the use of the multiplex ligation-dependent probe amplification method. The extension of the deletion varies from a relatively small size encompassing mainly the *TWIST1* gene up to a few megabases.

Table 3. *TWIST1* mutations in patients with SCS and related phenotypes

Nucleotide change[a],	Consequence at the protein level	Functional domain	n	Reference No.[c]
c.7C>T	Gln3X	5′ DNA binding	2	
c.61G>T	Glu21X	5′ DNA binding	1	
c.82C>T	Gln28X	5′ DNA binding	1	
c.106G>T	Gly36X	5′ DNA binding	3	
c.108delA	Gly36GlyfsX88	5′ DNA binding	1	
c.115C>G	p.Arg39Gly	NLS	1	
c.127_137del11	Arg43fsX233	5′ DNA binding	1	
c.128_138del 11	Arg44fsX233	5′ DNA binding	1	
c.181G>T	p.Gly61X	5′ DNA binding	1	
c.193G>T	p.Glu65X	5′DNA binding	4	
c.211C>T	p.Gln71X	5′DNA binding	2	110
c.230delA;c.232T>C	Lys77fsX124	5′ DNA binding	1	
c.263delG	Gly88fsX124	5′ DNA binding	1	111
c.272_273ins 10	Ser93fsX292	5′ DNA binding	1	
c.276_277dup21	Gly92_S93insGAGGGGG	5′ DNA binding	2	
c.283delAinsCG	Ser95fsX237	5′ DNA binding	1	
c.308_309insA	Tyr103X	5′ DNA binding	2	
c.309C>A/G	Tyr103X	5′ DNA binding	13	
c.309delC	Tyr103X	5′ DNA binding	2	
c.310G>T	Glu104X	5′ DNA binding	2	
c.326del17	p.Gln109fs	DNA binding	1	
Not referred	p.Gln109X	DNA binding	1	
c.336delG	p.Met112fsX12 ou	DNA binding	1	
c.340A>G	p.Asn114Asp	DNA binding	1	
Not referred	p.Asn114Ser	DNA binding	1	
c.346C>T	p.Arg116Trp	DNA binding	1	
Not referred	p.Arg116Gly	DNA binding	1	
c.348del17	p.Arg116fsX231	DNA binding	1	
c.352C>T	p.Arg118Cys	DNA binding	1	112
c.352_354del3	p.Arg118del	DNA binding	1	
c.353G>A	p.Arg118His	DNA binding	2	113
c.353G>C	p.Arg118Pro	DNA binding	1	
c.353_360del8	p.Arg118fsX234	DNA binding	1	
c.355C>T	p.Gln199X	DNA binding	2	
c.355delC	p.Gln119fsX124	DNA binding	1	
c.356A>C	p.Gln119Pro	DNA binding	1	
c.359G>C	p.Arg120Pro	DNA binding	1	
Not referred	p.Arg120Cys	DNA binding	1	
c.364C>T	p.Gln122X	helix I	2	
c.368C>A	p.Ser123X	helix I	3	
c.368C>G	p.Ser123Trp	helix I	3	

Table 3. (continued)

Nucleotide change[a],	Consequence at the protein level	Functional domain	n	Reference No.[c]
c.376G>T	p.Glu126X	helix I	4	
c.379G>A;c.398A>T	p.Ala127Thr/p.Lys133Ile	helix I	1	
c.379_381dup	p.Ala127_Phe128insA	helix I	1	
c.380C>A	p.Ala127Glu	helix I	1	
c.384_385insC	p.Ala129fsX237	helix I	1	
c.385G>C	p.Ala129Pro	helix I	1	
c.385_405dup	p.Ala129_Ile135insAALRKII	helix I	2	
c.392T>C	Leu131Pro	helix I	1	
c.395G>C	Arg132Pro	helix I	1	
c.397_417dup	p.Lys133_Pro139insKIIPTLP	helix I/loop	2	
c.402C>G	Ile134Met	helix I	1	
c.405_406dup21	Ile135_Pro136insAALRKII	helix I	2	
c.407C>T	Pro136Leu	helix I	2	
Not referred	Pro136Leu	helix I	1	
c.409A>C	Thr137Pro	helix I	1	
c.415C>T	Pro139Ser	loop	1	
c.416C>A	Pro139His	loop	1	
c.416C>T	Pro139Leu	loop	1	
c.416_417dup21	Pro139_Ser140insKIIPTLP	loop	7	
c.417_418dup21	Pro139_Ser140ins KIIPTLP	loop	3	
c.418_419dup21	Ser140X	loop	1	
c.420_421dup21	Ser140_Asp141insIIPTLPS	loop	2	
c.421G>T	Asp141Tyr	loop	2	
c.422A>G	Asp141Gly	loop	1	
c.423_424ins25	Asp141_Lys142insDHPHAALGfsX297	loop	1	
c.428delT	p.Leu143ArgfsX76	loop	1	
c.430A>C	Ser144Arg	loop	2	
c.433A>G	Lys145Glu	loop	1	
c.433_455del23	Lys145fsX229	loop	1	
c.435G>C	Lys145Asn	loop	1	
c.442A>G	Thr148Ala	loop	1	
c.443C>A	THr148Asn	loop	1	
c.443C>G	Thr148Ser	loop	1	
c.443C>T	Thr148Ile	loop	1	
c.445C>T	Leu149Phe	loop	2	
c.454G>C	Ala152Pro	loop	1	
c.455C>T	Ala152Val	loop	1	
c.460A>G	Arg154Gly	helix II	1	
c.460_461insA	Arg154fsX237	helix II	1	
c.464_469del5	Tyr155X	helix II	1	
c.465C>A	Tyr155X	helix II	1	

Table 3. (continued)

Nucleotide change[a],	Consequence at the protein level	Functional domain	n	Reference No.[c]
c.466A>G	Ile156Val	helix II	1	
c.470A>T	Asp157Val	helix II	1	
Not referred	Asp157Ala	helix III	1	
c.472T>C	Phe158Leu	helix II	2	
c.474C>G	Phe158Leu	helix II	2	
c.475C>T	Leu159Phe	helix II	1	
c.480C>G	Tyr160X	helix II	1	
c.481C>T	Gln161X	helix II	5	
c.481delC	Gln161fsX230	helix II	1	
c.482_488del7	Gln161fsX228	helix II	1	
c.485_488del4	Val162fsX229	helix II	1	
c.487delC	Leu163fsX230	helix II	1	
c.490C>T	Gln164X	helix II	1	
c.495ins10	p.Ala165fs	helix II	1	
c.541G>T	Glu181X	3′ helix II	1	
c.561C>G	Phe187Leu	TWIST box	1	
Deletion	entire gene	entire gene	20	

[a]Genomic sequence based on GenBank accession No. U80998; mutations are referred to as originally reported.

[b]Mutation nomenclature according to Den Dunnen and Antonarakis [114].

[c]All the original reports of the mutations are cited in this table except for the ones included in Jabs (115).

The rearrangement $(GGC)_5(CGC)(GGC)_5$ at nucleotides 244–276 was initially identified only among affected patients. Family and functional studies have demonstrated that it is not pathogenic. This polyglycine tract variation does not seem to modulate the phenotype when in *cis* with a pathogenic mutation in the *TWIST1* gene, but its effect in *trans* with a pathogenic mutation has not yet been functionally or phenotypically addressed [115].

Polymorphisms within the *TWIST1* gene have also been identified. No functional or systematic studies have yet been performed for this type of mutations, but they do apparently not influence the phenotype.

Effect of the Mutations in the Protein

The phenotypes caused by complete heterozygous deletions of the *TWIST1* gene in some SCS patients and of the *Twist1* null heterozygous (Twist+/−) mouse suggested that haploinsufficiency is the most likely disease-causing mechanism [116–118]. This assumption has been further reinforced by the observation that all pathogenic mutations so far identified in SCS patients lead to a similar phenotype [115–117].

Different mutational mechanisms in TWIST1 lead to haploinsufficiency in SCS. Nonsense mutations upstream or within the bHLH motif cause the synthesis of truncated proteins which are rapidly degraded, while missense mutations involving helix I or II regions create proteins that fail to heterodimerize and become abnormally located in the cytoplasm [119]. On the other hand, missense mutations in the loop-helix II junction region of the bHLH motif can lead to deficiency in protein-DNA interactions, while mutations in the middle of the loop seem to reduce heterodimerization with E12 protein and partial mislocalization of the protein [115]. Mutations in the TWIST1 box lead to abnormal interaction with RUNX2 while a naturally occurring mutation in one of the NLS domain leads to nuclear mislocalization of TWIST1 protein [110, 111]. Therefore, alterations in protein stability, dimerization deficiency, altered DNA-binding capacity or abnormal nuclear location can lead to TWIST loss of function.

Characterization of the breakpoints of some cytogenetically balanced translocations in SCS patients revealed that the coding region of *TWIST1* gene is preserved. Therefore, it is possible that the translocation breakpoints disrupt an important regulatory sequence of *TWIST1* or a second gene on 7p. Alternatively, the disease in these cases is caused by a positional effect on TWIST1 expression [115, 120].

Phenotype and Genotype Correlations

Large pedigrees segregating nonsense mutations or a deletion of the *TWIST1* gene and SCS have exemplified the great clinical intrafamilial variability of the syndrome, including low penetrance for craniosynostosis in one of these genealogies [115]. A remarkable interfamilial clinical variability in SCS has also been well documented [60, 115]. The molecular mechanisms that cause the extreme variation in the clinical outcome of the disease are unknown, and there is no evidence of a correlation between the phenotype and the nature or location of a specific point or small rearrangement mutations within the *TWIST1* gene. Physical findings in patients with large gene deletions also do not differ from those with small or point mutations. Although intellectual deficits are rarely seen in patients with point mutations, they are often found in those with deletions encompassing the gene, thus suggesting a correlation between *TWIST1* gene deletions and cognitive function. It is still unclear whether the degree of mental retardation in patients with a complete deletion of the *TWIST1* gene is related to the size and location of the molecular defect [115, 121]. A more systematic study including delineation of the breakpoints and a better definition of the cognitive deficit in a larger number of patients is necessary to draw final conclusions.

The expression level of TWIST1 protein and of those that dimerize with it is critical for the correct function of TWIST1. We could thus speculate that variation on the availability of the counterpart proteins that dimerize with Twist1, which can be dependent on genetic or environmental factors, may play a role in the determination of the expressivity of the disease.

Despite the lack of genotype-phenotype correlation for physical alterations, analysis of the *TWIST1* gene in a large set of craniosynostotic patients has contributed to a better delineation of the syndrome. Bifid halluces and unilateral radial aplasia are now part of the clinical spectrum of variability of SCS as it was shown that patients diagnosed with Robinow-Sorauf and Baller-Gerold syndromes carry mutations in *TWIST1* gene [115]. In contrast, very mild patients, nonsyndromic or in whom ptosis was the main clinical feature, have also been found to carry mutations in *TWIST1* [110, 115]. Therefore, the spectrum of clinical variability ranges from nonsyndromic or only ptosis to the full SCS phenotype, associated or not with bifid halluces and unilateral radial aplasia.

Some patients originally classified as SCS were found to have the p.Pro250Arg mutation at FGFR3 [109, 115], which is associated with Muenke syndrome. Therefore, it has been recommended that SCS patients negative for *TWIST1* mutations should be tested for this FGFR3 mutation. However, Kress et al. [110] argue that it is possible to clinically distinguish patients with SCS or Muenke syndrome. Based on the phenotype analysis of a large cohort of patients with *TWIST1* mutations or the p.Pro250Arg mutation in FGFR3, they suggested that low-set frontal hairline, gross ptosis of the eyelids, subnormal ear length, dilated parietal foramina, interdigital webbing, hallux valgus or broad great toe with bifid distal phalanx were significantly more prominent in patients with *TWIST1* mutations. In addition, intercranial hypertension as a consequence of early progressive multisutural fusion was a significant problem in SCS only, while mental delay and sensorineural hearing loss were associated with Muenke syndrome.

Several reports have shown that a few patients clinically classified as SCS do not harbor mutations either in the *TWIST1* gene or in the *FGFR* genes, suggesting genetic heterogeneity for the syndrome or a different mutational mechanism in these genes. No mutations have been found in potential candidate genes that are components of the same developmental pathway, including *SNAI1, SLUG* and *DERMO1* [109, 115].

Ephrin-B1 (EFNB1)

Gene and Protein Structure and Functions

Ephrins are one of the largest classes of membrane-bound ligands for Eph family receptor tyrosine kinases, which regulate cell adhesion and repulsion responses that guide the migration of cells and axons along specific pathways during animal development. The ephrins and Eph proteins are also known to have an important function to avoid mixing of cells across boundaries in embryo development. Eph/ephrin interactions lead to the generation of a bidirectional signal, in which both the Eph receptors and the ephrins activate downstream signaling cascades simultaneously. Eight ephrins belonging to two classes have been characterized: class A (EFNA1–A5) which are linked to the cell membrane by a glycosylphophatidylinositol anchor, and class B (EFNB1–B3) which are transmembrane proteins with intracellular region containing multiple tyrosine residues and a PDZ domain. Tyrosine phosphorylation and binding of PDZ-containing proteins are required for the function of transmembrane ephrins. The Eph receptors, 14 in number, are divided into EphA and EphB receptors, depending on their preferential affinity to ephrin-A or ephrin-B proteins [122–124].

Through linkage and positional candidate gene analysis it was demonstrated that mutations in one of the ephrin B genes, *EFNB1*, mapped at Xq13, cause a syndromic form of craniosynostosis, craniofrontonasal dysplasia [125, 126]. *EFNB1* contains 5 exons and encodes a protein of 346 aa.

Craniofrontonasal syndrome is an X-linked developmental disorder that shows greater severity in heterozygous females than in hemizygous males. Females present severe hypertelorism, coronal craniosynostosis either unilaterally or bilaterally, craniofacial asymmetry, frontal bossing, downslanting palpebral fissures, broad bifid nose, low posterior hairline with an anterior widow's peak, frizzy hair, and occasionally cleft lip or palate. Common extracranial features are sloping shoulders with dysplastic clavicles, mild cutaneous syndactyly, and characteristic longitudinal splitting of the nails, diaphragmatic hernia, and agenesis of corpus callosum. Males are rarely reported and paradoxically have a much milder phenotype, which includes hypertelorism and possibly cleft lip and/or palate [1, 125, 126]. Congenital diaphragmatic hernia can also be part of the phenotype in males, but its penetrance is still unknown [127].

EFNB1 Gene Mutations

Characterization and Distribution along the Gene

More than 70 different mutations distributed along the *EFNB1* gene have already been associated with craniofrontonasal syndrome; among these, 71 were intragenic and 3 were partial or complete gene deletions [125–130] (table 4). The intragenic mutations comprised 46 single-nucleotide and 1 double-nucleotide substitutions leading to missense or nonsense codons, splicing mutations or

Table 4. *EFNB1* mutations associated with craniofrontonasal dysplasia

Nucleotide change[a]	Exon (intron)	Consequence at mRNA or protein	Functional domain[b]	Cases n	Reference No.
4_4del	1	–	signal peptide	1	128
c.1A>G	1	p.Met1Val	signal peptide	1	125
c.30C>T[c]	1	p.Lys11SerfsX2	signal peptide	1	128
c.57G>A	1	p.Trp19X	signal peptide	1	125
c.80C>G	1	p.Pro27Arg	signal peptide	1	129
c.88_89delAA	1	p.Ala29fsX73	extracellular	1	129
c.109T>G	1	p.Trp37Gly	extracellular	2	128
c.110G>A	1	p.Trp37Gly	extracellular	1	128
c.123C>G	1	p.Asp41Lys	extracellular	1	128
c.146delG	2	p.Lys48fsX51	extracellular	1	129
c.151_153delGTG	2	p.Val51del	extracellular	1	127, 128
c.161C>T	2	p.Pro54Leu	extracellular	3	126, 128, 129
c.170_171GA>TT	2	p.Gly57Val	extracellular	1	128
c.185T>C	2	p.Ile62Thr	extracellular	1	125
c.191G>A	2	p.Cys64Tyr	extracellular	1	128
c.196delC	2	p.Arg66GlufsX93	extracellular	1	128
c.196C>T	2	p.Arg66X	extracellular	9	125, 128, 129
c.220G>T	2	p.Glu74X	extracellular	2	128, 129
c.229_232delAAGC	2	p.Tyr76fsX157	extracellular	1	129
c.233T>C	2	p.Leu78Pro	extracellular	1	128
c.246delG	2	p.Pro83fsX75	extracellular	1	125
c.258_261dupAGCT	2	p.Ala87fsX91	extracellular	1	129
c.265T>C	2	p.Cys89Arg	extracellular	1	128
c.266G>A	2	p.Cys89Tyr	extracellular	1	128
c.293T>C	2	p.Leu98Ser	extracellular	1	125
c.324_325insA	2	p.Ile108fsX131	extracellular	1	129
c.325delC	2	p.Ile108fsX158	extracellular	1	129
c.332C>T[d]	2	p.Thr111Ile	extracellular	1	126
c.339G>C	2	p.Lys113Asn	extracellular	1	128
c.344A>C	2	p.Gln115Pro	extracellular	1	128
c.346G>T	2	p.Glu116X	extracellular	1	129
c.355C>A	2	p.Pro119Thr	extracellular	1	125
c.355C>T	2	p.Pro119Ser	extracellular	1	129
c.355C>G	2	p.Pro119Ala	extracellular	1	128
c.356C>A	2	p.Pro119His	extracellular	2	125, 129
c.363C>A	2	p.Tyr121X	extracellular	1	128
c.368G>A	2	p.Gly123Asp	extracellular	1	128
c.377_384delTCAAGAAG	2	p.Glu125fsX128	extracellular	1	129
c.398delA	2	p.Tyr133SerfsX26	extracellular	1	128
c.406+1G>A	(2)	splice	extracellular	2	125, 128
c.407-1G>A	(2)	splice	extracellular	1	125
c.407-2A>G	(2)	splice	extracellular	1	129

Table 4. (continued)

Nucleotide change[a]	Exon (intron)	Consequence at mRNA or protein	Functional domain[b]	Cases n	Reference No.
c.407-2A>T	(2)	splice	extracellular	1	129
c.407C>T	3	p.Ser136Leu	extracellular	1	128
c.409A>G	3	p.Thr137Ala	extracellular	1	129
c.413C>T	3	p.Ser138Phe	extracellular	1	129
c.415delA	3	p.Ser138fsX158	extracellular	1	129
c.432delG	3	p.Leu145TrpfsX14	extracellular	2	127, 128
c.445G>T	3	p.Glu149X	extracellular	1	128
c.451G>A	3	p.Gly151Ser	extracellular	5	125, 128
c.452G>T	3	p.Gly151Val	extracellular	1	125
c.452G>A	3	p.Gly151Asp	extracellular	1	128
c.458G>A	3	p.Cys153Tyr	extracellular	1	129
c.458G>C	3	p.Cys153Ser	extracellular	2	125, 126
c.463A>C	3	p.Thr155Pro	extracellular	1	125
c.472A>G	3	p.Met158Val	extracellular	1	125
c.474G>T	3	p.Met158Ile	extracellular	1	125
c.496C>T	3	p.Gln166X	extracellular	1	128
c.500-2A>G	(3)	splicing	extracellular	1	128
c.546C>A	4	p.Ser182Arg	extracellular	1	129
c.550delG	4	p.Lys183fsX212	extracellular	1	129
c.564_565insT	4	p.Tyr189CysfsX10	extracellular	1	128
c.587delC	4	p.Pro196LeufsX17	extracellular	1	128
c.629-2A>G	(4)	splicing	extracellular	1	125
c.635_636delTG	5	p.Val212GlufsX19	extracellular	1	128
c.678_679insA	5	p.Ser226fsX231	extracellular	1	129
c.685_686insGG	5	p.Gly228fsX259	extracellular	1	129
c.685_686insG	5	p.Asp229GlyfsX31[e]	extracellular	1	130
c.969delC	5	p.Gly322fsX391	cytoplasmic (potential)	1	129
c.986delA	5	p.Val328fsX391	cytoplasmic (potential)	1	129
c.993_994insCT	5	p.Gln332LeufsX61	cytoplasmic (potential)	1	128
Deletion	1–5	no protein	entire gene	2	128
Deletion	1–3	no protein	entire gene	1	128
Deletion exons	2–5	no protein	entire gene	1	129

[a]Nomenclature according to GenBank accession No. NM_004429.
[b]Domains according to http://us.expasy.or.
[c]Mutation causes altered splicing.
[d]Published numbering incompatible with exon 2 sequence. c.332C>T corresponds to 1023C>T [129].
[e]Originally referred to as p.Gly230fsX.

alteration of the initiation codon; the remaining ones were frameshifting deletions, insertions or duplications and one in-frame deletion mutations. Of the 48 single nucleotide substitutions identified among 66 unrelated patients, only 2 mutations were more highly recurrent, respectively, at nucleotides c.196C (9/66) and c.451G (5/66); however, there is no evidence of a mutational hot spot along the gene. Nucleotide substitutions are located in exons 1–4 of the gene (encoding for the signal peptide/extracellular domains) while nearly 50% of the frameshift deletions/insertions occurred within the last two exons of the *EFNB1* gene (which encode part of the transmembrane and cytoplasmic domains).

Effect of the Mutation on the Protein

Missense mutations change highly conserved amino acid residues across species in the extracellular ephrin domain and are expected to disrupt protein folding or interaction sites for ephrin-B1 interacting partners (such as ephrin-B2 and EphB2), and thus correspond to loss-of-function mutations. The frameshift, nonsense and splice site mutations identified in exons 1–4 of the *EFNB1* gene generate premature termination codons that most likely elicit nonsense-mediated mRNA decay and therefore correspond to null mutants. Whether this also applies to the frameshift mutations in exon 5 is not quite clear, because premature termination occurs in the last exon of the gene. This may allow the synthesis of a truncated, soluble ephrin-B1 that could act in a dominant-negative fashion provided that it is properly processed and expressed as a stable polypeptide. Other frameshift mutations at the end of exon 5 change the reading frame and lead to the addition of several amino acids at the carboxyterminal part of ephrin-B1. These mutations are predicted to alter the structure of the cytoplasmic tail and disrupt the intracellular binding sites for Grb4 and PDZ-effector proteins, which are involved in ephrin-B1 reverse signaling. These C-terminal frameshifts may also impair bidirectional endocytosis of ephrin-B1 and EphB complexes, a mechanism that appears to regulate Eph-ephrin contact-mediated repulsion [125–129].

Genotype-Phenotype Correlations

Mutations in *EFNB1* have been found in the great majority of females (~95%) diagnosed with craniofrontonasal syndrome, thus suggesting genetic heterogeneity or a still unknown mutational mechanism in this gene in less than 10% of the cases [129].

There is great intrafamilial and interfamilial clinical variability among craniofrontonasal female subjects, including the extent of craniosynostosis and the occurrence of additional clinical features. No genotype-phenotype correlation is apparent in any of the studies, which implies that missense or frameshift changes cause a comparable disturbance of ephrin-B1 [125–129]. This X-linked disease has been a paradox in human genetics, as heterozygous female carriers of the mutation always present a more severe phenotype than hemizygous males. In addition, there is a significant excess of females.

It has been proposed that the phenotypic discrepancies between the sexes are due to cellular interference, a process associated with X inactivation. That is, in heterozygous females, there is a mosaic of cells expressing and not expressing ephrin-B1, which might interfere in the establishment of tissue boundaries during embryogenesis. On the other hand, as males will only have cells without ephrin-B1, no disruption in cell boundaries will occur and ligand/receptor promiscuity may explain the mild or absent manifestation of *EFNB1* mutations in hemizygotes [125, 126]. This hypothesis has been supported by the observation that mice harboring *Efnb1* null mutation show a similar paradoxical pattern of phenotypic severity, with heterozygous females consistently more severely affected than hemizygous males. In the heterozygous female mice, abnormal sorting of cells into ephrin-B1-expressing and ephrin-B1-nonexpressing patches was shown to correlate with the X-inactivation status of *Efnb1* [131]. However, this hypothesis does not explain the occurrence of congenital diaphragmatic hernia, as this malformation is present both in males and females with mutations in *EFNB1*. It is possible that ephrin-B1 does not have a nonredundant role in the development of the diaphragm [127].

The low proportion of affected males has been shown to be associated with the origin of the mutation, as 92% of the de novo mutations occur in the paternal germinative cells [128]. It is also of note that somatic mosaicism is quite high, accounting for 18.5% of the cases. These data have important implications for genetic counseling.

Final Considerations

The growth of the skull, which involves ossification and growth of the cranial plates and their fusion along the calvarial sutures, is very well coordinated with the growth of the developing brain and it might reflect an important evolutionary process. Identification of the molecular pathways involved in this developmental process will not only provide insights into the understanding of this process but will also have an important impact on diagnosis and genetic counseling.

Syndromic craniosynostosis is etiologically very heterogeneous and the involvement of several genes in the control of suture development is suggested by the diverse number of chromosomal abnormalities. This group of conditions is possibly caused by haploinsufficiency or gain-of-function mechanisms represented, respectively, by deletions and duplications. The identification of the genes within these chromosomal rearrangements involved with suture development remains a challenge.

The genes so far identified that, when mutated, unequivocally cause craniosynostosis belong to four functional groups: regulatory molecules at the DNA level: *TWIST1* and *MSX2*, tyrosine-kinase receptors: *FGFR1–3*, ligand receptors: *EFNB1* and *EFNA4*, and intracellular trafficking of membrane-associated protein: *RAB23*. RAB23 is the only one associated with an autosomal recessive condition, while mutations in the others cause autosomal dominant disorders. Five of these genes are involved in the process of cell proliferation and ossification and they seem to belong to a common molecular pathway. Gain-of-function mutations represent the main molecular mechanism causing the disorders, but loss of function can also lead to the phenotype. The association of ephrin genes with craniosynostosis has shed new light on the understanding of suture development, as they provided evidence that craniosynostosis, at least when involving coronal sutures, can be the result of a defect in the boundary formation between cellular compartments during suture formation. TWIST1, MSX2 and possibly FGFR2 may also be involved in this process, at least in tissues where these genes are coexpressed.

Although the number of patients with mutations in FBN1, TGFBR1 and 2 is still small and the penetrance of craniosynostosis is low, they provide insights into the importance of the extracellular matrix components and their signaling in suture development.

This is a very exciting field in human genetics and the molecular analysis in patients with craniosynostosis has made a major and significant contribution to the understanding of this complex mechanisms.

References

1 Cohen MM Jr, MacLean RE: Craniosynostosis: Diagnosis, Evaluation and Management, ed 2. New York, Oxford University Press, 2000.

2 Lajeunie E, Le Merrer M, Bonaiti-Pellie C, Marchac D, Renier D: Genetic study of nonsyndromic coronal craniosynostosis. Am J Med Genet 1995;55:500–504.

3 Lajeunie E, Le Merrer M, Bonaiti-Pellie C, Marchac D, Renier D: Genetic study of scaphocephaly. Am J Med Genet 1996;62:282–285.

4 Lajeunie E, Le Merrer M, Marchac D, Renier D: Syndromal and nonsyndromal primary trigonocephaly: analysis of a series of 237 patients. Am J Med Genet 1998;2:211–215.

5 Hennekam RCM, Van den Boogaard MJ: Autosomal dominant craniosynostosis of the sutura metopica. Clin Genet 1990;38:374–377.

6 Merrill AE, Bochukova EG, Brugger SM, Ishii M, Pilz DT, Wall SA, Lyons KM, Wilkie AO, Maxson RE Jr: Cell mixing at a neural crest-mesoderm boundary and deficient ephrin-Eph signaling in the pathogenesis of craniosynostosis. Hum Mol Genet 2006;15:1319–1328.

7 Jenkins D, Seelow D, Jehee FS, Perlyn CA, Alonso LG, Bueno DF, Donnai D, Josifiova D, Mathijssen IMJ, Morton JEV, Ørstavik KH, Sweeney E, Wall SA, Marsh JL, Nürnberg P, Passos-Bueno MR, Wilkie AOM: *RAB23* mutations in Carpenter syndrome imply an unexpected role for hedgehog signaling in cranial-suture development and obesity. Am J Hum Genet 2007;80:1162–1170.

8 Sood S, Eldadah ZA, Krause WL, McIntosh I, Dietz HC: Mutation in fibrillin-1 and the Marfanoid-craniosynostosis (Shprintzen-Goldberg) syndrome. Nat Genet 1996;12:209–211.

9 Flück CE, Tajima T, Pandey AV, Arlt W, Okuhara K, Verge CF, Jabs EW, Mendonca BB, Fujieda K, Miller WL: Mutant P450 oxidoreductase causes disordered steroidogenesis with and without Antley-Bixler syndrome. Nat Genet 2004;36:228–230.
10 Loeys BL, Chen J, Neptune ER, Judge DP, Podowski M, Holm T, Meyers J, Leitch CC, Katsanis N, Sharifi N, Xu FL, Myers LA, Spevak PJ, Cameron DE, De Backer J, Hellemans J, Chen Y, Davis EC, Webb CL, Kress W, Coucke P, Rifkin DB, De Paepe AM, Dietz HC: A syndrome of altered cardiovascular, craniofacial, neurocognitive and skeletal development caused by mutations in TGFBR1 or TGFBR2. Nat Genet 2005;37:275–281.
11 Cohen MM Jr: Sutural biology and the correlates of craniosynostosis. Am J Med Genet 1993;47:581–616.
12 Gajecka M, Yu W, Ballif BC, Glotzbach CD, Bailey KA, Shaw CA, Kashork CD, Heilstedt HA, Ansel DA, Theisen A, Rice R, Rice DP, Shaffer LG: Delineation of mechanisms and regions of dosage imbalance in complex rearrangements of 1p36 leads to a putative gene for regulation of cranial suture closure. Eur J Hum Genet 2005;13:139–149.
13 Van Buggenhout G, Van Ravenswaaij-Arts C, McMaas N, Thoelen R, Vogels A, Smeets D, Salden I, Matthijs G, Fryns JP, Vermeesch JR: The del(2)(q32.2q33) deletion syndrome defined by clinical and molecular characterization of four patients. Eur J Med Genet 2005;48:276–289.
14 Schwyzer U, Binkert F, Caflisch U, Baumgartner B, Schinzel A: Terminal deletion of the short arm of chromosome 3, del(3pter-p25): a recognizable syndrome. Helv Paediatr Acta 1987;42: 309–315.
15 Tipton RE, Berns JS, Johnson WE, Wilroy RS Jr, Summitt RL: Duplication 6q syndrome. Am J Med Genet 1979;3:325–330.
16 Van Buggenhout G, Maas NM, Fryns JP, Vermeesch JR: A dysmorphic boy with 4qter deletion and 4q32.3-34.3 duplication: clinical, cytogenetic, and molecular findings. Am J Med Genet 2004;131:186–189.
17 Zneimer SM, Cotter PD, Stewart SD: Telomere-telomere (end to end) fusion of chromosomes 7 and 22 with an interstitial deletion of chromosome 7p11.2→p15.1: phenotypic consequences and possible mechanisms. Clin Genet 2000;58:129–133.
18 Hinkel GK, Tolkendorf E, Bergan J: 7p-deletion syndrome (in German). Monatsschr Kinderheilkd 1988;136:824–827.
19 Fryns JP, Haspeslagh M, Agneessens A, van den Berghe H: De novo partial 2q3 trisomy/distal 7p22 monosomy in a malformed newborn with 7p deletion phenotype and craniosynostosis. Ann Genet 1985;28:45–48.
20 Morimoto M, An B, Ogami A, Shin N, Sugino Y, Sawai Y, Usuku T, Tanaka M, Hirai K, Nishimura A, Hasegawa K, Sugimoto T: Infantile spasms in a patient with williams syndrome and craniosynostosis. Epilepsia 2003;44:1459–1462.
21 Fryburg JS, Golden WL: Interstitial deletion of 8q13.3→22.1 associated with craniosynostosis. Am J Med Genet 1993;45:638–641.
22 Eshel G, Lahat E, Reish O, Barr J: Neurodevelopmental and behavioral abnormalities associated with deletion of chromosome 9p. J Child Neurol 2002;17:50–51.
23 Schimmenti LA, Higgins RR, Mendelsohn NJ, Casey TM, Steinberger J, Mammel MC, Wiesner GL: Monosomy 9p24→pter and trisomy 5q31→qter: case report and review of two cases. Am J Med Genet 1995;57:52–56.
24 Redon R, Baujat G, Sanlaville D, Le Merrer M, Vekemans M, Munnich A, Carter NP, Cormier-Daire V, Colleaux L: Interstitial 9q22.3 microdeletion: clinical and molecular characterisation of a newly recognised overgrowth syndrome. Eur J Hum Genet 2006;14:759–767.
25 Yatsenko SA, Cheung SW, Scott DA, Nowaczyk MJ, Tarnopolsky M, Naidu S, Bibat G, Patel A, Leroy JG, Scaglia F, Stankiewicz P, Lupski JR: Deletion 9q34.3 syndrome: genotype-phenotype correlations and an extended deletion in a patient with features of Opitz C trigonocephaly. J Med Genet 2005;42:328–335.
26 Francke U, Kernahan C, Bradshaw C: Del (10)p autosomal deletion syndrome: clinical, cytogenetic and gene marker studies. Humangenetik 1975;26:343–351.
27 Lukusa T, Smeets E, Vermeesch JR, Fryns JP: Small terminal 10q26 deletion in a male patient with Noonan-like stigmata: diagnosis by cytogenetic and FISH analysis. Genet Couns 2002;13:417–425.

28 Masuno M, Asano J, Yasuda K, Kondo T, Orii T: Balanced complex rearrangement involving chromosomes 8, 9, and 12 in a normal mother, derivative chromosome 9 with recombinant chromosome 12 in her daughter with minor anomalies. Am J Med Genet 1993;45:65–67.
29 Lemyre E, Lemieux N, Decarie JC, Lambert M: Del(14)(q22.1q23.2) in a patient with anophthalmia and pituitary hypoplasia. Am J Med Genet 1998;77:162–165.
30 Shur N, Cowan J, Wheeler PG: Craniosynostosis and congenital heart anomalies associated with a maternal deletion of 15q15-22.1. Am J Med Genet A 2003;120:542–546.
31 Fukushima Y, Wakui K, Nishida T, Nishimoto H: Craniosynostosis in an infant with an interstitial deletion of 15q [46,XY,del(15)(q15q22.1)]. Am J Med Genet 1990;36:209–213.
32 Thomas JA, Manchester DK, Prescott KE, Milner R, McGavran L, Cohen MM Jr: Hunter-McAlpine craniosynostosis phenotype associated with skeletal anomalies and interstitial deletion of chromosome 17q. Am J Med Genet 1996;62:372–375.
33 McDonald-McGinn DM, Gripp KW, Kirschner RE, Maisenbacher MK, Hustead V, Schauer GM, Keppler-Noreuil KM, Ciprero KL, Pasquariello P Jr, LaRossa D, Bartlett SP, Whitaker LA, Zackai EH: Craniosynostosis: another feature of the 22q11.2 deletion syndrome. Am J Med Genet A 2005;136:358–362.
34 Lucas J, Faivre J, Le Mee F, Hubert S, Pluquailec K, Picard F: De novo interstitial deletion of the long arm of chromosome 2: 46,XXX,del(2)(q14q21), associated with premature craniosynostosis (in French). Ann Genet 1987;30:33–38.
35 Gagnon JA, Richer CL, Lemieux N, Gauthier-Chouinard M: De novo appearance of a partial trisomy 1q in mosaic due to a 1;9 translocation (in French). Ann Genet 1984;27:33–37.
36 de Brasi D, Perone L, di Micco P, Andria G, Sebastio G, Iaccarino E, Pinto L, Aliberti F: Cloverleaf skull anomaly and de novo trisomy 4p. J Med Genet 1999;36:422–424.
37 Breslau-Siderius EJ, Wijnen JT, Dauwerse JG, de Pater JM, Beemer FA, Khan PM: Paternal duplication of chromosome 5q11.2-5q14 in a male born with craniostenosis, ear tags, kidney dysplasia and several other anomalies. Hum Genet 1993;92:481–485.
38 Shiihara T, Kato M, Kimura T, Hayasaka K, Yamamori S, Ogata T: Craniosynostosis with extra copy of MSX2 in a patient with partial 5q-trisomy. Am J Med Genet A 2004;128:214–216.
39 Odell JM, Siebert JR, Bradley C, Salk D: Duplication 7p in a family with t(7;11): association with anomalies of the anterior cranial base. Am J Med Genet 1987;27:687–692.
40 Seghezzi L, Maraschio P, Bozzola M, Maserati E, Tupler R, Marchi A, Tiepolo L: Ring chromosome 9 with a 9p22.3-p24.3 duplication. Eur J Pediatr 1999;158:791–793.
41 Yelavarthi KK, Zunich J: Familial interstitial duplication of 11q; partial trisomy (11)(q13.5q21). Am J Med Genet 2004;126A:423–426.
42 Babovic-Vuksanovic D, Westman JA, Jalal SM, Lindor NM: Clinical characteristics associated with dup17(q24q25.1) in a mosaic mother and two non-mosaic daughters. Clin Dysmorphol 1998;7:171–176.
43 Czako M, Riegel M, Morava E, Bajnoczky K, Kosztolanyi G: Opitz 'C' trigonocephaly-like syndrome in a patient with terminal deletion of 2p and partial duplication of 17q. Am J Med Genet A 2004;131:310–312.
44 Jehee FS, Rosenberg C, Krepischi-Santos AC, Kok F, Knijnenburg J, Froyen G, Vianna-Morgante AM, Opitz JM, Passos-Bueno MR: An Xq22.3 duplication detected by comparative genomic hybridization microarray (Array-CGH) defines a new locus (FGS5) for FG syndrome. Am J Med Genet A 2005;139:221–226.
45 Ward J, Vieto E, Lee D, Arosemena G: Acrocephalopolysyndactyly, pentalogy of Fallot, and hypoacusis in a patient with a de novo reciprocal translocation involving the short arm of chromosome 1 and the long arm of chromosome 18:46,XX,t(1;18)(p31;q11). J Med Genet 1993;30:438–439.
46 Hordnes K, Engebretsen LF, Knudtzon J: De novo balanced 5;21 translocation in a child with acrobrachycephaly, ventriculomegaly, pulmonary stenosis, ectopic anus and mental retardation. Clin Genet 1995;48:321–323.
47 Kaminker CP, Dain L, Lamas MA, Sanchez JM: Mosaic trisomy 9 syndrome with unusual phenotype. Am J Med Genet 1985;22:237–241.
48 Demyer W, Plamer C: Closed metopic suture with trigonocephaly in Down's syndrome. Neurology 1965;15:756–760.

49 Jehee FS, Bertola DR, Yelavarthi KK, Krepischi-Santos ACV, Vermeesch JR, Passos-Bueno MR: An 11q11-q13.3 duplication, including *FGF3* and *FGF4* genes, in a patient with syndromic multiple craniosynostosis. Am J Med Genet A, in press.
50 Brewer C, Holloway S, Zawalnyski P, Schinzel A, FitzPatrick D: A chromosomal deletion map of human malformations. Am J Hum Genet 1998;63:1153–1159.
51 Brewer C, Holloway S, Zawalnyski P, Schinzel A, FitzPatrick D: A chromosomal duplication map of malformations: regions of suspected haplo- and triplolethality – and tolerance of segmental aneuploidy – in humans. Am J Hum Genet 1999;64:1702–1708.
52 Huret JL, Leonard C, Forestier B, Rethoré MO, Lejeune J: Eleven new cases of del(9p) and features from 80 cases. J Med Genet 1988;25:741–749.
53 de Pater JM, Ippel PF, Bijlsma JB, Van Nieuwenhuizen O: Interstitial deletion 11q case report and review of the literature. Genet Couns 1997;4:335–339.
54 Christ LA, Crowe CA, Micale MA, Conroy J, Schwartz S: Chromosome breakage hotspots and delineation of the critical region for the 9p-deletion syndrome. Am J Hum Genet 1999;65: 1387–1395.
55 Leegde B, Kerstjens-Frederidse WS, Deelstra K, Begeer JH, Van Essen AJ: 11q-syndrome: three cases and a review of the literature. Genet Couns 1999;3:305–313.
56 Ornitz DM: FGFs, heparan sulfate and FGFRs: complex interactions essential for development. Bioessays 2000;22:108–112.
57 Givol D, Eswarakumar VP, Lonai P: The fibroblast growth factor signaling pathway; in Epstein CJ, Erickson RP, Wynshaw-Boris A (eds): Inborn Errors of Development. Oxford, Oxford University Press, 2004, pp 367–379.
58 Eswarakumar VP, Lax I, Schlessinger J: Cellular signaling by fibroblast growth factor receptors. Cytokine Growth Factor Rev 2005;16:139–149.
59 Ornitz DM, Xu J, Colvin JS, McEwen DG, MacArthur CA, Coulier F, Gao G, Goldfarb M: Receptor specificity of the fibroblast growth factor family. J Biol Chem 1996;271:15292–15297.
60 Cohen MM: FGFs/FGFRs and association disorders; in Epstein CJ, Erickson RP, Wynshaw-Boris A (eds): Inborn Errors of Development. Oxford, Oxford University Press, 2004, pp 380–400.
61 Roscioli T, Flanagan S, Kumar P, Masel J, Gattas M, Hyland VJ, Glass IA: Clinical findings in a patient with FGFR1 P252R mutation and comparison with the literature. Am J Med Genet 2000;93:228.
62 White KE, Cabral JM, Davis SI, Fishburn T, Evans WE, Ichikawa S, Fields J, Yu X, Shaw NJ, McLellan NJ, McKeown C, Fitzpatrick D, Yu K, Ornitz DM, Econs MJ: Mutations that cause osteoglophonic dysplasia define novel roles for FGFR1 in bone elongation. Am J Hum Genet 2005;76:361–367.
63 Wilkie AO: Bad bones, absent smell, selfish testes: the pleiotropic consequences of human FGF receptor mutations. Cytokine Growth Factor Rev 2005;16:187–203.
64 Priolo M, Lerone M, Baffico M, Baldi M, Ravazzolo R, Cama A, Capra V, Silengo M: Pfeiffer syndrome type 2 associated with a single amino acid deletion in the FGFR2 gene. Clin Genet 2000;58:81–83.
65 Lapunzina P, Fernandez A, Sanchez Romero JM, Delicado A, Saenz de Pipaon M, Lopez Pajares I, Molano J: A novel insertion in the FGFR2 gene in a patient with Crouzon phenotype and sacrococcygeal tail. Birth Defects Res A Clin Mol Teratol 2005;73:614.
66 Kress W, Collmann H, Büsse M, Halliger-Keller B, Mueller CR: Clustering of FGFR2 gene mutations in patients with Pfeiffer and Crouzon syndromes (FGFR2 associated craniosynostoses). Cytogenet Cell Genet 2000;91:1347.
67 Passos-Bueno MR, Sertie AL, Richieri-Costa A, Alonso LG, Zatz M, Alonso N, Brunoni D, Ribeiro SF: Description of a new mutation and characterization of FGFR1, FGFR2, and FGFR3 mutations among Brazilian patients with syndromic craniosynostoses. Am J Med Genet 1998;78: 237–241.
68 Lajeunie E, Heuertz S, El Ghouzzi V, Martinovic J, Renier D, Le Merrer M, Bonaventure J: Mutation screening in patients with syndromic craniosynostoses indicates that a limited number of recurrent FGFR2 mutations accounts for severe forms of Pfeiffer syndrome. Eur J Hum Genet 2006;14:289–298.

69 Gorry MC, Preston RA, White GJ, Zhang Y, Singhal VK, Losken HW, Parker MG, Nwokoro NA, Post JC, Ehrlich GD: Crouzon syndrome: mutations in two spliceoforms of FGFR2 and a common point mutation shared with Jackson-Weiss syndrome. Hum Mol Genet 1995;4:1387–1390.
70 Freitas EC, Nascimento SR, de Mello MP, Gil-da-Silva-Lopes VL: Q289P mutation in FGFR2 gene causes Saethre-Chotzen syndrome: some considerations about familial heterogeneity. Cleft Palate Craniofac J 2006;43:142–147.
71 Wilkie AO, Bochukova EG, Hansen RM, Taylor IB, Rannan-Eliya SV, Byren JC, Wall SA, Ramos L, Venancio M, Hurst JA, O'Rourke AW, Williams LJ, Seller A, Lester T: Clinical dividends from the molecular genetic diagnosis of craniosynostosis. Am J Med Genet A 2006;140:2631–2639.
72 Tartaglia M, Di Rocco C, Lajeunie E, Valeri S, Velardi F, Battaglia PA: Jackson-Weiss syndrome: identification of two novel FGFR2 missense mutations shared with Crouzon and Pfeiffer craniosynostotic disorders. Hum Genet 1997;101:47–50.
73 Park WJ, Meyers GA, Li X, Theda C, Day D, Orlow SJ, Jones MC, Jabs EW: Novel FGFR2 mutations in Crouzon and Jackson-Weiss syndromes show allelic heterogeneity and phenotypic variability. Hum Mol Genet 1995;4:1229–1233.
74 Meyers GA, Day D, Goldberg R, Daentl DL, Przylepa KA, Abrams LJ, Graham JM Jr, Feingold M, Moeschler JB, Rawnsley E, Scott AF, Jabs EW: FGFR2 exon IIIa and IIIc mutations in Crouzon, Jackson-Weiss, and Pfeiffer syndromes: evidence for missense changes, insertions, and a deletion due to alternative RNA splicing. Am J Hum Genet 1996;58:491–498.
75 Pulleyn LJ, Reardon W, Wilkes D, Rutland P, Jones BM, Hayward R, Hall CM, Brueton L, Chun N, Lammer E, Malcolm S, Winter RM: Spectrum of craniosynostosis phenotypes associated with novel mutations at the fibroblast growth factor receptor 2 locus. Eur J Hum Genet 1996;4:283–291.
76 Okajima K, Robinson LK, Hart MA, Abuelo DN, Cowan LS, Hasegawa T, Maumenee IH, Jabs EW: Ocular anterior chamber dysgenesis in craniosynostosis syndromes with a fibroblast growth factor receptor 2 mutation. Am J Med Genet 1999;85:160–170.
77 Everett ET, Britto DA, Ward RE, Hartsfield JK Jr: A novel FGFR2 gene mutation in Crouzon syndrome associated with apparent nonpenetrance. Cleft Palate Craniofac J 1999;36:533–541.
78 de Ravel TJ, Taylor IB, Van Oostveldt AJ, Fryns JP, Wilkie AO: A further mutation of the FGFR2 tyrosine kinase domain in mild Crouzon syndrome. Eur J Hum Genet 2005;13:503–505.
79 McGillivray G, Savarirayan R, Cox TC, Stojkoski C, McNeil R, Bankier A, Bateman JF, Roscioli T, Gardner RJ, Lamande SR: Familial scaphocephaly syndrome caused by a novel mutation in the FGFR2 tyrosine kinase domain. J Med Genet 2005;42:656–662.
80 Zankl A, Jaeger G, Bonafe L, Boltshauser E, Superti-Furga A: Novel mutation in the tyrosine kinase domain of FGFR2 in a patient with Pfeiffer syndrome. Am J Med Genet A 2004;131:299–300.
81 Schindler S, Friedrich M, Wagener H, Lorenz B, Preising MN: Heterozygous P250L mutation of fibroblast growth factor receptor 3 in a case of isolated craniosynostosis. J Med Genet 2002;39:764–766.
82 Tavormina PL, Shiang R, Thompson LM, Zhu YZ, Wilkin DJ, Lachman RS, Wilcox WR, Rimoin DL, Cohn DH, Wasmuth JJ: Thanatophoric dysplasia (types I and II) caused by distinct mutations in fibroblast growth factor receptor 3. Nat Genet 1995;9:321–328.
83 Shiang R, Thompson LM, Zhu YZ, Church DM, Fielder TJ, Bocian M, Winokur ST, Wasmuth JJ: Mutations in the transmembrane domain of FGFR3 cause the most common genetic form of dwarfism, achondroplasia. Cell 1994;78:335–342.
84 Bellus GA, McIntosh I, Smith EA, Aylsworth AS, Kaitila I, Horton WA, Greenhaw GA, Hecht JT, Francomano CA: A recurrent mutation in the tyrosine kinase domain of fibroblast growth factor receptor 3 causes hypochondroplasia. Nat Genet 1995;10:357–359.
85 Tavormina PL, Bellus GA, Webster MK, Bamshad MJ, Fraley AE, McIntosh I, Szabo J, Jiang W, Jabs EW, Wilcox WR, Wasmuth JJ, Donoghue DJ, Thompson LM, Francomano CA: A novel skeletal dysplasia with developmental delay and acanthosis nigricans is caused by a Lys650Met mutation in the fibroblast growth factor receptor 3 gene. Am J Hum Genet 1999;64:722–731.
86 Dode C, Levilliers J, Dupont JM, De Paepe A, Le Du N, Soussi-Yanicostas N, Coimbra RS, Delmaghani S, Compain-Nouaille S, Baverel F, Pecheux C, Le Tessier D, Cruaud C, Delpech M, Speleman F, Vermeulen S, Amalfitano A, Bachelot Y, Bouchard P, Cabrol S, Carel JC, Delemarre-van de Waal H, Goulet-Salmon B, Kottler ML, Richard O, Sanchez-Franco F, Saura R, Young J,

Petit C, Hardelin JP: Loss-of-function mutations in FGFR1 cause autosomal dominant Kallmann syndrome. Nat Genet 2003;33:463–465.
87 Shams I, Rohmann E, Eswakdkunar VP, Lew ED, Yuzawa S, Wollnik B, Schlessinger J, Lax I: LADD syndrome is caused by reduced activity of the FGF10-FGF receptor 2 signaling pathway. Mol Cell Biol 2007, E-pub ahead of print. DOI: 10.1128/MCB.00544–07.
88 Toydemir RM, Brassington AE, Bayrak-Toydemir P, Krakowiak PA, Jorde LB, Whitby FG, Longo N, Viskochil DH, Carey JC, Bamshad MJ: A novel mutation in FGFR3 causes camptodactyly, tall stature, and hearing loss (CATSHL) syndrome. Am J Hum Genet 2006;79:935–941.
89 Moloney DM, Slaney SF, Oldridge M, Wall SA, Sahlin P, Stenman G, Wilkie AO: Exclusive paternal origin of new mutations in Apert syndrome. Nat Genet 1996;13:48–53.
90 Glaser RL, Jiang W, Boyadjiev SA, Tran AK, Zachary AA, Van Maldergem L, Johnson D, Walsh S, Oldridge M, Wall SA, Wilkie AO, Jabs EW: Paternal origin of FGFR2 mutations in sporadic cases of Crouzon syndrome and Pfeiffer syndrome. Am J Hum Genet 2000;66:768–777.
91 Kan SH, Elanko N, Johnson D, Cornejo-Roldan L, Cook J, Reich EW, Tomkins S, Verloes A, Twigg SR, Rannan-Eliya S, McDonald-McGinn DM, Zackai EH, Wall SA, Muenke M, Wilkie AO: Genomic screening of fibroblast growth factor receptor 2 reveals a wide spectrum of mutations in patients with syndromic craniosynostosis. Am J Hum Genet 2002;70:472–486.
92 Morriss-Kay GM, Wilkie AO: Growth of the normal skull vault and its alteration in craniosynostosis: insights from human genetics and experimental studies. J Anat 2005;207:637–653.
93 Wilkie AO, Patey SJ, Kan SH, van den Ouweland AM, Hamel BC: FGFs, their receptors, and human limb malformations: clinical and molecular correlations. Am J Med Genet 2002;112:266–278.
94 Slaney SF, Oldridge M, Hurst JA, Moriss-Kay GM, Hall CM, Poole MD, Wilkie AO: Differential effects of FGFR2 mutations on syndactyly and cleft palate in Apert syndrome. Am J Hum Genet 1996;58:923–932.
95 Anderson J, Burns HD, Enriquez-Harris P, Wilkie AO, Heath JK: Apert syndrome mutations in fibroblast growth factor receptor 2 exhibit increased affinity for FGF ligand. Hum Mol Genet 1998;7:1475–1483.
96 Yu K, Herr AB, Waksman G, Ornitz DM: Loss of fibroblast growth factor receptor 2 ligand-binding specificity in Apert syndrome. Proc Natl Acad Sci USA 2000;97:14536–14541.
97 Ibrahimi OA, Zhang F, Eliseenkova AV, Itoh N, Linhardt RJ, Mohammadi M: Biochemical analysis of pathogenic ligand-dependent FGFR2 mutations suggests distinct pathophysiological mechanisms for craniofacial and limb abnormalities. Hum Mol Genet 2004;13:2313–2324.
98 Ibrahimi OA, Zhang F, Eliseenkova AV, Linhardt RJ, Mohammadi M: Proline to arginine mutations in FGF receptors 1 and 3 result in Pfeiffer and Muenke craniosynostosis syndromes through enhancement of FGF binding affinity. Hum Mol Genet 2004;13:69–78.
99 Oldridge M, Zackai EH, McDonald-McGinn DM, Iseki S, Morriss-Kay GM, Twigg SR, Johnson D, Wall SA, Jiang W, Theda C, Jabs EW, Wilkie AO: De novo alu-element insertions in FGFR2 identify a distinct pathological basis for Apert syndrome. Am J Hum Genet 1999;64:446–461.
100 Murre C, Murre C, Bain G, van Dijk MA, Engel I, Furnari BA, Massari ME, Matthews JR, Quong MW, Rivera RR, Stuiver MH: Structure and function of helix-loop-helix proteins. Biochim Biophys Acta 1994;1218:129–135.
101 Connerney J, Andreeva V, Leshem Y, Muentener C, Mercado MA, Spicer DB: Twist1 dimer selection regulates cranial suture patterning and fusion. Dev Dyn 2006;235:1345–1357.
102 Hamamori Y, Sartorelli V, Ogryzko V, Puri PL, Wu HY, Wang JY, Nakatani Y, Kedes L: Regulation of histone acetyltransferases p300 and PCAF by the bHLH protein twist and adenoviral oncoprotein E1A. Cell 1999;96:405–413.
103 Bialek P, Kern B, Yang X, Schrock M, Sosic D, Hong N, Wu H, Yu K, Ornitz DM, Olson EN, Justice MJ, Karsenty G: A twist code determines the onset of osteoblast differentiation. Dev Cell 2004;6:423–435.
104 Brueton LA, van Herwerden L, Chotai KA, Winter RM: The mapping of a gene for craniosynostosis: evidence for linkage of the Saethre-Chotzen syndrome to distal chromosome 7p. J Med Genet 1992;29:681–685.
105 Reid CS, McMorrow LE, McDonald-McGinn DM, Grace KJ, Ramos FJ, Zackai EH, Cohen MM Jr, Jabs EW: Saethre-Chotzen syndrome with familial translocation at chromosome 7p22. Am J Med Genet 1993;47:637–639.

106 Reardon W, McManus SP, Summers D, Winter RM: Cytogenetic evidence that the Saethre-Chotzen gene maps to 7p21.2. Am J Med Genet 1993;47:633–636.
107 van Herwerden L, Rose CS, Reardon W, Brueton LA, Weissenbach J, Malcolm S, Winter RM: Evidence for locus heterogeneity in acrocephalosyndactyly: a refined localization for the Saethre-Chotzen syndrome locus on distal chromosome 7p – and exclusion of Jackson-Weiss syndrome from craniosynostosis loci on 7p and 5q. Am J Hum Genet 1994;54:669–674.
108 Chen ZF, Behringer RR: Twist is required in head mesenchyme for cranial neural tube morphogenesis. Genes Dev 1995;9:686–699.
109 Paznekas WA, Cunningham ML, Howard TD, Korf BR, Lipson MH, Grix AW, Feingold M, Goldberg R, Borochowitz Z, Aleck K, et al: Genetic heterogeneity of Saethre-Chotzen syndrome, due to TWIST and FGFR mutations. Am J Hum Genet 1998;62:1370–1380.
110 Kress W, Schropp C, Lieb G, Petersen B, Busse-Ratzka M, Kunz J, Reinhart E, Schafer WD, Sold J, Hoppe F, Pahnke J, Trusen A, Sorensen N, Krauss J, Collmann H: Saethre-Chotzen syndrome caused by TWIST 1 gene mutations: functional differentiation from Muenke coronal synostosis syndrome. Eur J Hum Genet 2006;14:39–48.
111 Funato N, Twigg SR, Higashihori N, Ohyama K, Wall SA, Wilkie AO, Nakamura M: Functional analysis of natural mutations in two TWIST protein motifs. Hum Mutat 2005;25:550–556.
112 de Heer IM, de Klein A, van den Ouweland AM, Vermeij-Keers C, Wouters CH, Vaandrager JM, Hovius SE, Hoogeboom JM: Clinical and genetic analysis of patients with Saethre-Chotzen syndrome. Plast Reconstr Surg 2005;115:1894–1905.
113 De Heer IM, Hoogeboom AJ, Eussen HJ, Vaandrager JM, De Klein A: Deletion of the TWIST gene in a large five-generation family. Clin Genet 2004;65:396–399.
114 den Dunnen JT, Antonarakis SE: Nomenclature for the description of human sequence variations. Hum Genet 2001;109:121–124.
115 Jabs EW: TWIST and the Saethre-Chotzen syndrome; in Epstein C, Erickson R, Wynshaw-Boris A (eds): Inborn Errors of Development, ed 1. Oxford, Oxford University Press, 2004, pp 401–409.
116 El Ghouzzi V, Le Merrer M, Perrin-Schmitt F, Lajeunie E, Benit P, Renier D, Bourgeois P, Bolcato-Bellemin AL, Munnich A, Bonaventure J: Mutations of the TWIST gene in the Saethre-Chotzen syndrome. Nat Genet 1997;15:42–46.
117 Howard TD, Paznekas WA, Green ED, Chiang LC, Ma N, Ortiz de Luna RI, Garcia Delgado C, Gonzalez-Ramos M, Kline AD, Jabs EW: Mutations in TWIST, a basic helix-loop-helix transcription factor, in Saethre-Chotzen syndrome. Nat Genet 1997;15:36–41.
118 Bourgeois P, Bolcato-Bellemin AL, Danse JM, Bloch-Zupan A, Yoshiba K, Stoetzel C, Perrin-Schmitt F: The variable expressivity and incomplete penetrance of the twist-null heterozygous mouse phenotype resemble those of human Saethre-Chotzen syndrome. Hum Mol Genet 1998;7:945–957.
119 El Ghouzzi V, Legeai-Mallet L, Aresta S, Benoist C, Munnich A, de Gunzburg J, Bonaventure J: Saethre-Chotzen mutations cause TWIST protein degradation or impaired nuclear location. Hum Mol Genet 2000;9:813–819.
120 Krebs I, Weis I, Hudler M, Rommens JM, Roth H, Scherer SW, Tsui LC, Fuchtbauer EM, Grzeschik KH, Tsuji K, Kunz J: Translocation breakpoint maps 5 kb 3′ from TWIST in a patient affected with Saethre-Chotzen syndrome. Hum Mol Genet 1997;6:1079–1086.
121 Howard TD, Paznekas WA, Green ED, Chiang LC, Ma N, Ortiz de Luna RI, Garcia Delgado C, Gonzalez-Ramos M, Kline AD, Jabs EW: Mutations in TWIST, a basic helix-loop-helix transcription factor, in Saethre-Chotzen syndrome. Nat Genet 1997;15:36–41.
122 Holder N, Klein R: Eph receptors and ephrins: effectors of morphogenesis. Development 1999;126:2033–2044.
123 Wilkinson DG: Multiple roles of EPH receptors and ephrins in neural development. Nat Rev Neurosci 2001;2:155–164.
124 Murai KK, Pasquale EB: 'Eph'ective signaling: forward, reverse and crosstalk. J Cell Sci 2003;116:2823–2832.
125 Twigg SR, Kan R, Babbs C, Bochukova EG, Robertson SP, Wall SA, Morriss-Kay GM, Wilkie AO: Mutations of ephrin-B1 (EFNB1), a marker of tissue boundary formation, cause craniofrontonasal syndrome. Proc Natl Acad Sci USA 2004;101:8652–8657.

126 Wieland I, Jakubiczka S, Muschke P, Cohen M, Thiele H, Gerlach KL, Adams RH, Wieacker P: Mutations of the ephrin-B1 gene cause craniofrontonasal syndrome. Am J Hum Genet 2004;74:1209–1215.
127 Vasudevan PC, Twigg SR, Mulliken JB, Cook JA, Quarrell OW, Wilkie AO: Expanding the phenotype of craniofrontonasal syndrome: two unrelated boys with EFNB1 mutations and congenital diaphragmatic hernia. Eur J Hum Genet 2006;14:884–887.
128 Twigg SR, Matsumoto K, Kidd AM, Goriely A, Taylor IB, Fisher RB, Hoogeboom AJ, Mathijssen IM, Lourenco MT, Morton JE, et al: The origin of EFNB1 mutations in craniofrontonasal syndrome: frequent somatic mosaicism and explanation of the paucity of carrier males. Am J Hum Genet 2006;78:999–1010.
129 Wieland I, Reardon W, Jakubiczka S, Franco B, Kress W, Vincent-Delorme C, Thierry P, Edwards M, Konig R, Rusu C, et al: Twenty-six novel EFNB1 mutations in familial and sporadic craniofrontonasal syndrome (CFNS). Hum Mutat 2005;26:113–118.
130 Shotelersuk V, Siriwan P, Ausavarat S: A novel mutation in EFNB1, probably with a dominant negative effect, underlying craniofrontonasal syndrome. Cleft Palate Craniofac J 2006;43:152–154.
131 Compagni A, Logan M, Klein R, Adams RH: Control of skeletal patterning by ephrinB1-EphB interactions. Dev Cell 2003;5:217–230.

M.R. Passos-Bueno
Institute of Biosciences, University of São Paulo
Rua do Matão, 277
05508-900 São Paulo, SP (Brazil)
Tel. +55 11 30917740, E-Mail passos@ib.usp.br

Rice DP (ed): Craniofacial Sutures. Development, Disease and Treatment.
Front Oral Biol. Basel, Karger, 2008, vol 12, pp 144–159

Roles of FGFR2 and Twist in Human Craniosynostosis: Insights from Genetic Mutations in Cranial Osteoblasts

Pierre J. Marie, Karim Kaabeche, Hind Guenou

Laboratory of Osteoblast Biology and Pathology, INSERM U 606 and University Paris 7, Hôpital Lariboisière, Paris, France

Abstract

Recent advances in molecular genetics have led to a better understanding of the role of specific genes such as fibroblast growth factor receptor (FGFR) and Twist in cranial bone formation. Specifically, the analysis of osteoblast abnormalities induced by FGFR2 and Twist genetic mutations inducing craniosynostosis in humans has provided some insights into the role of these genes in the premature cranial suture formation in syndromic craniosynostosis. This also led to a better understanding of the cellular and molecular mechanisms that control osteoblast biology and pathology in humans. In this review paper, we summarize the effects of FGFR2 and Twist genetic mutations resulting in altered osteoblast phenotype and premature cranial fusion based on our analysis in human syndromic craniosynostosis.

Human Cranial Suture Formation

Most calvarial bones are formed by intramembranous ossification. During development, the condensation of mesenchymal cells is followed by their progressive differentiation into osteoblasts that form a mineralized matrix in ossification centers. These calvarial bones expand during development but do not fuse at the junction with other cranial bones, allowing skull expansion during growth [1, 2]. The junction between calvarial bones is a functional structure formed of two bone plates separated by cells with different functions. This structure, called a suture, is responsible for the maintenance of separation between the two membrane bones, and is essential for the growth of the skull. The formation and maintenance of the suture is a highly controlled process that is dependent on the recruitment, proliferation, differentiation and apoptosis of osteoprogenitor cells. Any perturbation

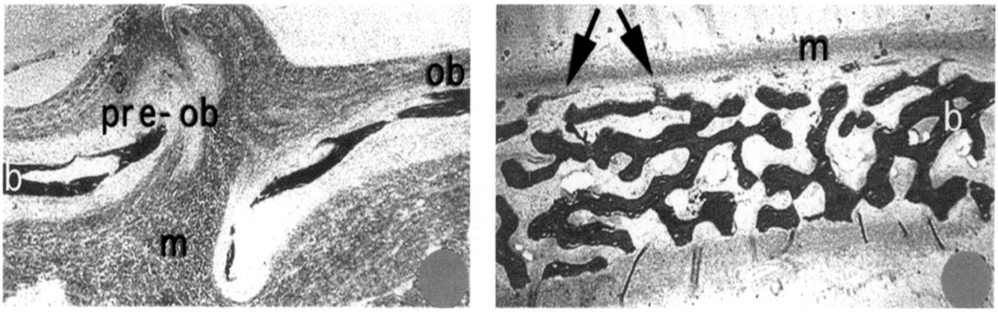

a *b*

Fig. 1. Photomicrographs showing the extensive periosteal bone matrix deposition (arrows) in a fused coronal suture (***b***) from a 26-week Apert fetus with a S252W-activating FGFR2 mutation compared to the normal coronal suture (***a***). m = Mesenchymal cells; pre-ob = preosteoblasts; ob = osteoblasts; b = bone.

between these processes induces premature or delayed fusion of the sutures and abnormal formation of cranial bones. Therefore, the events occurring at the suture level and controlling the cell behavior are important in the control of membranous ossification [2, 3]. Several cell types are involved in the control of suture formation. Most cells surrounding the suture are mesenchymal cells (fig. 1). In the vicinity of the suture, a minority of these cells differentiate into preosteoblasts. These cells then differentiate into mature osteoblasts which are found along the bone trabeculae that they are forming. At the end of the formation period, osteoblasts die by apoptosis or are embedded in the matrix, becoming osteocytes, which then undergo apoptosis at the end of their life [4]. The early commitment of mesenchymal stem cells into osteoblasts requires expression of Runx2, a master transcription factor that regulates several genes in osteoblasts, such as collagen type I (COLIA1), bone sialoprotein (BSP), osteopontin (OP), transforming growth factor (TGF-β) and osteocalcin (OC). In addition, other families of transcription factors, such as Msx2 and Dlx5, play important roles in osteoblast differentiation and cranial bone formation, in part by interacting with Runx2 [5].

The regulation of cranial suture by local factors has been extensively studied in rats and mice. Experimental studies in these models indicate that these events are under the control of several regulatory factors. Specifically, TGF-βs, bone morphogenetic proteins (BMPs), fibroblast growth factors (FGFs) and Wnt signaling were shown to act locally on cranial bone cells to regulate cell differentiation and survival [2, 6–10]. Most information on the control of membranous ossification by local factors was drawn, however, from experimental studies in rodents, and little is known about the regulation of osteoblast phenotype and cranial suture in humans.

Phenotype of Human Cranial Osteoblasts

Our laboratory has developed a series of studies with the aim of establishing the mechanisms of cranial osteoblastogenesis in humans [11]. We used bone cells derived from fetal or postnatal human calvaria which display characteristics of the osteoblast phenotype such as expression of osteoblast markers (alkaline phosphatase, type I collagen, osteonectin, osteopontin, osteocalcin) [12]. In addition to expressing osteoblast phenotypic characteristics, these human calvaria cells express functional receptors for parathyroid hormone-related peptide (PTHrP), fibroblast growth factor receptors (FGFRs) and BMP, and responsiveness to PTHrP, FGF2 and BMP-2, indicating that they are target cells for these factors [13–15]. Moreover, as discussed below, these human calvaria osteoblast cultures express a similar phenotype in vitro and in cranial sutures in vivo, which provides a unique model for analysis of the cellular and molecular mechanisms involved in human craniosynostosis [11].

Phenotype of Human Cranial Osteoblasts in Nonsyndromic Craniosynostosis

The pathogenesis of premature cranial suture ossification in humans remains largely unknown. One working hypothesis is that the premature fusion of cranial sutures results from an imbalance between cell proliferation and differentiation, leading to precocious osteoblast differentiation. We tested this hypothesis by evaluating the histological indices of bone formation and the characteristics of osteoblastic cells in infants and children with nonsyndromic craniosynostosis [16]. Histomorphometric parameters of bone formation are increased in fused sutures compared to nonaffected sutures, indicating that bone formation is increased in craniosynostosis. Consistently, analysis of cultured calvarial osteoblasts showed increased osteoblast differentiation markers (ALP activity, osteocalcin) in cells from fused sutures compared to normal sutures, whereas cell proliferation was unaltered [16]. Thus, the premature suture ossification in human nonsyndromic craniosynostosis results from premature maturation of osteoblastic cells, a feature which has been confirmed by other investigators [17]. As described below, correlations were found between the osteoblast phenotype in cultured calvaria cells and affected sutures in syndromic craniosynostosis [18, 19], indicating that the in vitro phenotype reflects the in vivo phenotype in craniosynostosis. These models are therefore useful to determine the mechanisms responsible for the abnormal cranial bone formation in human craniosynostosis.

Effects of FGFR2 Mutations on Human Cranial Osteoblast Phenotype

Activating FGFR2 Mutations Induce Craniosynostosis

During membranous bone formation, the proliferation, differentiation and apoptosis of cells of the osteoblastic lineage are dependent on the temporal expression and activity of high affinity FGFRs [9, 20, 21]. Studies of genetic models in mice and humans have provided evidence that mutations affecting FGF receptors are responsible for a number of syndromic craniosynostosis characterized by premature fusion of cranial sutures (craniosynostosis) [22]. Several gain-of-function FGFR mutations induce premature ossification of the cranial sutures and most mutations in the FGFR gene family are gain-of-function [21, 22]. In Apert syndrome, an autosomal dominant disorder characterized by coronal craniosynostosis, mutations in FGFR2 produce missense substitutions in the linker region between the second and third extracellular Ig domains. In vitro experimental studies indicate that Apert FGFR2 mutations induce ligand-independent activation of the receptor or alterations of ligand binding and signaling [23–28].

Activation of FGF signaling induces marked effects on skeletal cell proliferation, differentiation and apoptosis [29, 30]. Therefore, it is expected that activating FGFR2 mutations may alter the osteoblastic cell replication, differentiation or survival, resulting in premature suture fusion in craniosynostosis. Extensive studies have been conducted in genetically manipulated mice to determine the phenotypic consequences of FGFR signaling [31–36]. Activating FGFR2 mutations in mouse genetic models were found to induce positive, negative or null effects on cranial cell replication or differentiation, while apoptosis was mostly found to be increased. These divergent effects may in part be explained by the variable cellular responsiveness to FGFR activation which is dependent on the stage of osteoblast maturation [14, 31, 37]. FGF signaling is know to activate a variety of signaling pathways [38] that control a multitude of genes including transcription factors, soluble factors, membranous and matrix proteins [29, 30]. The variable response to FGFR activation may thus be related to the implication and interplay of multiple signal transducing molecules at different stages of differentiation [37, 39].

Activating FGFR2 Mutations Promote Human Cranial Osteoblast Differentiation

In order to determine the role of FGFR2 activation on cell proliferation, adhesion, differentiation or apoptosis in human craniosynostosis, we studied human cranial osteoblast cultures from unaffected and affected sutures in patients affected by the natural S252W and P253R Apert-activating FGFR2 mutations which are responsible for nearly all Apert cases [22]. We showed that the premature ossification induced by these mutations results from an increased extent of subperiosteal bone formation in vivo [18]. This effect results primarily from increased type 1 collagen by fetus or neonate osteoblasts, which was demonstrated in vitro and in vivo [18, 40]. Consistently, FGFR2 mutant osteoblasts showed increased osteocalcin and osteopontin expression associated with increased production of mineralized matrix in vitro, whereas cell growth was not affected in vitro or in vivo [18, 40]. Thus, activation of FGFR2 signaling in Apert syndrome results in premature calvaria cell differentiation, leading to increased subperiosteal bone matrix formation and accelerated calvaria ossification.

Several molecular mechanisms can contribute to the premature osteoblast differentiation in Apert syndrome. It has been suggested that Runx2, a master transcription factor that regulates the expression of several genes during osteogenesis [5], is a target gene for FGFR signaling. Craniosynostosis induced by the activating P250R mutation in FGFR1 in mice is associated with increased expression of Runx2 [34]. Consistently, a gain-of-function C342Y FGFR2 mutation enhances Runx2 expression and causes premature fusion of cranial sutures in mice [36]. The P253R and S252W FGFR2 mutations were also found to increase Runx2 expression in human calvarial osteoblasts from Apert patients [41, 42]. Conversely, disruption of FGFR2IIIC, the mesenchymal splice variant of FGFR2, decreases the transcription of Runx2 and retards ossification [33]. However, Runx2 expression was found to be unchanged in mouse osteoblastic cells expressing the C342Y or S252W FGFR2 mutations [31]. It is therefore unclear whether Runx2 directly or indirectly contributes to the osteoblast phenotype induced by FGFR activation.

Another mechanism may involve cell-cell interactions which are known to be essential for the early steps of cranial ossification [1]. Indeed, we found that the activating Apert FGFR2 mutations increase cell-cell aggregation in vitro, suggesting a role for cadherins in the phenotype induced by activated FGFR2 [40]. Indeed, FGFR2 mutant osteoblasts express increased N- and E-cadherin levels in vitro and in vivo, and inhibition of N-cadherin using antibodies or antisense RNA reduced osteoblast gene overexpression in mutant osteoblasts, suggesting that N-cadherin is involved in the abnormal phenotype induced by the mutation [40]. To gain further insight into the mechanisms involved in the effect of activating FGFR2 in cranial osteoblasts, we examined FGFR signaling in Apert osteoblasts. Apert mutant osteoblasts showed increased phospholipase C-γ, protein PKC-α phosphorylation and PKC activity [40]. Other studies showed that PKC-α expression [43, 44] was increased in primary Apert mutant osteoblasts. Strikingly, we found that inhibition of PKC activity in mutant osteoblasts can suppress N-cadherin as well as overexpression of osteoblast

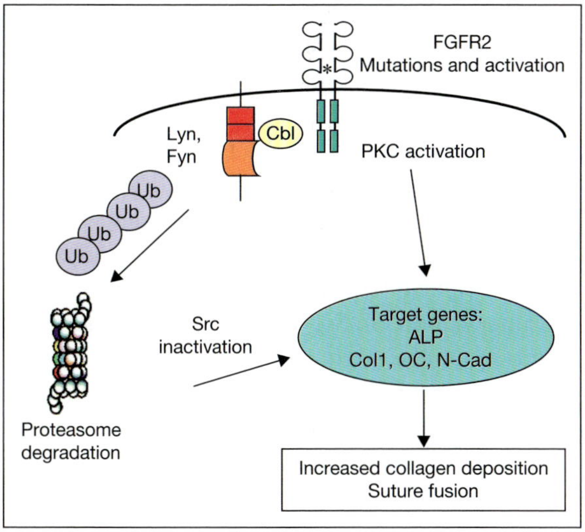

Fig. 2. Mechanisms and signaling pathways resulting from FGFR2 activation in human calvarial osteoblasts in Apert syndrome. PKC activation by the FGFR2 mutation enhances the expression of N-cadherin and osteoblast phenotypic genes. Additionally, FGFR2 activation induces Cbl-mediated Lyn and Fyn degradation by the proteasome, resulting in increased osteoblast gene expression.

marker genes in mutant cells, indicating that PKC signaling is involved in the increased osteoblast gene expression induced by the activating FGFR2 mutation in human calvaria osteoblasts [40] (fig. 2). This effect is consistent with the activation of PKC-mediated activation of N-cadherin synthesis by FGF2 in cranial osteoblasts [45], and with a role for PKC in N-cadherin-mediated aggregation and osteoblast differentiation in human cells [46].

Further studies indicate that other mechanisms, including FGFR2 downregulation, may be involved in the premature osteoblast differentiation in Apert osteoblasts. We found that constitutive activation of FGFR2 by the S252W FGFR2 mutation accelerates FGFR downregulation in mutant osteoblasts in vitro and in vivo [47]. Moreover, we found that FGFR2 downregulation in Apert osteoblasts results from receptor internalization rather than from changes in receptor mRNA. Ubiquitin-mediated proteasome degradation is an important mechanism controlling the degradation of many proteins [48]. Specifically, ubiquitin-dependent degradation of proteins involves the ubiquitination of the target protein followed by its degradation by the proteasome [49]. One ubiquitin ligase, Cbl, plays a major role in protein degradation through the proteasome pathway [50]. Interestingly, the ubiquitin ligase Cbl was found to control FGFR1 degradation after ligand activation [51]. In Apert osteoblasts, we found that the overactive FGFR2 mutation induces Cbl binding to the receptor, resulting in FGFR2 ubiquitination and proteasome degradation, which provides a mechanism by which FGFR2 is downregulated in response to constitutive activation of FGFR2. We also showed that FGFR2 activation induced by the overactive FGFR2 S252W mutation induces Cbl-mediated downregulation of the Src proteins Lyn and Fyn [52]. The molecular mechanisms for this tripartite molecular interaction may involve constitutive active FGFR2-dependent phosphorylation of Src family kinases leading to phosphorylation of Cbl, activation of the ubiquitin ligase activity of Cbl, resulting in ubiquitination and proteasome degradation of Lyn, Fyn and FGFR2. Strikingly, the Cbl-dependent downregulation of Lyn and Fyn induced by the overactive FGFR2 mutation results in increased expression of early markers of osteoblast differentiation [52]. Therefore, this mechanism contributes functionally to the premature osteoblast phenotype induced by the Apert FGFR2 mutation (fig. 2).

FGFR2 Mutations Affect Human Cranial Osteoblast Apoptosis

Apoptosis is essential for the elimination of osteoblasts during skeletal development as this phenomenon controls osteoblast lifespan and thereby tissue formation [53, 54]. In the mouse coronal suture, apoptotic cell death occurs at the same time and place as suture initiation, suggesting a role in suture development [55]. Because apoptosis normally occurs in the suture during development, perturbations in the number of apoptotic cells may lead to premature or delayed suture closure [2]. Several regulatory molecules are known to control osteoblast apoptosis [53, 54]. Among them, two groups found that FGF promotes apoptosis in mature osteoblasts [31, 56], suggesting a role for FGF signaling in the control of osteoblast apoptosis. Accordingly, constitutive activation of FGFR2 signaling by the C342Y Crouzon and the S252W Apert FGFR2 mutations was found to promote apoptosis in mouse osteoblasts [31, 34, 35]. Consistent with these mouse models, we found a greater number of apoptotic osteoblasts and osteocytes in the fused suture compared to the normal coronal suture in Apert syndrome [57]. Analysis of the underlying mechanisms revealed that activation of the FGFR2 receptor in Apert syndrome promotes apoptosis through activation of protein kinase C resulting in increased IL-1 and Fas, activation of caspase-8, increased Bax/Bcl-2 levels, increased effector caspases and DNA fragmentation [57] (fig. 2).

There is another mechanism by which activation of FGFR2 controls osteoblast survival. In fetal human Apert osteoblasts, we found that FGFR2 activation reduces osteoblast attachment on fibronectin and type I collagen in vitro, indicating that activation of FGFR2 controls osteoblast adhesion on bone matrix proteins. Specifically, FGFR2 activation specifically induced downregulation of α_5 integrin through Cbl-mediated α_5 integrin recruitment, ubiquitination and subsequent degradation via the proteasome [58]. This has functional consequence because the Cbl-dependent downregulation of α_5 integrin and subsequent reduction in cell attachment trigger caspase-dependent apoptosis through Bax/Bcl-2 and activation of the caspase-9-caspase-3 cascade [58]. Thus, Cbl-mediated ubiquitination of the α_5 integrin subunit contributes functionally to the osteoblast apoptosis induced by FGFR2 activation in osteoblasts. Whether the increased apoptosis in FGFR2 mutant osteoblasts plays a role in the premature suture closure remains to be determined. One hypothesis may be that apoptosis in mature osteoblasts may be a necessary event compensating for the accelerated osteoblast differentiation induced by FGFR2 signaling. Although we found that activation of FGFR2 promotes both osteoblast differentiation and apoptosis in Apert syndrome in vivo and in vitro, it is likely that the clinical syndrome of premature suture fusion is more related to the increased bone deposition [18, 22].

Twist Mutations Induce Craniosynostosis

Twist is a basic helix-loop-helix (bHLH) factor involved in mesodormal and myoblast differentiation [59]. In the mouse coronal suture, Twist expression occurs in early progenitors and decreases with osteogenesis [60], suggesting that Twist is a negative regulator of osteoblast differentiation. Mutations in the Twist gene in humans are associated with Saethre-Chotzen syndrome (SCS), an autosomal dominant hereditary disorder characterized by facial dysmorphism, digit defects and premature fusion of coronal sutures [61, 62], further revealing a role for Twist in cranial osteogenesis. Multiple mutations have been identified in the Twist gene, most of them being stop codons or missense mutations in the highly conserved bHLH domain, resulting in Twist haploinsufficiency [63, 64]. The phenotype in SCS patients with heterozygous deletion of Twist and of Twist-null heterozygous mice suggests that Twist haploinsufficiency is the causal mechanism of the disease. Twist is known to heterodimerize with the broadly expressed bHLH E proteins, which bind DNA canonical sequences called E boxes (CANNTG) which are consensus binding sites for bHLH proteins present in the promoter of target genes. In SCS, Twist mutations cause Twist protein degradation and loss of dimerization with E proteins, which abolish Twist binding activity to DNA [65, 66]. It is therefore expected that the decreased Twist ratio in the SCS may directly or indirectly induce alterations of phenotypic genes that are regulated by Twist.

Twist Haploinsufficiency Affects Human Cranial Osteoblast Differentiation

Using cranial osteoblasts derived from patients with SCS, we showed that Twist haploinsufficiency results in increased ALP and collagen expression, and increased osteogenic capability in vitro and in vivo [19], indicating that the reduced Twist dosage induces premature cranial ossification through increased bone deposition. The mechanisms by which Twist controls osteoblasts appear, however, to be complex. We found that deletion of bHLH in the Twist gene in postnatal human calvarial osteoblasts is associated with reduced expression of Runx2 and Runx2-regulated genes such as OP, BSP and OC [19, 67]. Moreover, TWIST inactivation alters Runx2 expression and binding ability to the osteocalcin promoter [67], indicating that Runx2 is a target gene for Twist in human osteoblasts [68]. It is intriguing to note that, in the developing mouse, Twist can inhibit the functional activity of Runx2 through a Twist box identified in the C-terminal domain of Twist [69], suggesting that Twist may interact with Runx2 independently of the bHLH domain during early stages of mouse skeletal development. These observations suggest that Twist may control the function of osteoblasts through distinct pathways depending on the physiological or developmental context.

Another mechanism by which Twist may control osteoblasts is through interaction with FGFR signaling. Studies in mice have suggested that Twist may interact with FGFR signaling in cranial bone [60, 70], suggesting links between Twist and FGFR signaling. In human osteoblasts from SCS patients, we found that the reduced Twist dosage reduces FGFR2 mRNA levels [71]. This may result from a direct effect of Twist since Twist binds to one region of the FGFR2 promoter that contains a CANNTG sequence [71]. Because FGF signaling is important for cranial suture formation and maintenance, the altered FGFR2 expression in Twist mutant osteoblasts may contribute to the abnormal osteoblast phenotype in the SC syndrome. Indeed, we showed that the altered Runx2 expression in Twist mutant osteoblasts results, in part, from the altered FGFR2 expression. Conversely, Runx2 may modulate the expression of FGFR2 through binding to one OSE2 site in the FGFR2 promoter [71]. Thus, Twist haploinsufficiency in SCS acts upstream of FGFR2 to reduce FGFR2 mRNA, which in turn affects Runx2 expression and downstream phenotypic markers in postnatal human cranial osteoblasts (fig. 3). The above conclusions arise from experiments using human postnatal osteoblasts directly derived from affected tissues and are therefore close to the in vivo situation in SCS. Nevertheless, Twist may control Runx2 differently at earlier stages of skeletal development. Indeed, in the developing mouse, Twist was found to transiently inhibit Runx2 activity [69]. Thus, Twist may control osteoblast differentiation by distinct molecular mechanisms at different stages of skeletal development.

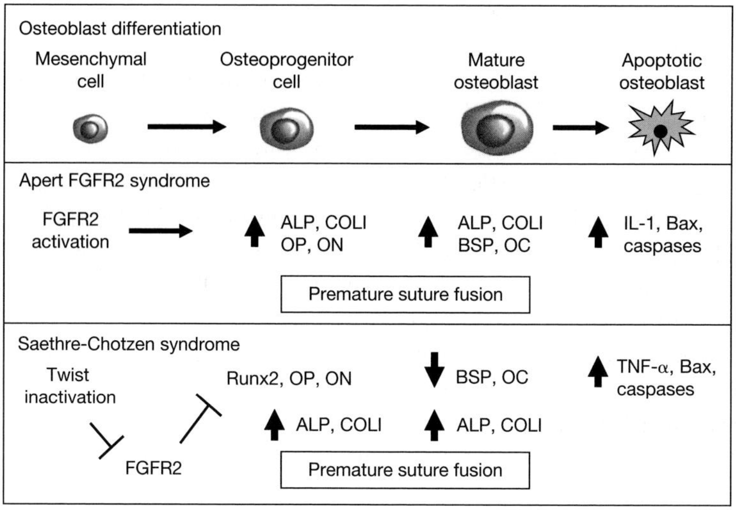

Fig. 3. Molecular mechanisms involved in the premature cranial fusion induced by FGFR2 and Twist mutations in human craniosynostosis. In Apert syndrome, FGFR2 activation results in increased osteoblast markers and collagen deposition in fetal or postnatal osteoblasts. In the Saethre-Chotzen syndrome, Twist haploinsufficiency results in altered FGFR2 and Runx2 expression, and increased collagen deposition in postnatal osteoblasts.

Overall, the premature suture closure resulting from Twist haploinsufficiency in humans is likely to result from several causes. One possible cause is the alteration of genes involved in osteogenesis, such as collagen synthesis which is increased in Twist human mutant osteoblasts. Because cranial osteoblast growth is increased in Twist mutant cells in SCS [19], we suggest that Twist haploinsufficiency expands osteogenic cells by keeping human calvarial cells in a premature stage characterized by low FGFR2 and Runx2 expression. In this context, cranial suture closure in SCS may result from an increased number of immature collagen-producing osteoblasts rather than from an increased differentiation rate of osteoblasts.

Twist Haploinsufficiency Promotes Human Cranial Osteoblast Apoptosis

A role of Twist in the control of cell survival was suggested by several findings. Twist-null mice show a massive wave of apoptosis during development [59]. Moreover, in vitro data indicate that ectopic Twist overexpression induces apoptosis [72], and Twist is involved in the antiapoptotic actions of the insulin-like growth factor-I receptor in vitro [73]. Consistently, we found that several mutations causing Twist haploinsufficiency in SCS increase osteoblast/osteocyte apoptosis both in vivo and in vitro in the SCS [74]. Several mechanisms may account for the increased osteoblast apoptosis induced by Twist haploinsufficiency. Using gene microarray analysis, we identified apoptotic-related genes that are constitutively overexpressed in Twist mutant cells [44]. Functional analyses in human mutant osteoblasts revealed that the reduced Twist dosage induces apoptosis by mechanisms implicating tumor necrosis factor-α (TNF-α) overexpression, resulting in activation of effector caspases, DNA degradation and cell death [74]. The interaction of Twist and cytokine signaling was confirmed by Sosic et al. [75] who reported that Twist proteins regulate cytokine signaling gene expression, including TNF-α, resulting in apoptosis in multiple tissues in mice. There are several potential molecular mechanisms by which Twist haploinsufficiency may induce TNF-α overexpression in mutant osteoblasts. Although Twist can inhibit apoptosis by antagonizing the p53 pathway [72], p53 does not appear to be implicated in apoptosis in Twist-lacking mice [75] or in human Twist mutant osteoblasts [74]. Twist can directly inhibit cytokine expression by acting on the promoter that contains E boxes [75]. Additionally, the increased expression of nuclear factor erythroid-related factor 1 (NRF1) in Twist mutant osteoblasts may activate TNF-α transcription [74]. Although these studies indicate that Twist controls apoptosis, it remains uncertain whether the increased osteoblast/osteocyte apoptosis in SCS plays a role in the premature suture ossification or whether this is a secondary event induced by Twist haploinsufficiency (fig. 3).

Concluding Remarks and Perspectives

The analysis of cranial skeletal dysplasias induced by genetic mutations proved to be useful to assess the mechanisms involved in human craniosynostosis. Specifically, our studies in human calvaria osteoblast models provided a cellular and molecular basis for the pathogenesis of craniosynostosis induced by FGFR2 and Twist mutations in humans. These models revealed some of the signaling mechanisms that play a role in the altered osteoblast differentiation and apoptosis in syndromic craniosynostosis. Moreover, this led to a more comprehensive view on the FGFR and Twist signaling mechanisms that control the osteoblast phenotype in humans (figs 2, 3).

Despite these significant advances in the role of FGFR2 and Twist in human craniosynostosis, several points remain to be addressed. First, we need to learn more about the specific role of FGFR signaling pathways that are involved in human craniosynostosis. Recent analysis of cell signaling in murine osteoblasts expressing FGFR2 mutations revealed that activation of FGFR downregulates Wnt target genes [76]. Future studies in human mutant osteoblasts may help to determine the implication of Wnt and other signaling pathways in the phenotype induced by FGFR2 activation in human craniosynostosis. Another important issue concerns the identification of other target genes that are targeted by genetic mutations in human craniosynostosis. Using microarray analyses, we and others found several target genes that are affected by FGFR and Twist genetic mutations in human or mouse craniosynostosis [44, 74, 76]. The identification of other functional target genes in FGFR2 and Twist mutant human osteoblasts may provide novel information on the molecular events that are involved in the premature cranial suture closure in human craniosynostosis.

Acknowledgments

The work of the authors was supported by grants from INSERM (PJM), French Minister of Research (KK) and Association Rhumatisme et Travail (HG). The authors thank past members of the group, as well as external collaborators (Dr. D. Renier, Dr. E. Lajeunie, Dr. V. El Ghouzzi, Dr. A. Munnich, Dr. J. Caverzasio and Dr. D. Bouvard) for their contributions to the work presented in this review paper.

References

1 Hall BK, Miyake T: All for one and one for all: condensations and the initiation of skeletal development. Bioessays 2000;22:138–147.
2 Opperman LA: Cranial sutures as intramembranous bone growth sites. Dev Dyn 2000;219: 472–485.
3 Cohen MM Jr: Perspectives on craniosynostosis. Am J Med Genet A 2005;136:313–326.
4 Marie PJ: The molecular genetics of bone formation: implications for therapeutic interventions in bone disorders. Am J Pharmacogenomics 2001;1:175–187.
5 Karsenty G, Wagner EF: Reaching a genetic and molecular understanding of skeletal development. Dev Cell 2002;2:389–406.
6 Greenwald JA, Mehrara BJ, Spector JA, Warren SM, Fagenholz PJ, Smith LE, Bouletreau PJ, Crisera FE, Ueno H, Longaker MT: In vivo modulation of FGF biological activity alters cranial suture fate. Am J Pathol 2001;158:441–452.
7 Kim H-J, Rice DPC, Kettunen PJ, Thesleff I: FGF-, BMP- and Shh-mediated signaling pathways in the regulation of cranial suture morphogenesis and calvaria bone development. Development 1998;125:1241–1251.
8 Morriss-Kay GM, Iseki S, Johnson D: Genetic control of the cell proliferation-differentiation balance in the developing skull vault: roles of fibroblast growth factor receptor signaling pathways. Novartis Found Symp 2001;232:102–116.
9 Dailey L, Ambrosetti D, Mansukhani A, Basilico C: Mechanisms underlying differential responses to FGF signaling. Cytokine Growth Factor Rev 2005;16:233–247.
10 Lenton KA, Nacamuli RP, Wan DC, Helms JA, Longaker MT: Cranial suture biology. Curr Top Dev Biol 2005;66:287–328.
11 Marie PJ, Debiais F, Hay E: Regulation of human cranial osteoblast phenotype by FGF-2, FGFR-2 and BMP-2 signaling. Histol Histopathol 2002;17:877–885.

12 de Pollak C, Arnaud E, Renier D, Marie PJ: Age-related changes in bone formation, osteoblastic cell proliferation, and differentiation during postnatal osteogenesis in human calvaria. J Cell Biochem 1997;64:128–139.
13 Lomri A, de Pollak C, Sebag M, Goltzman D, Kremer R, Marie PJ: Expression of parathyroid hormone-related peptide (PTHrP) and PTH/PTHrP receptor in newborn human calvaria osteoblastic cells. Eur J Endocrinol 1997;136:640–648.
14 Debiais F, Hott M, Graulet AM, Marie PJ: The effects of fibroblast growth factor-2 on human neonatal calvaria osteoblastic cells are differentiation stage specific. J Bone Miner Res 1998;13: 645–654.
15 Hay E, Hott M, Graulet AM, Lomri A, Marie PJ: Effects of bone morphogenetic protein-2 on human neonatal calvaria cell differentiation. J Cell Biochem 1999;72:81–93.
16 De Pollack C, Renier D, Hott M, Marie PJ: Increased bone formation and osteoblastic cell phenotype in premature cranial suture ossification (craniosynostosis). J Bone Miner Res 1996;11:401–407.
17 Shevde NC, Bendixen A, Maruyama M, Li BL, Billmire DA: Enhanced activity of osteoblast differentiation factor (PEBP2alphaA2/CBFa1) in affected sutural osteoblasts from patients with nonsyndromic craniosynostosis. Cleft Palate Craniofac J 2001;38:606–614.
18 Lomri A, Lemonnier J, Hott M, de Perseval N, Lajeunie E, Munnich A, Renier D, Marie PJ: Increased calvaria cell differentiation and bone matrix formation induced by fibroblast growth factor receptor-2 mutations in Apert syndrome. J Clin Invest 1998;101:1310–1317.
19 Yousfi M, Lasmoles F, Lomri A, Delannoy P, Marie PJ: Increased bone formation and decreased osteocalcin expression induced by reduced Twist dosage in the Saethre-Chotzen syndrome. J Clin Invest 2001;107:1153–1161.
20 Ornitz DM, Marie PJ: FGF signaling pathways in endochondral and intramembranous bone development and human genetic disease. Genes Dev 2002;16:1446–1465.
21 Ornitz DM: FGF signaling in the developing endochondral skeleton. Cytokine Growth Factor Rev 2005;16:205–213.
22 Wilkie AO: Bad bones, absent smell, selfish testes: the pleiotropic consequences of human FGF receptor mutations. Cytokine Growth Factor Rev 2005;16:187–203.
23 Anderson J, Burns HD, Enriquez-Harris P, Wilkie AOM, Heath JK: Apert syndrome mutations in fibroblast growth factor receptor 2 exhibit increased affinity for FGF ligand. Hum Mol Gen 1998;7:1475–1483.
24 Robertson SC, Meyer AN, Hart KC, Galvin BD, Webster MK, Gonoghue DJ: Activating mutations in the extracellular domain of the fibroblast growth factor 2 function by disruption of the disulfide bond in the third immunoglobulin-like domain. Proc Natl Acad Sci USA 1998;95:4567–4572.
25 Plotnikov AN, Hubbard SR, Schlessinger J, Mohammadi M: Crystal structures of two FGF-FGFR complexes reveal the determinants of ligand-receptor specificity. Cell 2000;101:413–424.
26 Ibrahimi OA, Eliseenkova AV, Plotnikov AN, Yu K, Ornitz DM, Mohammadi M: Structural basis for fibroblast growth factor receptor 2 activation in Apert syndrome. Proc Natl Acad Sci USA 2001;98:7182–7187.
27 Yu K, Herr AB, Waksman G, Ornitz DM: Loss of fibroblast growth factor receptor 2 ligand-binding specificity in Apert syndrome. Proc Natl Acad Sci USA 2000;97:14536–14541.
28 Yu K, Ornitz DM: Uncoupling fibroblast growth factor receptor 2 ligand binding specificity leads to Apert syndrome-like phenotypes. Proc Natl Acad Sci USA 2000;98:3641–3643.
29 Hurley MM, Marie PJ, Florkiewicz R: Fibroblast growth factor and fibroblast growth factor receptor families in bone; in Bilezikian J, Raisz LG, Rodan G (eds): Principles of Bone Biology. New York, Academic Press, 2002, pp 825–851.
30 Marie PJ: Fibroblast growth factor signaling controlling osteoblast differentiation. Gene 2003;316: 23–32.
31 Mansukhani A, Bellosta P, Sahni M, Basilico C: Signaling by fibroblast growth factors (FGF) and fibroblast growth factor receptor 2 (FGFR-2)-activating mutations blocks mineralization and induces apoptosis in osteoblasts. J Cell Biol 2000;149:1297–1308.
32 Zhou YX, Xu X, Chen L, Li C, Brodie SG, Deng CX: A Pro250Arg substitution in mouse Fgfr1 causes increased expression of Cbfa1 and premature fusion of calvarial sutures. Hum Mol Genet 2000;12:2001–2008.

33 Eswarakumar VP, Monsonego-Ornan E, Pines M, Antonopoulou I, Morriss-Kay GM, Lonai P: The IIIc alternative of Fgfr2 is a positive regulator of bone formation. Development 2002;129:3783–3793.
34 Chen L, Li D, Li C, Engel A, Deng CX: A Ser250Trp substitution in mouse fibroblast growth factor receptor 2 (Fgfr2) results in craniosynostosis. Bone 2003;33:169–178.
35 Yu K, Xu J, Liu Z, Sosic D, Shao J, Olson EN, Towler DA, Ornitz DM: Conditional inactivation of FGF receptor 2 reveals an essential role for FGF signaling in the regulation of osteoblast function and bone growth. Development 2003;130:3063–3074.
36 Eswarakumar VP, Horowitz MC, Locklin R, Morriss-Kay GM, Lonai P: A gain-of-function mutation of Fgfr2c demonstrates the roles of this receptor variant in osteogenesis. Proc Natl Acad Sci USA 2004;101:12555–12560.
37 Marie PJ, Coffin JD, Hurley MM: FGF and FGFR signaling in chondrodysplasias and craniosynostosis. J Cell Biochem 2005;96:888–896.
38 Eswarakumar VP, Lax I, Schlessinger J: Cellular signaling by fibroblast growth factor receptors. Cytokine Growth Factor Rev 2005;16:139–149.
39 Dailey L, Ambrosetti D, Mansukhani A, Basilico C: Mechanisms underlying differential responses to FGF signaling. Cytokine Growth Factor Rev 2005;16:233–247.
40 Lemonnier J, Hay E, Delannoy P, Lomri A, Modrowski D, Caverzasio J, Marie PJ: Role of N-cadherin and protein kinase C in osteoblast gene activation induced by the S252W fibroblast growth factor receptor 2 mutation in Apert craniosynostosis. J Bone Miner Res 2001;16:832–845.
41 Tanimoto Y, Yokozeki M, Hiura K, Matsumoto K, Nakanishi H, Matsumoto T, Marie PJ, Moriyama K: A soluble form of fibroblast growth factor receptor 2 (FGFR2) with S252W mutation acts as an efficient inhibitor for the enhanced osteoblastic differentiation caused by FGFR2 activation in Apert syndrome. J Biol Chem 2004;279:45926–45934.
42 Baroni T, Carinci P, Lilli C, Bellucci C, Aisa MC, Scapoli L, Volinia S, Carinci F, Pezzetti F, Calvitti M, Farina A, Conte C, Bodo M: P253R fibroblast growth factor receptor-2 mutation induces RUNX2 transcript variants and calvarial osteoblast differentiation. J Cell Physiol 2005;202:524–535.
43 Fragale A, Tartaglia M, Bernardini S, Michela Di Stasi AM, Di Rocco C, Velardi F, Teti A, Battaglia PA, Migliacco S: Decreased proliferation and altered differentiation in osteoblasts from genetically and clinically distinct craniosynostotic disorders. Am J Pathol 1999;154:1465–1477.
44 Lomri A, Lemonnier J, Delannoy P, Marie PJ: Increased expression of protein kinase Calpha, interleukin-1alpha, and RhoA guanosine 5′-triphosphatase in osteoblasts expressing the Ser252Trp fibroblast growth factor 2 receptor Apert mutation: identification by analysis of complementary DNA microarray. J Bone Miner Res 2001;16:705–712.
45 Debiais F, Lemonnier J, Hay E, Delannoy P, Caverzasio J, Marie PJ: Fibroblast growth factor-2 (FGF-2) increases N-cadherin expression through protein kinase C and Src-kinase pathways in human calvaria osteoblasts. J Cell Biochem 2001;81:68–81.
46 Delannoy P, Lemonnier J, Haÿ E, Modrowski D, Marie PJ: Protein kinase C-dependent upregulation of N-cadherin expression by phorbol ester in human calvaria osteoblasts. Exp Cell Res 2001;269:154–161.
47 Lemonnier J, Delannoy P, Hott M, Lomri A, Modrowski D, Marie PJ: The Ser252Trp fibroblast growth factor receptor-2 (FGFR-2) mutation induces PKC-independent downregulation of FGFR-2 associated with premature calvaria osteoblast differentiation. Exp Cell Res 2000;256:158–167.
48 Hochstrasser M: Ubiquitin, proteasomes, and the regulation of intracellular protein degradation. Curr Opin Cell Biol 1995;7:215–223.
49 Ciechanover A: Intracellular protein degradation: from a vague idea thru the lysosome and the ubiquitin-proteasome system and onto human diseases and drug targeting. Cell Death Differ 2005;12:1178–1190.
50 Sanjay A, Horne WC, Baron R: The Cbl family: ubiquitin ligases regulating signaling by tyrosine kinases. Sci STKE 2001;110:PE40.
51 Wong A, Lamothe B, Lee A, Schlessinger J, Lax I: FRS2 alpha attenuates FGF receptor signaling by Grb2-mediated recruitment of the ubiquitin ligase Cbl. Proc Natl Acad Sci USA 2002;99:6684–6689.
52 Kaabeche K, Lemonnier J, Le Mée S, Caverzasio J, Marie PJ: Cbl-mediated degradation of Lyn and Fyn induced by constitutive FGFR-2 activation supports osteoblast differentiation. J Biol Chem 2004;279:36259–36267.

53 Fromigue O, Modrowski D, Marie PJ: Apoptosis in membranous bone formation: role of fibroblast growth factor and bone morphogenetic protein signaling. Crit Rev Eukaryot Gene Expr 2005;15:75–92.
54 Xing L, Boyce BF: Regulation of apoptosis in osteoclasts and osteoblastic cells. Biochem Biophys Res Commun 2005;328:709–720.
55 Rice D, Kim H, Thesleff I: Apoptosis in murine calvarial bone and suture development. Eur J Oral Sci 1999;107:265–275.
56 Debiais F, Lefèvre G, Lemonnier J, Le Mée S, Lasmoles F, Mascarelli F, Marie PJ: Fibroblast growth factor-2 induces osteoblast survival through a phosphatidylinositol 3-kinase-dependent, -β-catenin-independent signaling pathway. Exp Cell Res 2004;297:235–246.
57 Lemonnier J, Haÿ E, Delannoy P, Fromigué O, Lomri A, Modrowski M, Marie PJ: Increased osteoblast apoptosis in Apert craniosynostosis: role of protein kinase C and interleukin-1. Am J Pathol 2001;158:1833–1842.
58 Kaabeche K, Guenou G, Bouvard D, Didelot N, Listrat A, Marie PJ: Cbl-mediated ubiquitination of alpha 5 integrin subunit mediates fibronectin-dependent osteoblast detachment and apoptosis induced by FGFR2 activation. J Cell Sci 2005;118:1223–1232.
59 Chen ZF, Behringer RR: Twist is required in head mesenchyme for cranial neural tube morphogenesis. Genes Dev 1995;9:686–699.
60 Johnson D, Iseki S, Wilkie AO, Morriss-Kay GM: Expression patterns of Twist and Fgfr1, -2 and -3 in the developing mouse coronal suture suggest a key role for twist in suture initiation and biogenesis. Mech Dev 2000;91:341–345.
61 Howard TD, Paznekas WA, Green ED, Chiang LC, Ma N, Ortiz De Luna RI, Garcia Delgado C, Gonzales-Ramos M, Kline AD, Jabs EW: Mutations in Twist, a basic helix-loop-helix transcription factor, in Saethre-Chotzen syndrome. Nat Genet 1997;15:36–41.
62 El Ghouzzi V, Le Merrer M, Perrin-Schmitt F, Lajeunie E, Benit P, Renier DC, Gonzales-Ramos M, Kline AD, Jabs EW: Mutations in Twist, a basic helix-loop-helix transcription factor, in Saethre-Chotzen syndrome. Nat Genet 1997;15:36–41.
63 Gripp K, Zackai E, Stolle C: Mutations in the human Twist gene. Hum Mut 2000;15:150–155.
64 El Ghouzzi V, Lajeunie E, Le Merrer M, Cormier-Daire V, Renier D, Munnich A, Bonaventure J: Mutations within or upstream of the basic helix-loop-helix domain of the Twist gene are specific to Saethre-Chotzen syndrome. Eur J Hum Genet 1999;7:27–33.
65 El Ghouzzi V, Legeai-Mallet L, Aresta S, Benoist C, Munnich A, de Gunzburg J, Bonaventure J: Saethre-Chotzen mutations cause Twist protein degradation or impaired nuclear location. Hum Mol Genet 2000;9:813–819.
66 El Ghouzzi V, Legeai-Mallet L, Benoist-Lasselin C, Lajeunie E, Renier D, Munnich A, Bonaventure J: Mutations in the basic domain and the loop-helix II junction of Twist abolish DNA binding in Saethre-Chotzen syndrome. FEBS Lett 2001;492:112–118.
67 Yousfi M, Lasmoles F, Marie PJ: TWIST inactivation reduces CBFA1/RUNX2 expression and DNA binding to the osteocalcin promoter in osteoblasts. Biochem Biophys Res Commun 2002;297:641–644.
68 Jabs EW: A TWIST in the fate of human osteoblasts identifies signaling molecules involved in skull development. J Clin Invest 2001;107:1075–1077.
69 Bialek P, Kern B, Yang X, Schrock M, Sosic D, Hong N, Wu H, Yu K, Ornitz DM, Olson EN, Justice MJ, Karsenty G: A twist code determines the onset of osteoblast differentiation. Dev Cell 2004;6:423–435.
70 Rice DP, Aberg T, Chan Y, Tang Z, Kettunen PJ, Pakarinen L, Maxson RE, Thesleff I: Integration of FGF and TWIST in calvarial bone and suture development. Development 2000;127:1845–1855.
71 Guenou H, Kaabeche K, Le Mee S, Marie PJ: A role for fibroblast growth factor receptor-2 in the altered osteoblast phenotype induced by Twist haploinsufficiency in the Saethre-Chotzen syndrome. Hum Mol Genet 2005;14:1429–1439.
72 Maestro R, Dei Tos AP, Hamamori Y, Krasnokutsky S, Sartorelli V, Kedes L, Doglioni C, Beach DH, Hannon GJ: Twist is a potential oncogene that inhibits apoptosis. Genes Dev 1999;13:2207–2217.
73 Dupont J, Fernandez AM, Glackin CA, Helman L, LeRoith D: Insulin-like growth factor 1 (IGF-1)-induced twist expression is involved in the anti-apoptotic effects of the IGF-1 receptor. J Biol Chem 2001;276:26699–26707.

74 Yousfi M, Lasmoles F, El Ghouzzi V, Marie PJ: Twist haploinsufficiency in Saethre-Chotzen syndrome induces calvaria osteoblast apoptosis due to increased TNFalpha expression and caspase-2 activation. Hum Mol Genet 2002;11:359–369.
75 Sosic D, Richardson JA, Yu K, Ornitz DM, Olson EN: Twist regulates cytokine gene expression through a negative feedback loop that represses NF-kappaB activity. Cell 2003;112:169–180.
76 Mansukhani A, Ambrosetti D, Holmes G, Cornivelli L, Basilico C: Sox2 induction by FGF and FGFR2 activating mutations inhibits Wnt signaling and osteoblast differentiation. J Cell Biol 2005;168:1065–1076.

Dr. P.J. Marie
INSERM Unité 606, Hôpital Lariboisière
2 rue Ambroise Paré
FR–75475 Paris Cedex 10 (France)
Tel. +33 1 49 95 63 58, Fax +33 1 49 95 84 52, E-Mail pierre.marie@larib.inserm.fr

Rice DP (ed): Craniofacial Sutures. Development, Disease and Treatment.
Front Oral Biol. Basel, Karger, 2008, vol 12, pp 160–177

Fibroblast Growth Factor Signaling in Cranial Suture Development and Pathogenesis

Mohammad K. Hajihosseini

School of Biological Sciences, University of East Anglia, Norwich, UK

Abstract

Apert, Pfeiffer and Crouzon syndromes are congenital craniosynostosis syndromes caused by mutations that perturb the level of fibroblast growth factor receptor (FGFR) signaling. The cellular and molecular impact of these mutations have been studied in vitro and in animal models in vivo. Here, I highlight the complexity of the FGF/FGFR signaling system and review the candidate modifiers responsible for regulating the levels of FGF/FGFR signaling in tissues. I also review what we have learned from the phenotypic analysis of mice that model these craniosynostosis syndromes and discuss some in vivo strategies for further understanding as well as alleviating the associated craniofacial defects.

Introduction

Interaction between epithelial and mesenchymal cells is vital to the normal development of the craniofacial skeleton. The critical involvement of fibroblast growth factor receptor (FGFR) signaling system in these interactions has been highlighted by the discovery that a set of congenital craniosynostosis syndromes – Apert, Pfeiffer, Crouzon and Jackson-Weiss – are caused by mutations in FGFR genes [1–4]. The affected children show premature fusion of sutures that separate the calvarial and facial bones and these may be accompanied by limb as well as sporadic visceral and neural anomalies [5, 6].

A series of studies have since dissected the role of FGF signaling in normal suture development and pathogenesis in craniosynostosis syndromes. For example, expression pattern analyses and loss-of-function studies in mice have identified some of the key FGF ligands and receptors that may regulate normal suture development [7–10]. Biochemical and crystallographic studies have furthered our understanding of mutant receptor structure and their mode of interactions with FGF ligands [11–13]. Introduction of FGFR mutations into cultured cells or the study of osteoblasts from affected patients has revealed the impact of aberrant FGF signaling on cell turnover and behavior [14, 15]. An important contribution has also been the generation of mice that model craniosynostosis syndromes (see below), where the impact and dynamics of aberrant FGF signaling can be analyzed in the appropriate temporal and spatial settings in vivo.

The anatomy and cell biology of sutures as well as advances in our understanding of the craniosynostosis syndromes have been reviewed in other chapters of this book and elsewhere [3, 16]. In this chapter, I shall review the complexity of the FGF/FGFR signaling system, providing an update on its regulators, and highlight what we have learned from the phenotypic analysis and manipulation of mice that model Apert, Pfeiffer and Crouzon syndromes.

FGF Signaling and Its Checkpoints: Overview of FGF Signaling

Genes encoding 22 Fgfs and five FGFRs (FGFR1–5) have been identified in mammals [17]. FGFs 11–14 show little interaction with cell surface FGFRs but appear to have important intracellular functions [18, 19]. The biological significance of FGFR5 [20], which lacks the classical tyrosine kinase domain, is yet to be determined. Hence, our current understanding is that the mammalian FGF signaling involves eighteen ligands and four receptors (FGFR1–4).

A typical FGFR molecule carries two or three extracellular immunoglobulin (Ig)-like domains harboring the ligand binding sites, and is anchored to the plasma membrane via a single pass transmembrane (TM) domain [reviewed by 21] (fig. 1). In addition, each receptor molecule possesses a juxtamembrane domain containing an FRS2 docking site and two split tyrosine kinase domains that become phosphorylated upon receptor activation. Receptor molecules are activated through homodimerization, a process that normally requires binding to FGF ligands in the presence of sulfated proteoglycans. Activated receptors recruit several cytoplasmic proteins whose phosphorylation leads to the activation of MAP kinase, PI3 kinase and PLC-γ signaling pathways, culminating in changes in nuclear gene expression profile and/or rearrangement of cell cytoskeleton. FGF signaling regulates a diverse set of cellular functions – from proliferation and differentiation to migration and adhesion – depending on the cell type and the intersection of FGF signaling with other signaling pathways, such as Wnts, BMPs, or Hedgehog [see reviews in 22–24].

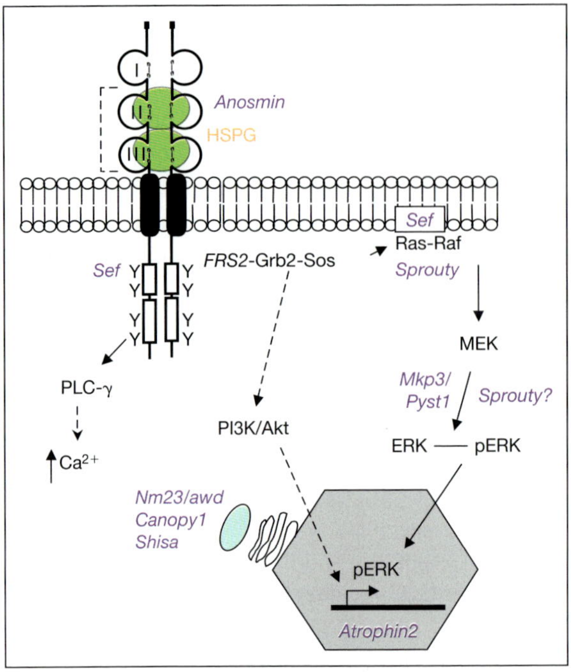

Fig. 1. Schematic representation of FGFR structure, its intracellular signaling mediators and modulators. The three principle pathways, MAP kinase, PI3 kinase and PLC-γ, are shown in black; modulators are shown in pink. Green represents FGF ligands bound to the receptor; solid boxes represent the transmembrane domain. Y = Tyrosine residues in the intracellular domain of the receptor molecule.

FGFR Diversity, Ligand Binding Specificity and Tissue Distribution

Mammalian FGFRs are typically encoded by 18–19 exons, but a multitude of receptor isoforms are generated through alternative splicing of the transcripts or use of different translation initiation sites [21]. These products can be broadly categorized into three groups.

The first and least understood are soluble FGFR isoforms. Examples include a molecule that specifically lacks the TM domain or truncated receptor molecules that harbor the IgII and the N-terminal half of IgIII, with or without fusion to the first 3 amino acids of TM domain (fig. 2a).

The second relates to the inclusion or exclusion of two consecutive amino acids, valine (428) and threonine (429), in the juxtamembrane region of FGFRs 1–3 (i.e. the so-called VT+ or VT− isoforms; fig. 2b). In the case of

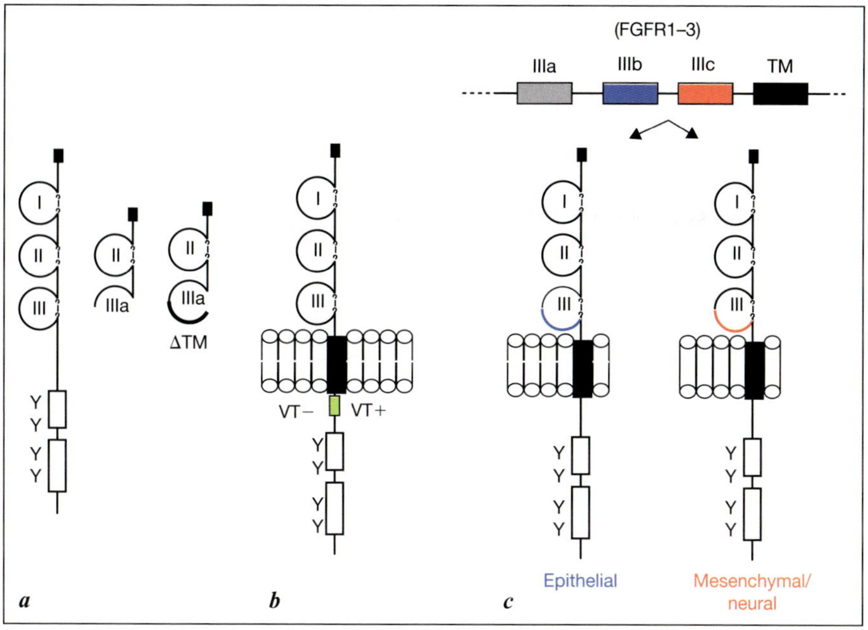

Fig. 2. FGFR variants produced by alternative splicing or use of alternative translation sites. ***a*** Soluble FGFRs. ***b*** VT+ and VT− isoforms. ***c*** IIIb and IIIc isoforms and their tissue distributions (for FGFR2).

FGFR1, these isoforms can influence its interaction with specific signaling pathways [25]. The third group is the so-called IIIb and IIIc isoforms in FGFRs 1–3, which arise from alternative splicing of exons that contribute to the C terminal half of IgIII domain (fig. 2c). The most studied prototypes of these splice variants are FGFR2-IIIb and FGFR2-IIIc [26–28].

FGFR2-IIIb arises from inclusion of exon 8 [i.e. spliced exons 7(IIIa)-8(IIIb)-10(TM)] and is expressed predominantly in epithelial cells. It acts as the receptor for FGFs 3, 7, 10 and 22, which are synthesized by cells of mesenchymal origin. By contrast, FGFR2-IIIc is a 7(IIIa)-9(IIIc)-10(TM) splice product expressed predominantly by mesenchymal (and neural cells) and binds FGFs 2, 4, 6, 8, 9 and 18, ligands that are generally synthesized by epithelial cells [29]. FGF1 (acidic FGF) can activate all FGF receptors/receptor isoforms. Superimposed on an anatomical juxtapositioning of epithelial and mesenchymal cells, this mutually exclusive pattern of FGF and FGFR2 isoform expression allows a unidirectional cross talk between these two cell types (fig. 4a).

Combined evidence from gene expression pattern and gene targeting studies suggests that during *early* development of certain tissues, FgfR2-IIIb's functional counterpart in mesenchymal cells is FgfR1-IIIc rather than FgfR2-IIIc [28]. For example, the *early* growth of lung, limb and palatine shelves, which relies on epithelial mesenchymal interactions, is arrested by the loss of FGFR2-IIIb, but not FGFR2-IIIc function [7, 30]. Later in development, however, as in the lung, FgfR2-IIIb and IIIc isoforms may become mutual partners in the cross talk between epithelial and mesenchymal cells [28]. Conversely, there are situations where functional signaling through FgfR2-IIIc in mesenchymal cells does not temporally coincide with a requirement for FgfR2-IIIb function in epithelial cells, despite the presence of FgfR2-IIIb and its activating ligands. The coronal sutures that separate the developing frontal and parietal bones in the skull provide an example of this scenario, where FgfR2-IIIc is strongly expressed by a cluster of neural crest-derived mesenchymal cells that act as progenitors for calvarial osteoblasts [31]. Accordingly, embryonic calvarial growth/ossification is significantly retarded by the loss of FgfR2-IIIc, or its ligand FGF18, but apparently not FgfR2-IIIb, or its ligand, Fgf10 [7, 10, 30, 32]. Fgf10/FgfR2-IIIb signaling may have a role in *postnatal* bone growth/function but currently these putative roles remain undefined because both Fgf10 and FgfR2-IIIb null mice lack lungs and die at birth [30, 32].

Critical Requirement for Control of FGF Signaling Levels

A series of phenotypes have been observed in transgenic mice that harbor hypo- or hypermorphic alleles of distinct FGFs or FGFRs [e.g. 33–35], and this has made it abundantly clear that the level of FGF signaling experienced by target cells is as important as the signal itself. Moreover, it has been suggested that FGF signaling can operate both in a morphogen/gradient-like mechanism and a gene-dosage/threshold-dependent manner [e.g. 36, 37]. Hence, much work has focused on characterizing the factors and mechanisms that fine-tune the level of FGF signaling in different tissues. These can be broadly classified into extracellular and intracellular factors.

In the extracellular environment, the level of signaling may be controlled by the range and bioavailability of FGF ligands, their interaction with the type and amount of FGFRs expressed on the cell surface, and the presence of distinct sulfated proteoglycans that would be needed to facilitate these interactions. Members of the matrix metalloprotease family (the MMPs and ADAMS) may play critical roles here as they could act to release extracellularly stored FGF ligands and/or cleave receptor molecules to attenuate signaling [38, 39]. Indeed, a chromosomal translocation which upregulates MMP23 causes craniosynostosis [38].

The level of signaling may also be controlled by the action of soluble antagonists and protagonists. The EGF, Wnts and Bmp signaling systems are inhibited by Argos, sFRP and Noggin, respectively [40–43], while LRP family members act as extracellular cofactors for Wnt signaling [44]. Soluble antagonists of FGFR signaling have not been identified but could include truncated FGFR species (fig. 2a). However, FGFR1 signaling can be facilitated by the molecule Anosmin, the product of the Kallmann gene [45].

A host of TM and intracellular regulators and checkpoints have now been identified (listed in table 1). The majority of these were discovered through genetic screening for mutant *Drosophila*, zebrafish or *Xenopus laevis* but subsequent studies have revealed the existence of homologues in chick, mouse and human. In general, these modulators participate in a positive feedback loop such that their genes are upregulated in response to FGFR signaling itself. They vary in their mode of action. Molecules such as Shisa and Canopy 1 play a role in the retention and maturation/glycosylation of FGFRs within the endoplasmic retricular (ER) compartment, thereby controlling the rate of receptor expression and turnover [46, 47]. Mkp3 and Sef, by contrast, are involved in direct inhibition and uncoupling of activated receptors or components of the MAP kinase pathway [48–52]. Other modulators have been shown to have a dual role. For example, phosphorylation of FRS2alpha can culminate in both positive and negative regulation of FGFR signaling, through the activation of the MAP kinase pathway, and the ubiquitination and subsequent degradation of activated FGFRs (and phosphorylated FRS2a), respectively [22, 53].

Yet other molecules serve to modulate multiple signaling pathways in a tissue/stage-specific manner. This is exemplified by the ability of some Sprouty family members to regulate EGFR and GDNF signaling [54], and that of Shisa, in regulating Wnt as well as FGF signaling [47]. Finally, members of the FLRT family appear to play a role in selective cell-cell adhesion, which may not be coupled to their ability to promote FGFR signaling [55, 56].

It is not clear whether these molecules modulate the activity of all or just a subset of FGFR species. Moreover, their involvement in modulation of FGFR signaling during craniofacial development remains to be determined.

Mouse Models of Apert, Pfeiffer and Crouzon Syndromes

In recent years, a number of researchers have modeled in mice the FGFR (1 and 2) mutations that give rise to Apert, Pfeiffer and Crouzon syndromes (table 2), in order to dissect the mode of action of these mutations, and explore potential therapeutic strategies for alleviating the related phenotypes. Phenotypic analysis of these mice has provided novel insights into the precise

Table 1. Molecules that modulate FGFR signaling

Gene/gene product	General features and mode of action	Selected Ref. No.
Anosmin/Kal1	Product of Kallmann syndrome gene that acts as an extracellular coactivator of FGFR1	45
Atrophin 2	A transcriptional corepressor of sef. Its mutation results in loss-of-Fgf8-like phenotypes in zebrafish	72
Awd/Nm23	A tumor suppressor gene that regulates the level of cell-surface-expressed FGFRs through control of vesicular transport. Has multiple isoforms, some of which are expressed predominantly in the developing brain	73, 74
Canopy1	One of four family members conserved across species. An ER-bound saposin-like protein capable of interacting with extracellular domain of FGFR1. Thought to regulate the maturation or modification of FGFRs and/or composition of lipid rafts which are important for RTK signaling	46
FLRTs (fibronectin-leucine-rich transmembrane proteins)	Three-member-strong family that is upregulated by and promotes FGFR signaling. May also have a role in cell adhesion and sorting processes	55, 56, 75
FRS2 (FGFR substrate 2)	A docking protein family member that becomes phosphorylated by activated FGFRs. Plays a feedback regulatory role: its tyrosine phosphorylation recruits a set of proteins that activates the MAP kinase and PI3 kinase pathways, while its threonine phosphorylation inhibits this process	22, 53
Mkp3/Pyst1/dup6 (MAP kinase phosphatase 3)	Negatively regulates FGFR signaling by binding to and dephosphorylating activated MAP kinase proteins. Its expression is positively regulated by FGFR signaling in multiple embryonic organs	48, 50, 76
Shisa	Can negatively regulate FGFR signaling by retaining FGFRs within the ER compartment and/or suppressing their N-linked sugar modification. Expression pattern is conserved in early mouse and chick embryos (also an inhibitor of Wnt signaling)	47, 77
Sef (similar expression to FGF)	A negative regulator that acts at multiple sites of FGFR signal transduction; prevents phosphorylation of FGFRs and separately, the activation and functioning of the Ras-MEK-ERK pathway. Two human isoforms identified	49, 51, 78

Table 1. (continued)

Gene/gene product	General features and mode of action	Selected Ref. No.
Sproutys	Four-member-strong family of negative regulators of FGFR signaling. Genes are induced by and proteins are recruited to the plasma membrane in response to FGFR signaling. Some phosphorylated Sprys prevent the activation of Ras and nonphosphorylated Sprys inhibit Raf1. Effects can be cell type- and stage-specific. Can also modulate EGF, VEGF and GDNF signaling	24, 79, 80

Table 2. Mouse models of Apert, Pfeiffer and Crouzon syndromes

Syndrome	Human mutations	Mouse models/mutations	Ref. No.
Apert	$FGFR2^{+/S252W}$; $FGFR2^{+/P253A}$ FGFR2 (rare) heterozygous *Alu* insertions in and around exon 9 (IIIc); upregulation of FgfR2-IIIb in mesenchymal cells	$FgfR2^{+/S252W}$ FgfR2-$IIIc^{+/\Delta}$ Upregulation of FgfR2-IIIb in mesenchymal and neural cells upon deletion of exon 9 (IIIc)	59, 60 57
Crouzon	FGFR2 (a host of heterozygous mutations in the extracellular domain) Most prominent: +/C278F +/C342Y +/S347C	$FgfR2^{+/C342Y}$	81
Pfeiffer	FGFR2 (a host of heterozygous mutations in the extracellular and cytoplasmic domains) $FGFR1^{+/P250Arg}$	$FGFR1^{+/P250Arg}$ $FGFR1^{+/+}$; plus 2 or 4 copies of BAC-encoded $FgfR1^{P252Arg}$ integrated into chromosome 4	82 37

range of defects (cranial and non-cranial), harbored by the affected patients, as well as the role of FGFR1 and FGFR2 signaling in mammalian organogenesis. A few examples are highlighted below.

The first Apert mouse model arose serendipitously through a *loxP*-Cre-mediated heterozygous deletion of FgfR2-exon 9 (the IIIc-encoding exon; red box fig. 1c) [57]. It was discovered that in these FgfR2-$IIIc^{+/\Delta}$ mice (here on abbreviated to $IIIc^{+/\Delta}$), FgfR2-IIIb becomes ectopically expressed alongside FgfR2-IIIc in mesenchymal and neural tissues, reminiscent of a rare heterozygous Apert syndrome mutation that disrupts the normal slicing of exon IIIc [58].

As discussed above, mesenchymal cells predominantly express FgfR2-IIIc and therefore respond only to its cognate ligands. In $IIIc^{+/\Delta}$ mice, mesenchymal tissues become responsive to *both* IIIb- and IIIc-activating ligands and because these isoforms share an identical cytoplasmic domain, a net gain-of-FGFR2 function ensues. Indeed, a host of such ligands have been found to be expressed in the developing mouse coronal sutures [8] and $IIIc^{+/\Delta}$ mice develop fusion of the coronal sutures [57].

By and large, the $IIIc^{+/\Delta}$ mutation recapitulates the effect/s of more common Apert mutations – FGFR2 S252W and P253R – as these were recently shown to lose their ligand binding specificity and respond to both IIIb- and IIIc-activating ligands [12]. Not surprisingly, there is a large phenotypic overlap between $IIIc^{+/\Delta}$ and $FgfR2^{+/S252W}$ mice [59, 60]. However, the $IIIc^{+/\Delta}$ phenotype appears to be more severe such that invariably $IIIc^{+/\Delta}$ mice show postnatal growth retardation and die within a week of birth [57].

As well as coronal craniosynostosis, Apert syndrome patients show a truncated maxilla (midface) and bulgy eyes (occular proptosis). Analysis of $IIIc^{+/\Delta}$ mice suggested that the latter phenotypes arise from the arrested growth of maxillary-premaxillay and zygomatic arch bones due to premature fusion of their intervening joints/sutures (fig. 3). Zygomatic arch bones form the lower rim of the eye socket and so their growth arrest would create a shallow eye orbit that cannot fully accommodate the eye.

$FgfR2^{+/S252W}$ mice also show the ectopic formation of cartilage within the developing sagittal sutures [60]. Interestingly, overexpression of Fgf9, an FgfR2-IIIc ligand, can also induce abnormal cartilage formation in calvarial primorida [61].

$IIIc^{+/\Delta}$, and indeed $FgfR2^{+/S252W}$ mice, also show premature ossification of the intersternebral cartilage, as well as a host of visceral and neural defects that are sporadically observed in Apert syndrome patients [5, 6]. It will be important to determine and compare the molecular basis of these abnormalities with those underlying the cranial defects. For example, perturbed Wnt signaling underlies the Apert-like lung defects in $IIIc^{+/\Delta}$ mice [62] and interestingly, experimental elevation of Wnt signalling levels through genetic disruption of its negative regulator, Axin2, can yield coronal craniosynostosis [63].

Apert and Pfeiffer syndrome patients also carry distal limb defects but these are not observed in mice that harbor heterozygous Apert or Pfeiffer syndrome-like (FGFR1 and FGFR2) mutations. Possible explanations include differences in gene dosage requirement and/or potential differences in the

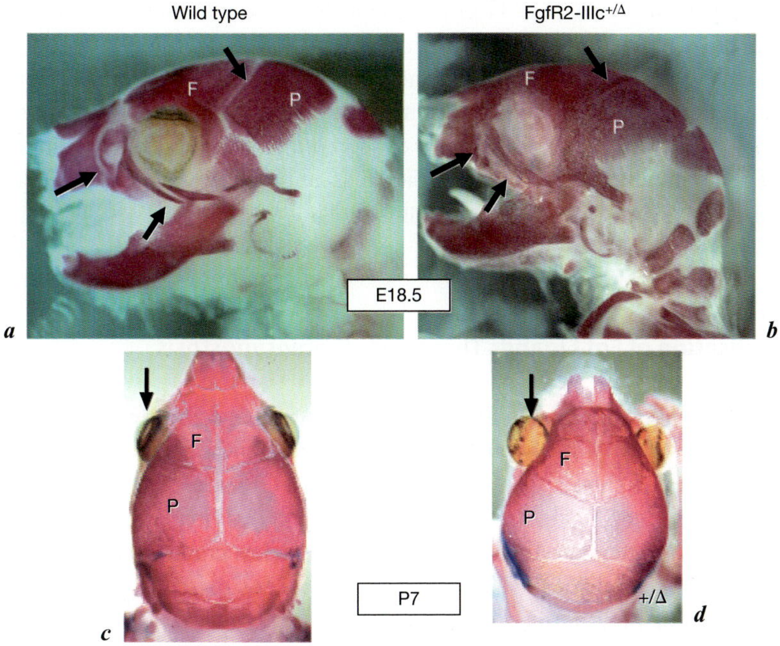

Fig. 3. Apert-like craniofacial defects in FgfR2-IIIc$^{+/\Delta}$ mice. Alizarin-red-stained heads of wild-type (***a***, ***c***) and IIIc$^{+/\Delta}$ (***b***, ***d***) mice. ***a***, ***b*** Arrows point to sutures and joints separating the frontal (F) and parietal bones (P), zygomatic arch and maxilla-premaxillary bones. ***c***, ***d*** Dorsal view of the skulls to show abnormal protrusion of eyes in IIIc$^{+/\Delta}$ mice.

temporal and spatial distribution of the ligands that activate the mutant FGFRs in the two species.

However, the analysis of mice that harbor a tandem of two BAC-encoded hypermorphic FgfR1 mutation (Pfeiffer Pro252Arg) on chromosome 4 has shed some light on this enigma [37]. In addition to the BAC mutation, these mice carry two wild-type endogenous copies of FgfR1 on chromosome 8 and show fusion of frontal sutures but lack the Pfeiffer-like digit-I-specific defects. When the wild type to mutant receptor ratio is raised to 2:4 through selective breeding, the craniofacial phenotypes (fusion of frontal, zygomatic arch and maxilla-premaxiallary sutures/joints) are exacerbated and surprisingly, these are then accompanied by digit-I-specific limb defects. Moreover, these limb defects disappear in the offspring when the 2 (wild type):2 mutant FgfR1 ratio is restored.

The analysis of 4-BAC-FgfR1 embryos has revealed that the digit-I defect involves a downregulation of the canonical Wnt signaling inhibitor, Dkk1, accompanied by an upregulation of ligand, Wnt5a [37]. One conclusion from this work has been that while the development of cranial sutures follows a morphogen-like gradient of FGF signaling – exacerbating with increasing amount of BAC-FgfR1 mutation, that of distal limbs is regulated by a gene dosage-dependent threshold-responsive mechanism.

Identification of Fgf Ligands That Cause Craniosynostosis

Structural and biochemical studies show that Apert and Pfeiffer syndrome mutations induce their gain-of-function activity in a ligand-dependent manner. RT-PCR analysis has shown that a wide variety of FGFs are expressed in the developing mouse coronal sutures [37]. It follows that hyperactive FGFR signaling could be attenuated, so as to prevent or delay craniosynostosis, by knocking down the levels of Fgf/s that cause craniosynostosis. Critically, these ligands should not play a role in normal embryonic calvarial development, but they could be either IIIb- or IIIc-activating ligands. FGF18 for example can be excluded from this list because its loss retards the growth of calvarial bones [10].

One strategy for definitive identification of such ligands is the generation of double mutant mice that carry the Apert or Pfeiffer mutations but are also deficient in gene/s encoding the candidate ligand/s. Rescue of craniosynostosis in these mice would implicate the ligand in its cause. Our preliminary studies show that a genetic abrogation of Fgf10, a major FgfR2-IIIb-activating ligand, is sufficient to rescue the coronal and facial suture fusions in $IIIc^{+/\Delta}$ mice. This concurs with the biochemical data that highlighted Fgf10 as a putative candidate with which mutant Apert receptors aberrantly interact [12]. However, even a partial knockdown of Fgf10, as in $IIIc^{+/\Delta}$; $Fgf10^{+/-}$ mice, can lead to a rescue of craniosynostosis and this dramatic observation supports the notion that the development and possibly the pathogenic fusion of craniofacial sutures occurs in a morphogen-like manner, where the bioavailability of ligands is one way in which FGFR signaling is regulated in the sutures.

A similar strategy can be used to definitively identify the IIIc-activating ligand/s that – besides Fgf18 – may contribute to the net gain-of-FGFR2 function in $IIIc^{+/\Delta}$ or $FgfR2^{+/S252W}$ coronal sutures. Fgf2 would be a strong candidate. It is expressed in these sutures [8]; application of excess FGF2 results in coronal fusion [64] and targeted disruption of Fgf2 in mice neither retards nor accelerates coronal suture development [65].

All Gain or Some Loss?

Accumulating evidence is challenging the view that a gain-of-FGFR2 function underlies *all* of the phenotypes observed in Apert, Pfeiffer and Crouzon syndromes, or indeed is the consequence of all such mutations. Some may result from loss-of-FGFR2 function, either directly, or as a secondary consequence of the gain-of-FGFR function.

The more direct effect is exemplified by the Crouzon FGFR2 C342Y and C278F mutations, which lack a cysteine residue in the extracellular IgIII domain, and unlike the Apert or Pfeiffer mutations, undergo ligand-independent receptor dimerization [66]. Recent biochemical data show that the Crouzon-type autophosphorylation occurs both in cell surface-bound mutant receptors and during their passage through the ER compartment. In addition, Crouzon-type FGFR2 molecules fail to undergo proper N-glycosylation within the ER compartment [67]. A combination of these two effects is thought to destine a significant proportion of mutant receptors for degradation within the proteosomes, in a cell type-dependent manner [67]. The net effect of this perturbed receptor trafficking would be dramatically reduced or complete loss-of-FGFR2 function in osteoblasts, leading to their premature differentiation and hence craniosynostosis. Indeed, craniosynostosis can also result from loss-of-FgfR2 function, as observed in FgfR2-IIIc$^{-/-}$ mice [7].

Our own preliminary observations have raised the possibility that some phenotypes in Apert syndrome may arise from loss-of-FGFR2 function in the epithelial compartment, secondary to a gain-of-FgfR2 function in mesenchymal cells. Cleft palate is an example.

IIIc$^{+/\Delta}$ mice (described above) show a mild delay in the fusion of palatine shelves. However, when the Fgf10 gene dosage is halved in this background, i.e. in IIIc$^{+/\Delta}$; Fgf10$^{+/-}$ double mutant mice, a significant number develop full cleft palate. This phenotype cannot be due to loss of FgfR2-IIIc per se in mesenchyme, because it is not observed in FgfR2-IIIc$^{-/-}$ mice [7]. Yet, invariably, cleft palate does occur in mice that lack FgfR2-IIIb or its ligand Fgf10 [30, 68].

The molecular basis of gain-of-FgfR2 function in IIIc$^{+/\Delta}$ mice is the ectopic expression of FgfR2-IIIb in the mesenchyme, the receptor for Fgf10, and in principle this ectopic receptor could compete with the epithelially-expressed FGFR2-IIIb, for limited amounts of Fgf10 (fig. 4b). This may be of little consequence when Fgf10 is at 'saturating' levels in IIIc$^{+/\Delta}$ mice (i.e. IIIc$^{+/\Delta}$; Fgf10$^{+/+}$). However, when this competition is accentuated by lowering the Fgf10 gene dosage in IIIc$^{+/\Delta}$; Fgf10$^{+/-}$ mice, occasionally this competition may deprive the epithelial FgfR2-IIIb from Fgf10 and in effect yield a Fgf10$^{-/-}$ or FgfR2-IIIb$^{-/-}$-like phenotype, such as cleft palate.

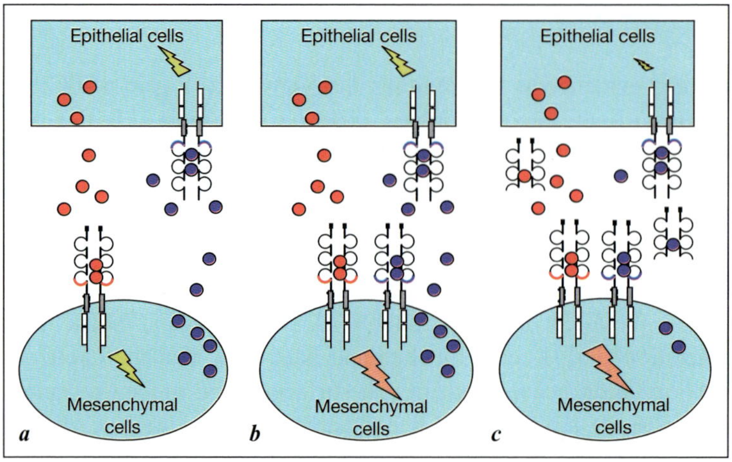

Fig. 4. Impact of Apert-like mutations on FgfR2 signaling within mesenchymal and epithelial cells. ***a*** Normal epithelial and mesenchymal cell interactions rely on the mutually exclusive expression of FgfR2-IIIb (blue) and IIIc (red) isoforms, together with their respective activating ligands (blue and red circles). This results in a particular level of FgfR2 signaling in each compartment (yellow sparks). ***b*** Apert mutations work primarily by raising the level of FgfR2 signaling in mesenchymal cells (orange sparks) – either through the aberrant interaction of mutant receptors with inappropriate ligands or through the upregulation of FgfR2-IIIb in this tissue compartment. ***c*** Mutant receptors may enter a competition with epithelially expressed FgfR2-IIIb for its activating ligands, which may result in reduced or loss of FgfR2-IIIb signaling in epithelial cells. Truncated receptors such as IIIa-TM may also participate in this competition.

Two independent lines of FgfR2$^{+/S252W}$ mutant mice have been generated, but only one of these lines develops a mild palatal defect. In Apert patients, cleft palate is associated more with the FGFR2$^{+/S252W}$ mutation but is not observed in all such individuals [58]. These variations could be explained in terms of the genetic background in which an Apert syndrome mutation finds itself, or possibly the way a gain-of-FgfR2 function affects the level of expression of Fgf10 or its related ligands in the mesenchyme (fig. 4c). Future work will help resolve these postulated relationships and differences.

A third mechanism through which a partial loss-of-FGFR2 function may arise in Apert and/or Pfeiffer syndrome patients is the upregulation/stabilization of soluble FGFR isoforms. Both IIIc$^{+/\Delta}$ mice [57] and some mutant-FGFR2-bearing Pfeiffer patients, additionally harbor an exon 8 (IIIa) to exon 10 (TM) spliced transcript [69, 70]. This aberrant splicing introduces a frame shift mutation and a premature termination codon (PTC) in exon 10, and so the translated product would be a soluble FGFR2 receptor, composed of Ig domains I, II and IIIa, fused to the first 3 amino acids of TM domain (fig. 2a). This transcript is not detected in wild-type mice or normal individuals, possibly because as a PTC-bearing molecule it would be destroyed by the nonsense-mediated decay pathway [71]. We have termed this molecule IIIa-TM and in recent work have discovered that when overexpressed, it can bind FGF ligands and attenuate FGF signaling in vitro and in vivo [Wheldon et al., unpubl. data]. The exact level of contribution of IIIa-TM to Apert/Pfeiffer-like phenotypes remains to be determined. Nonetheless, these findings warrant a detailed examination of the range of splice variants that may be upregulated in these patients.

Concluding Remarks

Much of what we know about the role of FGF signaling in the development of the mammalian craniofacial skeleton is derived from studying Apert, Crouzon and Pfeiffer craniosynostosis syndromes. Mouse models have, and will continue to make a significant contribution to this understanding. The emerging view is that a given FGFR mutation impacts different parts of the craniofacial skeleton in different ways. The future challenge is to understand the molecular basis of these differences. In due course, we are likely to learn more about the complexity of FGFR signaling itself and come up with strategies that can help alleviate distinct phenotypes associated with these congenital syndromes.

References

1 Lajeunie E, Ma HW, Bonaventure J, Munnich A, Le Merrer M, Renier D: FGFR2 mutations in Pfeiffer syndrome. Nat Genet 1995;9:108.

2 Muenke M, Schell U, Hehr A, Robin NH, Losken HW, Schinzel A, Pulleyn LJ, Rutland P, Reardon W, Malcolm S, et al: A common mutation in the fibroblast growth factor receptor 1 gene in Pfeiffer syndrome. Nat Genet 1994;8:269–274.

3 Ornitz DM, Marie PJ: FGF signaling pathways in endochondral and intramembranous bone development and human genetic disease. Genes Dev 2002;16:1446–1465.

4 Wilkie AO: Bad bones, absent smell, selfish testes: the pleiotropic consequences of human FGF receptor mutations. Cytokine Growth Factor Rev 2005;16:187–203.

5 Cohen MM Jr, Kreiborg S: An updated pediatric perspective on the Apert syndrome. Am J Dis Child 1993;147:989–993.

6 Cohen MM Jr, Kreiborg S: Visceral anomalies in the Apert syndrome. Am J Med Genet 1993;45:758–760.

7 Eswarakumar VP, Monsonego-Ornan E, Pines M, Antonopoulou I, Morriss-Kay GM, Lonai P: The IIIc alternative of Fgfr2 is a positive regulator of bone formation. Development 2002;129: 3783–3793.

8 Hajihosseini MK, Heath JK: Expression patterns of fibroblast growth factors-18 and -20 in mouse embryos is suggestive of novel roles in calvarial and limb development. Mech Dev 2002;113: 79–83.

9 Liu Z, Xu J, Colvin JS, Ornitz DM: Coordination of chondrogenesis and osteogenesis by fibroblast growth factor 18. Genes Dev 2002;16:859–869.
10 Ohbayashi N, Shibayama M, Kurotaki Y, Imanishi M, Fujimori T, Itoh N, Takada S: FGF18 is required for normal cell proliferation and differentiation during osteogenesis and chondrogenesis. Genes Dev 2002;16:870–879.
11 Anderson J, Burns HD, Enriquez-Harris P, Wilkie AO, Heath JK: Apert syndrome mutations in fibroblast growth factor receptor 2 exhibit increased affinity for FGF ligand. Hum Mol Genet 1998;7:1475–1483.
12 Ibrahimi OA, Zhang F, Eliseenkova AV, Itoh N, Linhardt RJ, Mohammadi M: Biochemical analysis of pathogenic ligand-dependent FGFR2 mutations suggests distinct pathophysiological mechanisms for craniofacial and limb abnormalities. Hum Mol Genet 2004;13: 2313–2324.
13 Yu K, Herr AB, Waksman G, Ornitz DM: Loss of fibroblast growth factor receptor 2 ligand-binding specificity in Apert syndrome. Proc Natl Acad Sci USA 2000;97:14536–14541.
14 Lemonnier J, Hay E, Delannoy P, Fromigue O, Lomri A, Modrowski D, Marie PJ: Increased osteoblast apoptosis in apert craniosynostosis: role of protein kinase C and interleukin-1. Am J Pathol 2001;158:1833–1842.
15 Mansukhani A, Bellosta P, Sahni M, Basilico C: Signaling by fibroblast growth factors (FGF) and fibroblast growth factor receptor 2 (FGFR2)-activating mutations blocks mineralization and induces apoptosis in osteoblasts. J Cell Biol 2000;149:1297–1308.
16 Nie X, Luukko K, Kettunen P: FGF signalling in craniofacial development and developmental disorders. Oral Dis 2006;12:102–111.
17 Ornitz DM, Itoh N: Fibroblast growth factors. Genome Biol 2001;2:3005.
18 Lou JY, Laezza F, Gerber BR, Xiao M, Yamada KA, Hartmann H, Craig AM, Nerbonne JM, Ornitz DM: Fibroblast growth factor 14 is an intracellular modulator of voltage-gated sodium channels. J Physiol 2005;569:179–193.
19 Olsen SK, Garbi M, Zampieri N, Eliseenkova AV, Ornitz DM, Goldfarb M, Mohammadi M: Fibroblast growth factor (FGF) homologous factors share structural but not functional homology with FGFs. J Biol Chem 2003;278:34226–34236.
20 Sleeman M, Fraser J, McDonald M, Yuan S, White D, Grandison P, Kumble K, Watson JD, Murison JG: Identification of a new fibroblast growth factor receptor, FGFR5. Gene 2001;271: 171–182.
21 McKeehan WL, Wang F, Kan M: The heparan sulfate-fibroblast growth factor family: diversity of structure and function. Prog Nucleic Acid Res Mol Biol 1998;59:135–176.
22 Eswarakumar VP, Lax I, Schlessinger J: Cellular signaling by fibroblast growth factor receptors. Cytokine Growth Factor Rev 2005;16:139–149.
23 Thisse B, Thisse C: Functions and regulations of fibroblast growth factor signaling during embryonic development. Dev Biol 2005;287:390–402.
24 Tsang M, Dawid IB: Promotion and attenuation of FGF signaling through the Ras-MAPK pathway. Sci STKE 2004;2004:pe17.
25 Burgar HR, Burns HD, Elsden JL, Lalioti MD, Heath JK: Association of the signaling adaptor FRS2 with fibroblast growth factor receptor 1 (Fgfr1) is mediated by alternative splicing of the juxtamembrane domain. J Biol Chem 2002;277:4018–4023.
26 Miki T, Bottaro DP, Fleming TP, Smith CL, Burgess WH, Chan AM, Aaronson SA: Determination of ligand-binding specificity by alternative splicing: two distinct growth factor receptors encoded by a single gene. Proc Natl Acad Sci USA 1992;89:246–250.
27 Orr-Urtreger A, Bedford MT, Burakova T, Arman E, Zimmer Y, Yayon A, Givol D, Lonai P: Developmental localization of the splicing alternatives of fibroblast growth factor receptor-2 (FGFR2). Dev Biol 1993;158:475–486.
28 Peters KG, Werner S, Chen G, Williams LT: Two FGF receptor genes are differentially expressed in epithelial and mesenchymal tissues during limb formation and organogenesis in the mouse. Development 1992;114:233–243.
29 Zhang X, Ibrahimi OA, Olsen SK, Umemori H, Mohammadi M, Ornitz DM: Receptor specificity of the fibroblast growth factor family. The complete mammalian FGF family. J Biol Chem 2006;281:15694–15700.

30 De Moerlooze L, Spencer-Dene B, Revest J, Hajihosseini M, Rosewell I, Dickson C: An important role for the IIIb isoform of fibroblast growth factor receptor 2 (FGFR2) in mesenchymal-epithelial signalling during mouse organogenesis. Development 2000;127: 483–492.
31 Rice DP, Rice R, Thesleff I: Fgfr mRNA isoforms in craniofacial bone development. Bone 2003;33:14–27.
32 Min H, Danilenko DM, Scully SA, Bolon B, Ring BD, Tarpley JE, DeRose M, Simonet WS: Fgf-10 is required for both limb and lung development and exhibits striking functional similarity to Drosophila branchless. Genes Dev 1998;12:3156–3161.
33 Carlton MB, Colledge WH, Evans MJ: Crouzon-like craniofacial dysmorphology in the mouse is caused by an insertional mutation at the Fgf3/Fgf4 locus. Dev Dyn 1998;212:242–249.
34 Meyers EN, Lewandoski M, Martin GR: An Fgf8 mutant allelic series generated by Cre- and Flp-mediated recombination. Nat Genet 1998;18:136–141.
35 Partanen J, Schwartz L, Rossant J: Opposite phenotypes of hypomorphic and Y766 phosphorylation site mutations reveal a function for Fgfr1 in anteroposterior patterning of mouse embryos. Genes Dev 1998;12: 2332–2344.
36 Delfini MC, Dubrulle J, Malapert P, Chal J, and Pourquie O: Control of the segmentation process by graded MAPK/ERK activation in the chick embryo. Proc Natl Acad Sci USA 2005;102: 11343–11348.
37 Hajihosseini MK, Lalioti MD, Arthaud S, Burgar HR, Brown JM, Twigg SR, Wilkie AO, Heath JK: Skeletal development is regulated by fibroblast growth factor receptor 1 signalling dynamics. Development 2004;131:325–335.
38 Gajecka M, Yu W, Ballif BC, Glotzbach CD, Bailey KA, Shaw CA, Kashork CD Heilstedt HA, Ansel DA, Theisen A, Rice R, Rice DP, Shaffer LG: Delineation of mechanisms and regions of dosage imbalance in complex rearrangements of 1p36 leads to a putative gene for regulation of cranial suture closure. Eur J Hum Genet 2005;13:139–149.
39 Peduto L, Reuter VE, Shaffer DR, Scher HI, Blobel CP: Critical function for ADAM9 in mouse prostate cancer. Cancer Res 2005;65: 9312–9319.
40 Bafico A, Gazit A, Pramila T, Finch PW, Yaniv A, Aaronson SA: Interaction of frizzled related protein (FRP) with Wnt ligands and the frizzled receptor suggests alternative mechanisms for FRP inhibition of Wnt signaling. J Biol Chem 1999;274:16180–16187.
41 Canalis E, Economides AN, Gazzerro E: Bone morphogenetic proteins, their antagonists, and the skeleton. Endocr Rev 2003;24:218–235.
42 Klein DE, Nappi VM, Reeves GT, Shvartsman SY, Lemmon MA: Argos inhibits epidermal growth factor receptor signalling by ligand sequestration. Nature 2004;430:1040–1044.
43 Warren SM, Brunet LJ, Harland RM, Economides AN, Longaker MT: The BMP antagonist noggin regulates cranial suture fusion. Nature 2003;422: 625–629.
44 He X, Semenov M, Tamai K, Zeng X: LDL receptor-related proteins 5 and 6 in Wnt/beta-catenin signaling: arrows point the way. Development 2004;131:1663–1677.
45 Gonzalez-Martinez D, Kim SH, Hu Y, Guimond S, Schofield J, Winyard P, Vannelli GB, Turnbull J, Bouloux PM: Anosmin-1 modulates fibroblast growth factor receptor 1 signaling in human gonadotropin-releasing hormone olfactory neuroblasts through a heparan sulfate-dependent mechanism. J Neurosci 2004;24:10384–10392.
46 Hirate Y, Okamoto H: Canopy1, a novel regulator of FGF signaling around the midbrain-hindbrain boundary in zebrafish. Curr Biol 2006;16:421–427.
47 Yamamoto A, Nagano T, Takehara S, Hibi M, Aizawa S: Shisa promotes head formation through the inhibition of receptor protein maturation for the caudalizing factors, Wnt and FGF. Cell 2005; 120:223–235.
48 Eblaghie MC, Lunn JS, Dickinson RJ, Munsterberg AE, Sanz-Ezquerro JJ, Farrell ER, Mathers J, Keyse SM, Storey K, Tickle C: Negative feedback regulation of FGF signaling levels by Pyst1/MKP3 in chick embryos. Curr Biol 2003;13:1009–1018.
49 Furthauer M, Lin W, Ang SL, Thisse B, Thisse C: Sef is a feedback-induced antagonist of Ras/MAPK-mediated FGF signalling. Nat Cell Biol 2002;4:170–174.
50 Kawakami Y, Rodriguez-Leon J, Koth CM, Buscher D, Itoh T, Raya A, Ng JK, Esteban CR, Takahashi S, Henrique D, Schwarz MF, Asahara H, Izpisua Belmonte JC: MKP3 mediates the cellular response to FGF8 signalling in the vertebrate limb. Nat Cell Biol 2003;5:513–519.

51 Tsang M, Friesel R, Kudoh T, and Dawid IB, et al: Identification of Sef, a novel modulator of FGF signalling. Nat Cell Biol 2002;4:165–169.
52 Zhou B, Wang ZX, Zhao Y, Brautigan DL, Zhang ZY: The specificity of extracellular signal-regulated kinase 2 dephosphorylation by protein phosphatases. J Biol Chem 2002;277:31818–31825.
53 Lax I, Wong A, Lamothe B, Lee A, Frost A, Hawes J, Schlessinger J: The docking protein FRS2alpha controls a MAP kinase-mediated negative feedback mechanism for signaling by FGF receptors. Mol Cell 2002;10:709–719.
54 Basson MA, Watson-Johnson J, Shakya R, Akbulut S, Hyink D, Costantini FD, Wilson PD, Mason IJ, Licht JD: Branching morphogenesis of the ureteric epithelium during kidney development is coordinated by the opposing functions of GDNF and Sprouty1. Dev Biol 2006;299:466–477.
55 Bottcher RT, Pollet N, Delius H, Niehrs C: The transmembrane protein XFLRT3 forms a complex with FGF receptors and promotes FGF signalling. Nat Cell Biol 2004;6:38–44.
56 Karaulanov EE, Bottcher RT, Niehrs C: A role for fibronectin-leucine-rich transmembrane cell-surface proteins in homotypic cell adhesion. EMBO Rep 2006;7:283–290.
57 Hajihosseini MK, Wilson S, De Moerlooze, Dickson C: A splicing switch and gain-of-function mutation in FgfR2-IIIc hemizygotes causes Apert/Pfeiffer-syndrome-like phenotypes. Proc Natl Acad Sci USA 2001;98:3855–3860.
58 Oldridge M, Zackai EH, McDonald-McGinn DM, Iseki S, Morriss-Kay GM Twigg SR, Johnson D, Wall SA, Jiang W, Theda C, Jabs EW, Wilkie AO: De novo alu-element insertions in FGFR2 identify a distinct pathological basis for Apert syndrome. Am J Hum Genet 1999;64: 446–461.
59 Chen L, Li D, Li C, Engel A, Deng CX: A Ser250Trp substitution in mouse fibroblast growth factor receptor 2 (Fgfr2) results in craniosynostosis. Bone 2003;33:169–178.
60 Wang Y, Xiao R, Yang F, Karim BO, Iacovelli AJ, Cai J, Lerner CP, Richtsmeier JT, Leszl JM, Hill CA, Yu K, Ornitz DM, Elisseeff J, Huso DL, Jabs EW: Abnormalities in cartilage and bone development in the Apert syndrome FGFR2+/S252W mouse. Development 2005;132:3537–3548.
61 Govindarajan V, Overbeek PA: FGF9 can induce endochondral ossification in cranial mesenchyme. BMC Dev Biol 2006;6:7.
62 De Langhe SP, Carraro, G Warburton D, Hajihosseini MK, Bellusci S: Levels of mesenchymal FGFR2 signaling modulate smooth muscle progenitor cell commitment in the lung. Dev Biol 2006;299:52–62.
63 Liu B, Yu HM, Hsu W: Craniosynostosis caused by Axin2 deficiency is mediated through distinct functions of beta-catenin in proliferation and differentiation. Dev Biol 2007;30:298–308.
64 Iseki S, Wilkie AO, Morriss-Kay GM: Fgfr1 and Fgfr2 have distinct differentiation- and proliferation-related roles in the developing mouse skull vault. Development 1999;126:5611–5620.
65 Dono R, Faulhaber J, Galli A, Zuniga A, Volk T, Texido G, Zeller R, Ehmke H: FGF2 signaling is required for the development of neuronal circuits regulating blood pressure. Circ Res 2002;90: E5–E10.
66 Mangasarian K, Li Y, Mansukhani A, Basilico C: Mutation associated with Crouzon syndrome causes ligand-independent dimerization and activation of FGF receptor-2. J Cell Physiol 1997; 172:117–125.
67 Hatch NE, Hudson M, Seto ML, Cunningham ML, Bothwell M: Intracellular retention, degradation, and signaling of glycosylation-deficient FGFR2 and craniosynostosis syndrome-associated FGFR2C278F. J Biol Chem 2006;281: 27292–27305.
68 Rice R, Spencer-Dene B, Connor EC, Gritli-Linde A, McMahon AP, Dickson C, Thesleff I, Rice DP: Disruption of Fgf10/Fgfr2b-coordinated epithelial-mesenchymal interactions causes cleft palate. J Clin Invest 2004;113:1692–1700.
69 Tsukuno M, Suzuki H, Eto Y: Pfeiffer syndrome caused by haploinsufficient mutation of FGFR2. J Craniofac Genet Dev Biol 1999;19:183–188.
70 Wilkie AO: Abnormal spliceform expression associated with splice acceptor mutations in exon IIIc of FGFR2. Am J Med Genet 2002;111:105.
71 Maquat LE: Nonsense-mediated mRNA decay in mammals. J Cell Sci 2005;118:1773–1776.
72 Asai Y, Chan DK, Starr CJ, Kappler JA, Kollmar R, Hudspeth AJ: Mutation of the atrophin2 gene in the zebrafish disrupts signaling by fibroblast growth factor during development of the inner ear. Proc Natl Acad Sci USA 2006;103:9069–9074.

73 Amrein L, Barraud P, Daniel JY, Perel Y, Landry M: Expression patterns of nm23 genes during mouse organogenesis. Cell Tissue Res 2005;322:365–378.
74 Dammai V, Adryan B, Lavenburg KR, Hsu T: Drosophila awd, the homolog of human nm23, regulates FGF receptor levels and functions synergistically with shi/dynamin during tracheal development. Genes Dev 2003;17: 2812–2824.
75 Haines BP, Wheldon LM, Summerbell D, Heath JK, Rigby PW: Regulated expression of FLRT genes implies a functional role in the regulation of FGF signalling during mouse development. Dev Biol 2006;297:14–25.
76 Dickinson RJ, Eblaghie MC, Keyse SM, Morriss-Kay GM: Expression of the ERK-specific MAP kinase phosphatase PYST1/MKP3 in mouse embryos during morphogenesis and early organogenesis. Mech Dev 2002;113:193–196.
77 Filipe M, Goncalves L, Bento M, Silva AC, Belo JA: Comparative expression of mouse and chicken Shisa homologues during early development. Dev Dyn 2006;235:2567–2573.
78 Kovalenko D, Yang X, Chen PY, Nadeau RJ, Zubanova O, Pigeon K, Friesel R: A role for extracellular and transmembrane domains of Sef in Sef-mediated inhibition of FGF signaling. Cell Signal 2006;18:1958–1966.
79 Hacohen N, Kramer S, Sutherland D, Hiromi Y, Krasnow MA: sprouty encodes a novel antagonist of FGF signaling that patterns apical branching of the Drosophila airways. Cell 1998;92:253–263.
80 Mason JM, Morrison DJ, Basson MA, Licht JD: Sprouty proteins: multifaceted negative-feedback regulators of receptor tyrosine kinase signaling. Trends Cell Biol 2006;16:45–54.
81 Eswarakumar VP, Horowitz MC, Locklin R, Morriss-Kay GM, Lonai P: A gain-of-function mutation of Fgfr2c demonstrates the roles of this receptor variant in osteogenesis. Proc Natl Acad Sci USA 2004;101:12555–12560.
82 Zhou YX, Xu X, Chen L, Li C, Brodie SG, Deng CX: A Pro250Arg substitution in mouse Fgfr1 causes increased expression of Cbfa1 and premature fusion of calvarial sutures. Hum Mol Genet 2000;9:2001–2008.

Dr. Mohammad K. Hajihosseini
School of Biological Sciences, University of East Anglia
Norwich NR4 7TJ (UK)
Tel. +44 1603 591318, Fax +44 1603 592250, E-Mail m.k.h@uea.ac.uk

Rice DP (ed): Craniofacial Sutures. Development, Disease and Treatment.
Front Oral Biol. Basel, Karger, 2008, vol 12, pp 178–196

Tgf-β Regulation of Suture Morphogenesis and Growth

Joseph T. Rawlins, Lynne A. Opperman

Department of Biomedical Sciences, Baylor College of Dentistry, Texas A&M Health Science Center, Dallas, Tex., USA

Abstract

Premature suture obliteration results in an inability of cranial and facial bones to grow, with resulting craniofacial dysmorphology requiring surgical correction. Understanding the biological signaling associated with suture morphogenesis will enable less invasive treatment of patients with fused sutures, combined with therapy using biological molecules. While a number of advances have been made in identifying the genetic etiologies of various craniosynostotic syndromes, the pathogenesis of this condition is still not completely understood. Recently, it has been shown that differential expression of various transforming growth factor-β (Tgf-β) isoforms plays a crucial role in regulating suture patency once the sutures have formed. It has also been shown that differential expression of Tgf-β isoforms may also play a role in craniosynostosis by altering proliferation, differentiation, and apoptosis within the suture. This chapter focuses on the role of Tgf-β in suture morphogenesis and growth, exploring Tgf-β biology, receptors, signaling pathways, animal models, and expression in both normal and pathological sutures.

Introduction

Cranial suture morphogenesis is a lengthy developmental process initiated during early embryogenesis and completed upon fusion of adjacent bones during adulthood. Abnormal suture development can evolve from several possible causes. Failure of bone fronts to approximate one another will result in the absence of suture formation and wide-open fontanels, such as seen in cleidocranial dysplasia. Bony obliteration of the suture site can also result from an inability of bone fronts to appropriately overlap or butt up against one another during early suture formation. Lastly, an inability to sustain a suture once it is formed will result in premature osseous obliteration of the suture site.

There are several craniofacial pathologies with abnormal cranial suture biology. These pathologies can result from either prematurely obliterated sutures or as wide-open midline defects and are known to be associated with several genetic mutations. Known mutations include various regions of the *fibroblast growth factor (FGF) receptor* genes and a variety of transcription factors which include *MSX2, TWIST*, and *RUNX2*. The extent of these mutations and resulting sutural defects has been addressed extensively in other chapters.

Growth factors such as transforming growth factor beta (Tgf-β), Fgfs, and bone morphogenic proteins (Bmps) are known to be involved in cranial suture morphogenesis [1–4]. In response to extracellular signals, growth factors are manufactured by cells and normally secreted in an inactive propeptide form associated with a latency binding protein. The growth factors remain in the local environment, bind to their associated receptors, trigger an intracellular signaling cascade, and increase transcriptional activity. This chapter will focus on the role of Tgf-βs in cranial suture morphogenesis and growth.

Tgf-β Biology

The Tgf-β superfamily consists of a large family of structurally related polypeptide growth factors. Based on structural and functional criteria, these can be divided into two main groups: the Tgf-β/activin and Bmp/growth and differentiation factor (Gdf) branches [5]. Five distinct Tgf-β genes have been identified in vertebrates and three of these (Tgf-β1, Tgf-β2, and Tgf-β3) are expressed in mammals. Each of the three isoforms has been highly conserved throughout evolution, suggesting specific developmental roles for each [6, 7]. Family members are involved in many key areas of growth and development, including cell proliferation, organization, differentiation, motility, and death. Cranial suture research has focused primarily on the effects of the three mammalian isoforms – Tgf-β1, Tgf-β2, and Tgf-β3 – along with Bmps on suture morphogenesis and growth. In sutures, each isoform is differentially expressed at various stages of development and binds with different affinities to their receptors [4, 8]. Recently, mutations in the human TGF-β type 1 (TGFBRI) and type 2 (TGFBRII) receptors were shown to phenotypically resemble marfanoid craniosynostosis syndrome [9]. However, no mutations in the three TGF-β isoforms present in humans have been described that present cranial suture abnormalities in humans. There is good evidence that Tgf-β1, Tgf-β2, and Tgf-β3 play crucial roles in regulating suture patency once the sutures have formed.

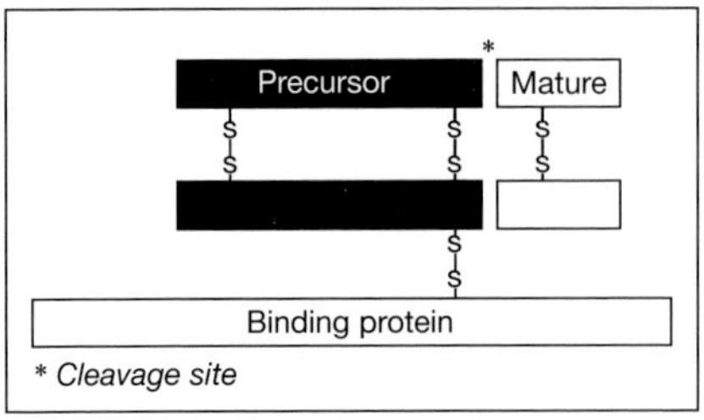

Fig. 1. Diagram of Tgf-β bound to its latency binding protein. Latent Tgf-β is a homodimer that consists of a mature Tgf-β noncovalently associated with a precursor or latency-associated peptide (LAP), which in turn is linked by a disulfide linkage to a latent Tgf-β binding protein (Ltbp). Ltbp has no covalent linkage with mature Tgf-β and is not needed to confer latency on the complex [modified from 69]. * = Cleavage site for activating Tgf-β.

Tgf-β1, Tgf-β2, and Tgf-β3 are 25-kDa homodimeric polypeptides, exhibit 70–82% sequence identity, and transduce their signals by binding and bringing together TgfbrI and TgfbrII. Most of the work in animal models and cell culture regarding Tgf-β secretion and latency binding proteins has been done using the Tgf-β1 isoform. However, it is likely that similar mechanisms apply to all three isoforms. Cells secrete Tgf-β as a 290-kD high-molecular-mass latent Tgf-β complex that contains a 190-kD latent Tgf-β binding protein (Ltbp) linked by a disulfide bridge to the Tgf-β precursor [10–12] (fig. 1). However, bone cells are unique in that at least 50% of their latent Tgf-β is secreted as a 100-kD latent complex that lacks Ltbp and consists only of the mature 25-kD Tgf-β homodimer noncovalently associated with a 70-kD precursor homodimer known as latency-associated protein (Lap). The absence of Ltbp may help to segregate secreted Tgf-β into free pools available for activation, and Ltbp-bound Tgf-β may be destined for bone matrix storage [13].

Release of Tgf-β from latent complexes is thought to involve changes in the balance of several components of the plasmin activation system, and the extent to which plasmin activity is maintained may be controlled by the amount of active Tgf-β [14]. After release from inactive complexes or from the bone matrix, intact Tgf-β dimers are active, and induce their biological effects by binding to cell surface receptors.

Tgf-β Receptors

The Tgf-β superfamily members have several different cell surface receptors. These receptors have a characteristic three-finger toxin fold in the ligand-binding extracellular domain, a single transmembrane domain, and an intracellular serine-threonine kinase domain [5]. The receptors are divided into two groups, designated as type I and type II receptors. There are multiple subgroups within these two receptor types that vary due to sequence variations and dominant ligand interactions. Traditionally, Tgf-βs bind to the constitutively active TgfbrII, which then recruits the TgfbrI. This results in the transphosphorylation of the TgfbrI receptor and activation of downstream signaling cascades [5].

Other cell surface proteins interact with Tgf-β and may be required in addition to the traditional TgfbrI/TgfbrII-ligand interactions. The most abundant cell surface Tgf-β binding protein in many cell types is betaglycan or type III Tgf-β receptor (TgfbrIII). TgfbrIII is a transmembrane protein that is heavily glycosylated and has a large extracellular domain and short cytoplasmic tail that lacks kinase activity. Initially, it was believed that TgfbrIII was mostly involved in concentrating Tgf-β ligand before presentation of the ligand to the signaling receptors TgfbrI and TgfbrII [15]. Recent data suggests that the cytoplasmic tail of TgfbrIII is required to support Tgf-β2 signaling but is not required to promote binding of Tgf-β2 to the signaling receptor complex [16]. This finding leads to the suggestion that TgfbrIII plays an additional role in the regulation of Tgf-β signaling to the traditional growth factor presentation role [16].

The presence of Tgf-βs and their receptors was first described in bone cells derived from fetal rat calvaria [17]. Changes in TgfbrI and TgfbrII immunoreactivity were noted in actively fusing rat posterior interfrontal sutures when compared with fully mature nonfusing sagittal sutures [18]. Moreover, the numbers of TgfbrI-expressing osteoblasts and osteocytes in the bone fronts lining fusing sutures increased compared to nonfusing sutures, while addition of Tgf-β3 to calvaria in culture decreased the number of TgfbrI-expressing cells during rescue of sutures from obliteration [19]. One mechanism by which Tgf-βs may regulate suture patency is by regulating tissue responsiveness to other Tgf-β family members by regulating their access to receptors. Tgf-β2 and Tgf-β3 use the same cell surface receptors yet have opposite effects on suture patency, cellular proliferation, and apoptosis within the suture [20]. Since Tgf-β3 rescue of sutures is accompanied by a decrease in TgfbrI-expressing cells, one mechanism by which Tgf-β3 might promote suture patency could be by decreasing the number of TgfbrI accessible to Tgf-β2.

Conditional knockout mice for *Tgfbr2* show complete cleft secondary palate, calvaria agenesis, and other skull defects [21]. The cleft palate in these *Tgfbr2* knockouts results from a cell proliferation defect within the palatal mesenchyme. Similarly during skull development, disruption of Tgf-β signaling in the cranial neural crest cells severely impairs cell proliferation in the dura mater, consequently resulting in calvaria agenesis [21]. Additionally, Loeys et al. [9] recently showed that heterozygous mutations in TGFBRI and TGFBRII result in altered craniofacial and skeletal development that resembles marfanoid craniosynostosis syndrome.

Intracellular Signaling

Tgf-β signal transduction has been studied extensively in many cell types. However, intracellular signaling pathways downstream of Tgf-β receptors have not been well studied in craniofacial suture development and maintenance. As discussed in the previous section, Tgf-β family members bind to TgfbrII serine/threonine kinase receptors, followed by heteromeric binding with TgfbrI [5]. This association of TgfbrI with TgfbrII results in the phosphorylation of TgfbrI by TgfbrII, resulting in receptor activation and the transduction of downstream signals through a variety of transcription factor phosphorylation events. The major Tgf-β signaling pathway involves several Smad proteins (the name is derived from the homologous *Drosophila* gene *mad*, which stands for 'mothers against decapentaplegic').

There are three types of Smad proteins: common partner Smads (Co-Smads), receptor-regulated Smads (R-Smads), and inhibitory Smads (I-Smads). Two main groups of R-Smads are activated by different sets of type I receptors and activate distinct downstream responses [22]. These include Bmp receptor-activated Smad1, Smad5, and Smad8, and the Tgf-β/activin-activated Smads, Smad2 and Smad3 [22, 23]. As soon as the R-Smads are phosphorylated as a result of activation of the cell surface receptor, they form a complex with the Co-Smad, Smad4. The R-Smad/Smad4 complex then translocates to the nucleus and binds DNA directly or indirectly to regulate transcription of a variety of different gene targets to regulate proliferation, differentiation, and apoptosis in the suture.

Much of what is known about Tgf-β signaling in craniofacial sutures is based on experiments in other cell types. However, it is known that Tgf-β2 and Tgf-β3 use the serine/threonine kinase Smad2/Smad3 signaling pathway [17, 22]. Smad3 appears to be important for regulating the mucosal immune response, while Smad2 has been associated with craniofacial development [24]. If Smads have differential roles for regulating the way different tissues respond to Tgf-β signaling, then it is possible that other signaling pathways are required for differential responses to Tgf-β1, Tgf-β2, and Tgf-β3 by the same tissues.

Given the critical role of the Tgf-β signaling pathway in controlling diverse cellular functions, it should be of little surprise that additional intracellular regulatory mechanisms for Tgf-β exist. There is now substantial evidence that Tgf-β family members, – both Tgf-βs and Bmps – also signal via tyrosine kinase mitogen-activated protein kinase (Mapk) pathways. This signaling can occur in both Smad-dependent and Smad-independent ways. For Smad-dependent signaling, Smads can be either upstream or downstream of the Mapk pathways. For example, Yu et al. [25] showed that Tgf-β1 phosphorylated Smad1 downstream of signaling via the Ras/Mek pathway, while Tgf-β1 activation of Atf2 was upstream of and dependent on Smad4 activation of p38 [26]. Furthermore, Erk1/2 and p38 were shown to differentially regulate Bmp2- and Tgf-β1-mediated osteoblast function in a Smad4-dependent fashion [27]. In Smad-independent signaling Tgf-β was shown to activate Jnk signaling via a Rho-dependent pathway to activate AP-1 [28], c-Jun, and Atf-2 function [29, 30], and mobilization of the actin cytoskeleton [31]. This Smad-independent signaling was also found to be pathway specific in that Bmp2-induced apoptosis was PKC-dependent, but PKA-, p38- and Erk/Mek-independent [32].

While Smad2 but not Smad3 has been shown to be required for early craniofacial development [24], the signaling pathways required for Tgf-β2 regulation of later events such as suture development and growth are unclear. As described earlier, alterations in TGFBRII signaling induced by gene mutations has been associated with cranial suture defects [9], and several pathways could be responsible for transducing the signal initiated by Tgf-β2 binding to this receptor. Erk1/2 signaling has been shown to be critical for normal expression of the osteoblast phenotype [27]. The Erk1/2 pathway is central to signaling by growth factors such as Egf and Fgf, the former which requires Erk1/2 signaling to inhibit palatal closure [33, 34]. The Erk1/2 pathway is also critical for Fgf2-stimulated premature cranial suture closure, as blocking Erk1/2 phosphorylation prevents Fgf2-induced suture closure [35]. Recent data demonstrates that Tgf-β2-induced suture closure also occurs via an Erk1/2-dependent signaling pathway [36]. Using a calvarial explant assay, it was demonstrated that Tgf-β2 both phosphorylated Erk1/2 and upregulated Erk1/2 protein expression. Further, blocking Erk1/2 phosphorylation prevented Tgf-β2-induced suture closure, inhibited Erk1/2 protein expression, and induced Smad2/3 expression [36]. Based on these findings, a model for Tgf-β2-responsive signaling pathways responsible for Tgf-β regulation of suture patency was proposed (fig. 2).

In this model, Tgf-β2 induces suture closure through both direct and indirect mechanisms. Tgf-β2 works directly to induce suture closure by phosphorylating Erk1/2. Tgf-β2 also works via Erk1/2 phosphorylation to indirectly affect suture closure. The indirect effects are boosting Erk1/2 protein expression, increasing a major substrate for the Fgf2-induced suture closure signaling pathway, and by inhibiting Smad2/3 protein expression, reducing a Tgf-β3 signaling pathway substrate, potentially involved in Tgf-β3 rescue of sutures from obliteration. Interestingly, blocking Erk1/2 phosphorylation not only prevented Tgf-β2-induced suture closure, but it also reversed Tgf-β2 inhibition of Smad2/3 expression, strengthening the argument for a role for Smad2/3 in maintaining suture patency.

The indirect effect of Tgf-β2 on Fgf2 signaling was demonstrated by showing that pretreating sutures with Tgf-β2 for 3 days increased Fgf2-induced

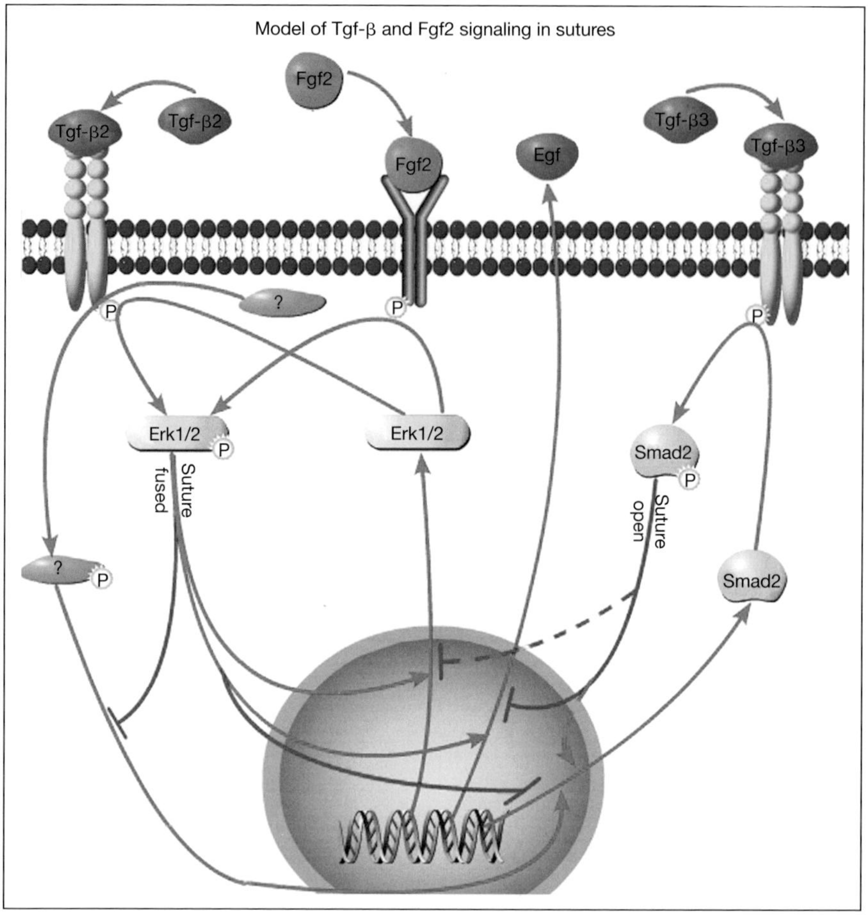

Fig. 2. Diagram of a model showing cell signaling pathways regulating suture patency. The question marks indicate as yet unidentified signaling molecules involved in a pathway identified by experimental data. Solid lines indicate known signaling events. Dashed lines indicate predicted signaling events based on the model. For clarity, molecules upstream and downstream of Erk1/2 and Smad2 have not been included in the model. Nuclear events shown in this model are for expression or inhibition of Erk1/2, Egf and Smad2 proteins. Phosphorylation events are shown in response to growth factor receptor binding [reprinted with permission from 36].

Erk1/2 phosphorylation [36]. Furthermore, blocking Tgf-β2 activity with neutralizing antibodies reversed Fgf2-induced suture closure [Opperman, unpubl. data], suggesting a significant role for Tgf-β2 in regulating Fgf2 activity in sutures.

Tgf-β Distribution in Sutures and Perisutural Tissues

Differential staining patterns are observed for the different Tgf-β isoforms in fusing and nonfusing sutures. All three Tgf-βs are present in the dura and periosteum of cranial bones throughout suture morphogenesis [4, 37]. However, Tgf-βs are distributed differently within the suture matrix and bone fronts during initial suture formation, when the suture is fully formed, and during suture obliteration. During initial suture formation and in patent sutures, Tgf-βs are absent from or low in the suture matrix, while the suture matrix of fusing sutures contains high levels of Tgf-β1 and Tgf-β2 [4, 37, 38]. On either side of the suture, the osteogenic bone fronts are immunoreactive for Tgf-β1 and Tgf-β3 during initial suture formation, and all three Tgf-βs are present in the bone fronts of fully formed sutures. However, Tgf-β3 is absent from the bone fronts of fusing sutures [4, 37].

Similar to the rat and mouse sutures, Tgf-β isoform immunoreactivity showed differential staining patterns between wild-type and synostosed perisutural tissues in a naturally occurring craniosynostotic rabbit model [39]. In wild type, patent suture immunoreactivity for Tgf-β1 and Tgf-β3 was greater than Tgf-β2. In synostosed sutures, the opposite pattern was observed, with Tgf-β2 immunoreactivity greater than Tgf-β1 and Tgf-β3 in the osteogenic fronts, dura mater, and periosteum.

Several in vivo and in vitro model systems have been used to examine the effects of Tgf-β1, Tgf-β2, and Tgf-β3 on calvarial osteoblasts and suture cells. These systems include cell and tissue culture, as well as a variety of animal models, which are described in the next section.

In vitro Models for Studying Tgf-β Effects on Osteoblasts and Suture Cells

Cell Culture

Osteoblasts which are the cells responsible for formation of new bone are directly affected by Tgf-β, which can induce differentiation or proliferation, depending on the osteoblastic cell type examined. Suture cells are thought to be osteogenic progenitor cells, and can be isolated from sutures microdissected from the surrounding bones, and their response to Tgf-βs examined in cell culture. Understanding the factors that regulate proliferation and differentiation of osteogenic cells has been significantly enhanced by the isolation and culture of bone- and suture-derived cell populations. Cell populations enriched in osteoblasts and their immediate precursors have been isolated from fetal or neonatal rodent calvariae [40]. These isolated osteoblast-like cell populations have been extensively characterized and shown to be enriched in alkaline phosphatase-positive cells and to synthesize type I collagen [41]. When calvarial-derived cell populations were maintained for extended periods in the presence of serum and ascorbic acid, cell proliferation continued postconfluence in foci scattered throughout the monolayer. With continued culture these foci formed mineralized nodules that stained positive for alkaline phosphatase [41, 42].

Although Tgf-β inhibited the growth of many types of cells, it appears to be a biphasic stimulator of mitogenic activity of primary calvarial osteoblasts [43]. Tgf-β has multiple effects on bone cells depending on their phenotype, stage of differentiation, and concentration of Tgf-β; Tgf-β stimulates chemotaxis, DNA synthesis and cell division [44]. At higher concentrations of Tgf-β1, the mitogenic activity is decreased and there is an increased synthesis of type I collagen and bone matrix proteins. Tgf-β1 added to confluent calvarial osteoblast cultures inhibited the formation of bone nodules; both the number and total area of the nodules were completely inhibited by Tgf-β1 [45].

In calvarial osteoblast cell culture, exogenous application of Tgf-β2 to the media resulted in an isoform-specific regulation of osteoblastic gene expression. Tgf-β2 treatment caused increased Tgf-β1 and osteopontin expression, decreased alkaline phosphatase expression, and suppression of osteocalcin expression [46]. Recently, Premaraj et al. [47] demonstrated that a dense collagen gel can be used as a vehicle for sustained transient delivery of plasmid DNA encoding Tgf-β3 in rat calvarial osteoblasts. The transfected calvarial osteoblasts resulted in prolonged and elevated growth factor production. It was then confirmed using the same collagen gel vehicle that plasmids could be delivered in the same manner in calvarial organ culture [47]. Together, these results suggest that the use of a collagen gel as a vehicle may provide a strategy to achieve localized and controlled, nonviral gene delivery in vivo. These results also suggest that research done at the cellular level and techniques developed on in vitro models can eventually be translated to use in tissues and organs.

Tissue and Organ Culture

The mechanisms by which Tgf-βs regulate suture patency are beginning to be elucidated. Knowledge of the biological role of TGF-β in suture morphogenesis and growth has also been advanced through in vitro calvarial culture models. The posterior frontal suture in the Sprague-Dawley rat fuses from 12 to 20 days of age, whereas all other cranial sutures remain patent. Calvaria can be dissected from various aged fetal and postnatal animals, and cultured in serum-free medium. These calvarial organ culture systems are excellent models where suture fusion versus patency can be studied. Suture patency and fusion can be examined by monitoring the distribution of target genes during critical time points by immunohistochemistry. Growth factors like TGF-β can also be added or neutralized so that the morphological and biological effects on cranial sutures can be discovered. Additionally, contributions to suture morphogenesis by the surrounding tissues such as the periosteum and dura mater can be examined by removal of these tissue layers prior to transplantation. Understanding the role of these tissues in regulating suture morphogenesis and patency provides the basis for understanding the effects of soluble growth factors such as Tgf-βs that are secreted by these tissues, and whose receptors are present on the surfaces of cells within the tissue matrices.

Early experiments examined the role that the dura mater played in suture development and in maintaining suture patency. Removal of fetal dura mater from beneath the suture before explanting the calvaria into tissue culture initially resulted in the normal overlap of the bone fronts. In the absence of dura mater, however, the newly formed sutures were unable to sustain themselves and became obliterated by bone [2]. Furthermore, as coronal sutures continued to develop they were found to be able to sustain themselves in culture even in the absence of dura mater. These results indicated that dura mater is permissive for suture formation, but that an inductive stimulus from dura mater is required during suture formation before the suture is able to maintain patency independent of the surrounding tissues.

From these experiments, it was hypothesized that during initial suture formation, inductive signals from the approaching bone fronts allowed sutures to form normally [48]. Once the bone fronts overlapped one another, a signal or signals from the dura mater is required to stabilize the newly formed suture (fig. 3b). After the suture becomes stable, it produces and osteoinhibitory signal within the dura mater (fig. 3c). Failure of suture stabilization or failure to produce an osteoinhibitory signal by the suture would then result in suture obliteration (fig. 3d). There is a good possibility that Tgf-β1 and Tgf-β3 can act as inductive or stabilizing signals, regulating the Tgf-β2 signal responsible for stimulating bone growth at the suture edges.

This idea is supported by recent studies suggesting that regionally differentiated dura mater regulates cranial suture fate by secreting growth factors such as Tgf-βs and Fgfs [9, 49, 50]. For example, dura mater from underneath the naturally fusing rodent posterior frontal suture enhanced expression of osteogenic genes to a greater extent than dura mater from beneath normally patent sagittal suture [50]. This data suggests that depending on the status of the suture, different signals are received by the dura mater, which responds by producing and releasing different levels of growth factors to act on the osteogenic cells of the suture.

The in vitro calvarial culture model has been used to test the effect of Tgf-βs and other growth factors on suture morphogenesis and patency. Adding Tgf-β2 protein or neutralizing antibodies to Tgf-β3 to cultures of fetal rat calvariae

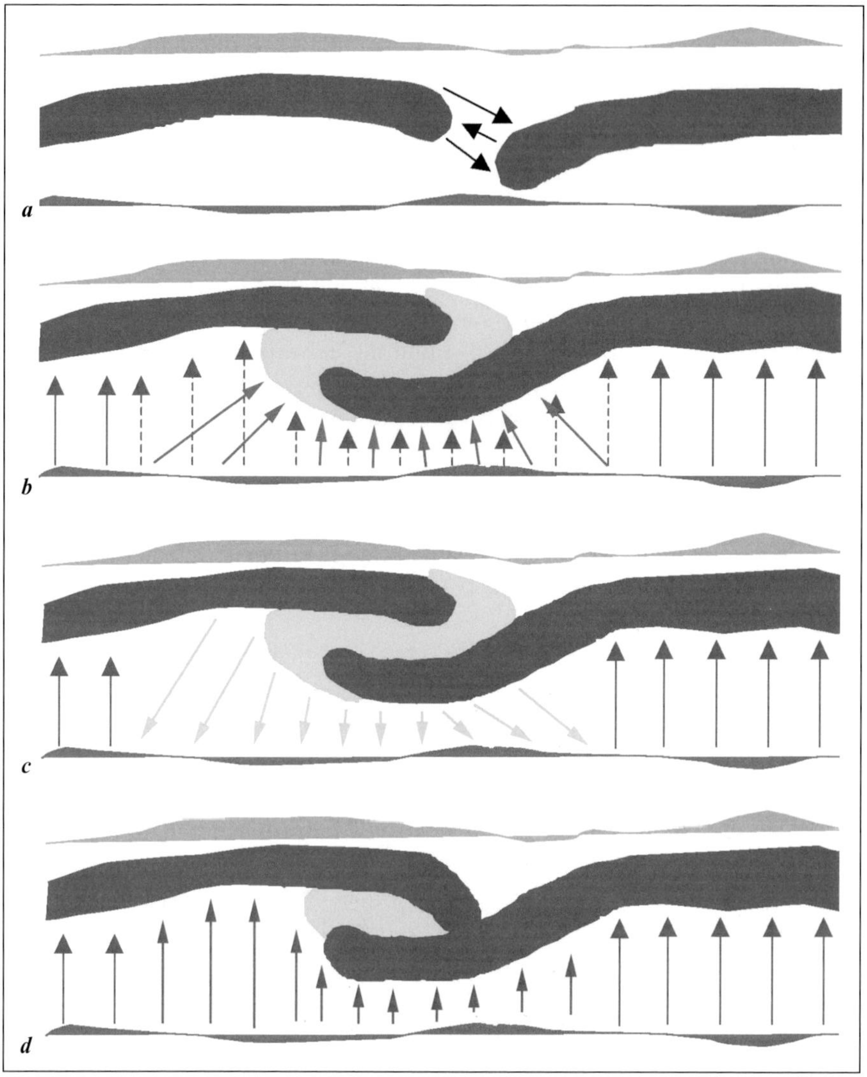

Fig. 3. Diagrammatic representation of various stages of suture morphogenesis (***a–c***) and suture fusion (***d***). ***a*** Inductive signals (arrows) arising from the approaching bone fronts allow the bone fronts to deflect away from each other or butt up against each other without obliterating the suture. These signals are independent of signals from the dura mater or periosteum. ***b*** Once the bone fronts have overlapped one another, a signal (arrows) arising from the dura mater maintains the presence of the newly formed suture. Osteogenic signals (arrows) from the dura mater cause the bones to become thickened by depositing and mineralizing new osteoid on the periosteal surface. These osteogenic signals may be continuous along the dura mater prior to formation of the suture (dotted arrows). ***c*** Once the suture is stabilized, it signals (arrows) the

resulted in suture obliteration with elevated levels of cell proliferation preceding sutural obliteration [20, 51]. Alternatively, rescue of sutures from obliteration occurs by addition of Tgf-β3 or removal of Tgf-β2 activity with neutralizing antibodies. Tgf-β3 rescue is accompanied by decreased cell proliferation [20]. Supporting evidence was found when anti-Tgf-β2 was injected subperiosteally over the posterior frontal suture in calvaria organ culture and caused a reduction in the percent of bony bridging [52]. In contrast to their effects on proliferation, Tgf-β2 decreased levels of apoptosis within the suture matrix in culture, while sutures rescued from obliteration by Tgf-β3 had elevated levels of apoptosis in the suture matrix [20]. This data provides good evidence that Tgf-βs regulate suture morphogenesis by controlling cell numbers within the suture matrix and bone fronts by regulating the amounts of proliferation and apoptosis of sutural and perisutural cells. It is therefore apparent that altering the balance between the different Tgf-β isomers or between Tgf-βs and other growth factors alters the equilibrium between proliferation and apoptosis and can result in suture obliteration.

Tgf-β Animal Models

In order to delineate and define the specific roles of each mammalian Tgf-β isoform, transgenic null mutant mice have been constructed. Transgenic null mice have been created for Tgf-β1, Tgf-β2, Tgf-β3, TgfbrI, TgfbrII, TgfbrIII, and some of their associated intracellular signaling pathway genes, like Smad2 and Erk1/2. In addition to transgenic mice, a congenital rabbit model with bilateral coronal suture synostosis has proved very useful in determining the role of Tgf-β in the craniosynostosis pathway [39, 53, 54].

Although the *Tgf-β1* homozygous null mutation causes some intrauterine lethality due to defective hematopoiesis and defective yolk sac vasculature, more than one third of the fetuses develop to term and appear clinically normal at birth [55]. After 2 weeks, these mice develop a wasting syndrome and die about 1–2 weeks later with no apparent craniofacial defects [56–60].

Tgf-β2 null mice exhibit perinatal mortality and a wide range of developmental defects that include craniofacial, axial and appendicular skeletal, heart, eye, ear, and urogenital tract organ defects. Craniofacial defects include retrognathia, dysmorphic calvariae, reduction in bone size and cranial ossification with resultant enlarged fontanels (fig. 4). Additionally, morphological

local underlying dura mater not to produce osteogenic signals. ***d*** In the absence of osteoinhibitory signals from the suture, the underlying dura mater remains continuously osteogenic (arrows), overriding signals within the suture and resulting in osseous obliteration of the suture. Periosteum is adjacent [reprinted with permission from 48].

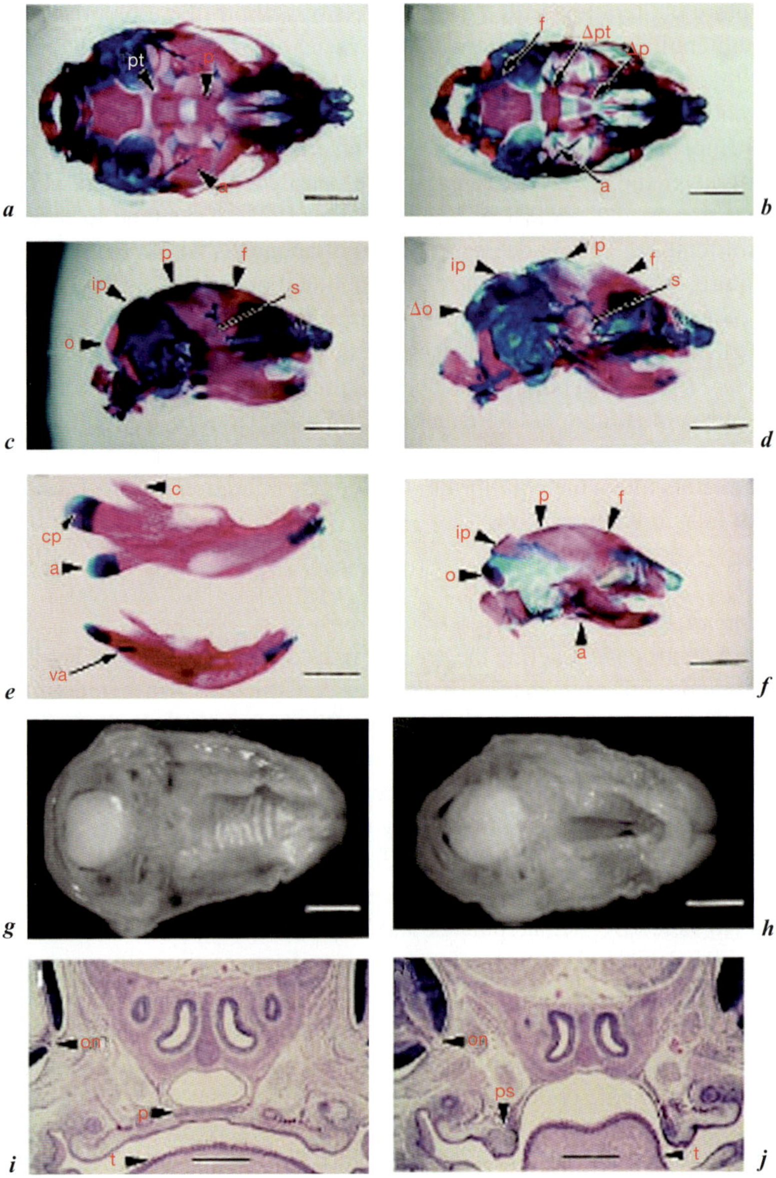

Fig. 4. Craniofacial defects of TGF-β2 null mice. ***a*** Ventral view of Alcian blue (cartilage) and alizarin red (bone) staining of E18.5 skull from sibling wild-type animal. a = Alisphenoid; p = palatine bone; pt = pterygoid bone. Bar: 2.2 mm. ***b*** Ventral view of null sibling skull with cleft palate showing generally reduced ossification and the absence of the alisphenoid, pterygoid process and palatine bones. f = Fusion of exoccipital and basisphenoid bones; Δp = deleted palatine bone; Δpt = deleted pterygoid process. Bar:

defects in the mandible are fully penetrant, along with cleft palate in 23% of null animals [61].

Mice lacking the *Tgf-β3* gene die within 24 h after birth due to abnormal lung development and feeding problems associated with a cleft palate [62, 63]. The unique feature of *Tgf-β3* knockout mice is that no other visible morphological anomalies occur in the craniofacial region or in other organs, with the exception of the lung. It has since been suggested that Tgf-β3 may regulate palatal fusion by inducing filopodia on the outer cell membrane of the palatal medial edge epithelia prior to and to facilitate shelf contact [64].

Both *TgfbrI* and *TgfbrII* null mutations result in early embryonic lethality in part due to vascular defects in the yolk sac, making it impossible to investigate the functional significance in palatogenesis and cranial suture development [65]. However, Ito et al. [21] found that conditional inactivation of *TgfbrII* in cranial neural crest cells resulted in complete clefting of the secondary palate, calvaria agenesis, and other skull defects. Calvaria agenesis was found to be the due to a disruption of Tgf-β signaling in cranial neural crest cells which resulted in impaired cell proliferation in the dura mater. *TgfbrIII* null embryos are also not viable, and the embryos die between gestation day 16.5 and birth with defects in hepatic and cardiovascular development. Fibroblasts derived from *TgfbrIII* null embryos exhibited significantly reduced sensitivity to Tgf-β2 resulting in growth inhibition, changes in reporter gene activation, and decreased Smad2 nuclear localization [66].

With the majority of the homozygous null Tgf-β-associated genes resulting in early embryonic lethality, the congenital bilateral coronal suture synostotic rabbit model has proven to be a valuable model to investigate Tgf-β signaling and surgical correction [67]. Overexpression of Tgf-β2, either in isolation or in association with an underexpression of Tgf-β1 and Tgf-β3, may be related to premature suture fusion in this pathological rabbit model [39].

2.2 mm. ***c*** Lateral view of wild-type E18.5 skull. f = Frontal bone; ip = interparietal bone; o = occipital bone; p = parietal bone; s = squamous bone. Bar: 2.2 mm. ***d*** Lateral view of null E18.5 skull showing reduced ossification of the interparietal, occipital, parietal, frontal and squamous bones. Δo = Deleted occipital bone. Bar: 2.2 mm. ***e*** Mandibles from E18.5 siblings. a = Angle; cp = condylar process; c = coronoid process; va = vestigial angle. Bar: 1.36 mm. ***f*** Lateral view of E17.5 skull from an HET animal used as a less mature growth control for ***a–d*** above. Bar: 2.2 mm. ***g*** Palate from a wild-type E18.5 mouse. Bar: 2.2 mm. ***h*** Cleft palate from a null E18.5 mouse. Bar: 2.2 mm. ***i*** Transverse histology section of wild-type E18.5 palate. on = Optic nerve; p = palate; t = tongue. Bar: 550 μm. ***j*** Transverse histology section of a sibling null E18.5 mouse with cleft palate showing vertical palatal shelves (ps). Bar: 550 μm [reprinted from 61].

Previous developmental studies in rodents showed that low levels of Tgf-β3 are associated with the normal fusion of the posterior frontal suture [37]. Addition of Tgf-β3 using a slow-absorbing collagen gel delivery system prevented posterior interfrontal suture fusion in vivo in a dose-dependent manner [68]. In a similar experiment using the collagen gel delivery system, Tgf-β3 rescued coronal suture fusion in the congenital rabbit model [53]. These results suggest that there is a dose-dependent effect of Tgf-β3 on suture morphology in both normal and pathological suture fusion. Taken together, these results also suggest that manipulation of growth factors such as TGF-βs may have clinical applications in the treatment of craniosynostosis.

Conclusions, Future Studies, and Direction

Craniosynostosis is a frequently occurring condition, whose etiology is multifactorial and which exhibits genetic heterogeneity. Maintenance of suture patency depends on the regulation of a complex array of factors that include tissue interactions, mechanical influences, and biochemical signaling. For this reason, it is important to understand the links between different transcription factors, growth factors, and their receptors so that molecular intervention could limit the need for gross surgical repair.

Understanding how factors such as Tgf-βs, Fgfs, Bmps, and other factors are regulated within the suture will clarify how membranous bone growth occurs at the suture while keeping the suture in an unossified state. One of the complicating factors is establishing the expression levels of these factors during normal suture morphogenesis and growth and what constitutes sufficiently altered levels to result in suture obliteration. Some studies use normal animal models to determine expression levels, whereas others rely on transgenic models. As knowledge from these models begins to emerge, progress will continue to be made to develop biologically based therapies that are combined with traditional surgical repair.

References

1 Kim HJ, Rice DP, Kettunen PJ, Thesleff I: FGF-, BMP- and Shh-mediated signalling pathways in the regulation of cranial suture morphogenesis and calvarial bone development. Development 1998;125:1241–1251.

2 Opperman LA, Passarelli RW, Morgan EP, Reintjes M, Ogle RC: Cranial sutures require tissue interactions with dura mater to resist osseous obliteration in vitro. J Bone Miner Res 1995;10:1978–1987.

3 Opperman LA, Sweeney TM, Redmon J, Persing JA, Ogle RC: Tissue interactions with underlying dura mater inhibit osseous obliteration of developing cranial sutures. Dev Dyn 1993;198:312–322.

4 Roth DA, Longaker MT, McCarthy JG, Rosen DM, McMullen HF, Levine JP, et al: Studies in cranial suture biology. 1. Increased immunoreactivity for TGF-beta isoforms (beta 1, beta 2, and beta 3) during rat cranial suture fusion. J Bone Miner Res 1997;12:311–321.
5 de Caestecker M: The transforming growth factor-beta superfamily of receptors. Cytokine Growth Factor Rev 2004;15:1–11.
6 Massague J, Cheifetz S, Boyd FT, Andres JL: TGF-beta receptors and TGF-beta binding proteoglycans: recent progress in identifying their functional properties. Ann NY Acad Sci 1990;593:59–72.
7 Roberts AB, Flanders KC, Heine UI, Jakowlew S, Kondaiah P, Kim SJ, et al: Transforming growth factor-beta: multifunctional regulator of differentiation and development. Philos Trans R Soc Lond B Biol Sci 1990;327:145–154.
8 Opperman LA, Chhabra A, Nolen AA, Bao Y, Ogle RC: Increased cell proliferation and altered collagen production precede rat cranial suture fusion in vitro. Mol Biol Cell 1997;8:329a.
9 Loeys BL, Chen J, Neptune ER, Judge DP, Podowski M, Holm T, et al: A syndrome of altered cardiovascular, craniofacial, neurocognitive and skeletal development caused by mutations in TGFBR1 or TGFBR2. Nat Genet 2005;37:275–281.
10 Centrella M, Horowitz MC, Wozney JM, McCarthy TL: Transforming growth factor-beta gene family members and bone. Endocr Rev 1994;15:27–39.
11 Kanzaki T, Olofsson A, Moren A, Wernstedt C, Hellman U, Miyazono K, et al: TGF-beta 1 binding protein: a component of the large latent complex of TGF-beta 1 with multiple repeat sequences. Cell 1990;61:1051–1061.
12 Tsuji T, Okada F, Yamaguchi K, Nakamura T: Molecular cloning of the large subunit of transforming growth factor type beta masking protein and expression of the mRNA in various rat tissues. Proc Natl Acad Sci USA 1990;87:8835–8839.
13 Bonewald LF, Wakefield L, Oreffo RO, Escobedo A, Twardzik DR, Mundy GR: Latent forms of transforming growth factor-beta (TGF beta) derived from bone cultures: identification of a naturally occurring 100-kDa complex with similarity to recombinant latent TGF beta. Mol Endocrinol 1991;5:741–751.
14 Allan EH, Zeheb R, Gelehrter TD, Heaton JH, Fukumoto S, Yee JA, et al: Transforming growth factor beta inhibits plasminogen activator (PA) activity and stimulates production of urokinase-type PA, PA inhibitor-1 mRNA, and protein in rat osteoblast-like cells. J Cell Physiol 1991;149:34–43.
15 Lopez-Casillas F, Cheifetz S, Doody J, Andres JL, Lane WS, Massague J: Structure and expression of the membrane proteoglycan betaglycan, a component of the TGF-beta receptor system. Cell 1991;67:785–795.
16 Blobe GC, Schiemann WP, Pepin MC, Beauchemin M, Moustakas A, Lodish HF, et al: Functional roles for the cytoplasmic domain of the type III transforming growth factor beta receptor in regulating transforming growth factor beta signaling. J Biol Chem 2001;276:24627–24637.
17 Centrella M, Ji C, Casinghino S, McCarthy TL: Rapid flux in transforming growth factor-beta receptors on bone cells. J Biol Chem 1996;271:18616–18622.
18 Mehrara BJ, Steinbrech DS, Saadeh PB, Gittes GK, Longaker MT: Expression of high-affinity receptors for TGF-beta during rat cranial suture fusion. Ann Plast Surg 1999;42:502–508.
19 Opperman LA, Galanis V, Williams AR, Adab K: Transforming growth factor-beta3 (Tgf-β3) down-regulates Tgf-β receptor type I (Tβr-I) during rescue of cranial sutures from osseous obliteration. Orthod Craniofac Res 2002;5:5–16.
20 Opperman LA, Adab K, Gakunga PT: Transforming growth factor-beta 2 and TGF-beta 3 regulate fetal rat cranial suture morphogenesis by regulating rates of cell proliferation and apoptosis. Dev Dyn 2000;219:237–247.
21 Ito Y, Yeo JY, Chytil A, Han J, Bringas P Jr, Nakajima A, et al: Conditional inactivation of Tgfbr2 in cranial neural crest causes cleft palate and calvaria defects. Development 2003;130:5269–5280.
22 Massague J, Wotton D: Transcriptional control by the TGF-beta/Smad signaling system. EMBO J 2000;19:1745–1754.
23 Chen RH, Su YH, Chuang RL, Chang TY: Suppression of transforming growth factor-beta-induced apoptosis through a phosphatidylinositol 3-kinase/Akt-dependent pathway. Oncogene 1998;17:1959–1968.

24 Weinstein M, Yang X, Deng C: Functions of mammalian Smad genes as revealed by targeted gene disruption in mice. Cytokine Growth Factor Rev 2000;11:49–58.

25 Yue J, Hartsough MT, Frey RS, Frielle T, Mulder KM: Cloning and expression of a rat Smad1: regulation by TGFbeta and modulation by the Ras/MEK pathway. J Cell Physiol 1999;178: 387–396.

26 Simeone DM, Zhang L, Graziano K, Nicke B, Pham T, Schaefer C, et al: Smad4 mediates activation of mitogen-activated protein kinases by TGF-beta in pancreatic acinar cells. Am J Physiol Cell Physiol 2001;281:C311–C319.

27 Lai CF, Cheng SL: Signal transductions induced by bone morphogenetic protein-2 and transforming growth factor-beta in normal human osteoblastic cells. J Biol Chem 2002;277:15514–15522.

28 Engel ME, McDonnell MA, Law BK, Moses HL: Interdependent SMAD and JNK signaling in transforming growth factor-beta-mediated transcription. J Biol Chem 1999;274:37413–37420.

29 Hocevar BA, Brown TL, Howe PH: TGF-beta induces fibronectin synthesis through a c-Jun N-terminal kinase-dependent, Smad4-independent pathway. EMBO J 1999;18:1345–1356.

30 Rousse S, Lallemand F, Montarras D, Pinset C, Mazars A, Prunier C, et al: Transforming growth factor-beta inhibition of insulin-like growth factor-binding protein-5 synthesis in skeletal muscle cells involves a c-Jun N-terminal kinase-dependent pathway. J Biol Chem 2001;276: 46961–46967.

31 Edlund S, Landstrom M, Heldin CH, Aspenstrom P: TGF-beta-induced mobilisation of the actin cytoskeleton requires signalling by the small GTPases Cdc42 and RhoA. Mol Biol Cell 2002;13: 902–914.

32 Hay E, Lemonnier J, Fromigue O, Marie PJ: Bone morphogenetic protein-2 promotes osteoblast apoptosis through a Smad-independent, protein kinase C-dependent signaling pathway. J Biol Chem 2001;276:29028–29036.

33 Marshall CJ: Specificity of receptor tyrosine kinase signaling: transient versus sustained extracellular signal-regulated kinase activation. Cell 1995;80:179–185.

34 Yamamoto T, Cui XM, Shuler CF: Role of ERK1/2 signaling during EGF-induced inhibition of palatal fusion. Dev Biol 2003;260:512–521.

35 Kim HJ, Lee MH, Park HS, Park MH, Lee SW, Kim SY, et al: Erk pathway and activator protein 1 play crucial roles in FGF2-stimulated premature cranial suture closure. Dev Dyn 2003;227: 335–346.

36 Opperman LA, Fernandez CR, So S, Rawlins JT: Erk1/2 signaling is required for Tgf-beta2-induced suture closure. Dev Dyn 2006;235:1292–1299.

37 Opperman LA, Nolen AA, Ogle RC: TGF-beta 1, TGF-beta 2, and TGF-beta 3 exhibit distinct patterns of expression during cranial suture formation and obliteration in vivo and in vitro. J Bone Miner Res 1997;12:301–310.

38 Most D, Levine JP, Chang J, Sung J, McCarthy JG, Schendel SA, et al: Studies in cranial suture biology: up-regulation of transforming growth factor-beta1 and basic fibroblast growth factor mRNA correlates with posterior frontal cranial suture fusion in the rat. Plast Reconstr Surg 1998;101:1431–1440.

39 Poisson E, Sciote JJ, Koepsel R, Cooper GM, Opperman LA, Mooney MP: Transforming growth factor-beta isoform expression in the perisutural tissues of craniosynostotic rabbits. Cleft Palate Craniofac J 2004;41:392–402.

40 Rodan GA, Heath JK, Yoon K, Noda M, Rodan SB: Diversity of the osteoblastic phenotype. Ciba Found Symp 1988;136:78–91.

41 Nefussi JR, Boy-Lefevre ML, Boulekbache H, Forest N: Mineralization in vitro of matrix formed by osteoblasts isolated by collagenase digestion. Differentiation 1985;29:160–168.

42 Sudo H, Kodama HA, Amagai Y, Yamamoto S, Kasai S: In vitro differentiation and calcification in a new clonal osteogenic cell line derived from newborn mouse calvaria. J Cell Biol 1983;96:191–198.

43 ten Dijke P, Iwata KK, Goddard C, Pieler C, Canalis E, McCarthy TL, et al: Recombinant transforming growth factor type beta 3: biological activities and receptor-binding properties in isolated bone cells. Mol Cell Biol 1990;10:4473–4479.

44 Pfeilschifter J, Wolf O, Naumann A, Minne HW, Mundy GR, Ziegler R: Chemotactic response of osteoblastlike cells to transforming growth factor beta. J Bone Miner Res 1990;5:825–830.

45 Harris SE, Bonewald LF, Harris MA, Sabatini M, Dallas S, Feng JQ, et al: Effects of transforming growth factor beta on bone nodule formation and expression of bone morphogenetic protein 2, osteocalcin, osteopontin, alkaline phosphatase, and type I collagen mRNA in long-term cultures of fetal rat calvarial osteoblasts. J Bone Miner Res 1994;9:855–863.
46 Fagenholz PJ, Warren SM, Greenwald JA, Bouletreau PJ, Spector JA, Crisera FE, et al: Osteoblast gene expression is differentially regulated by TGF-beta isoforms. J Craniofac Surg 2001;12: 183–190.
47 Premaraj S, Mundy B, Parker-Barnes J, Winnard PL, Moursi AM: Collagen gel delivery of Tgf-beta3 non-viral plasmid DNA in rat osteoblast and calvarial culture. Orthod Craniofac Res 2005;8:320–322.
48 Opperman LA: Cranial sutures as intramembranous bone growth sites. Dev Dyn 2000;219: 472–485.
49 Mathy JA, Lenton K, Nacamuli RP, Fong KD, Song HM, Fang TD, et al: FGF-2 stimulation affects calvarial osteoblast biology: quantitative analysis of nine genes important for cranial suture biology by real-time reverse transcription polymerase chain reaction. Plast Reconstr Surg 2003;112: 528–539.
50 Warren SM, Greenwald JA, Nacamuli RP, Fong KD, Song HJ, Fang TD, et al: Regional dura mater differentially regulates osteoblast gene expression. J Craniofac Surg 2003;14:363–370.
51 Greenwald JA, Mehrara BJ, Spector JA, Warren SM, Crisera FE, Fagenholz PJ, et al: Regional differentiation of cranial suture-associated dura mater in vivo and in vitro: implications for suture fusion and patency. J Bone Miner Res 2000;15:2413–2430.
52 Moursi AM, Winnard PL, Fryer D, Mooney MP: Delivery of transforming growth factor-beta2-perturbing antibody in a collagen vehicle inhibits cranial suture fusion in calvarial organ culture. Cleft Palate Craniofac J 2003;40:225–232.
53 Chong SL, Mitchell R, Moursi AM, Winnard P, Losken HW, Bradley J, et al: Rescue of coronal suture fusion using transforming growth factor-beta 3 (Tgf-beta 3) in rabbits with delayed-onset craniosynostosis. Anat Rec A Discov Mol Cell Evol Biol 2003;274:962–971.
54 Mooney MP, Moursi AM, Opperman LA, Siegel MI: Cytokine therapy for craniosynostosis. Expert Opin Biol Ther 2004;4:279–299.
55 Dickson MC, Martin JS, Cousins FM, Kulkarni AB, Karlsson S, Akhurst RJ: Defective haematopoiesis and vasculogenesis in transforming growth factor-beta 1 knock out mice. Development 1995;121:1845–1854.
56 Boivin GP, O'Toole BA, Orsmby IE, Diebold RJ, Eis MJ, Doetschman T, et al: Onset and progression of pathological lesions in transforming growth factor-beta 1-deficient mice. Am J Pathol 1995;146:276–288.
57 DeWees S, Geiger JH: Structural studies of the Msx-1 homeodomain-DNA complex I. Acta Crystallogr D Biol Crystallogr 1999;55:2039–2040.
58 Kulkarni AB, Huh CG, Becker D, Geiser A, Lyght M, Flanders KC, et al: Transforming growth factor beta 1 null mutation in mice causes excessive inflammatory response and early death. Proc Natl Acad Sci USA 1993;90:770–774.
59 Kulkarni AB, Ward JM, Yaswen L, Mackall CL, Bauer SR, Huh CG, et al: Transforming growth factor-beta 1 null mice. An animal model for inflammatory disorders. Am J Pathol 1995;146: 264–275.
60 Shull MM, Ormsby I, Kier AB, Pawlowski S, Diebold RJ, Yin M, et al: Targeted disruption of the mouse transforming growth factor-beta 1 gene results in multifocal inflammatory disease. Nature 1992;359:693–699.
61 Sanford LP, Ormsby I, Gittenberger-de Groot AC, Sariola H, Friedman R, Boivin GP, et al: TGFbeta2 knockout mice have multiple developmental defects that are non-overlapping with other TGFbeta knockout phenotypes. Development 1997;124:2659–2670.
62 Kaartinen V, Voncken JW, Shuler C, Warburton D, Bu D, Heisterkamp N, et al: Abnormal lung development and cleft palate in mice lacking TGF-beta 3 indicates defects of epithelial-mesenchymal interaction. Nat Genet 1995;11:415–421.
63 Proetzel G, Pawlowski SA, Wiles MV, Yin M, Boivin GP, Howles PN, et al: Transforming growth factor-beta 3 is required for secondary palate fusion. Nat Genet 1995;11:409–414.

64 Taya Y, O'Kane S, Ferguson MW: Pathogenesis of cleft palate in TGF-beta3 knockout mice. Development 1999;126:3869–3879.
65 Oshima M, Oshima H, Taketo MM: TGF-beta receptor type II deficiency results in defects of yolk sac hematopoiesis and vasculogenesis. Dev Biol 1996;179:297–302.
66 Stenvers KL, Tursky ML, Harder KW, Kountouri N, Amatayakul-Chantler S, Grail D, et al: Heart and liver defects and reduced transforming growth factor beta2 sensitivity in transforming growth factor beta type III receptor-deficient embryos. Mol Cell Biol 2003;23:4371–4385.
67 Mooney MP, Losken HW, Tschakaloff A, Siegel MI, Losken A, Lalikos JF: Congenital bilateral coronal suture synostosis in a rabbit and craniofacial growth comparisons with experimental models. Cleft Palate Craniofac J 1993;30:121–128.
68 Opperman LA, Moursi AM, Sayne JR, Wintergerst AM: Transforming growth factor-beta 3(Tgf-beta3) in a collagen gel delays fusion of the rat posterior interfrontal suture in vivo. Anat Rec 2002;267:120–130.
69 Dallas SL, Miyazono K, Skerry TM, Mundy GR, Bonewald LF: Dual role for the latent transforming growth factor-beta binding protein in storage of latent TGF-beta in the extracellular matrix and as a structural matrix protein. J Cell Biol 1995;131:539–549.

Dr. Lynne A. Opperman
Department of Biomedical Sciences, Baylor College of Dentistry
Texas A&M Health Science Center
PO Box 660677
Dallas, TX 75266-0677 (USA)
Tel. +1 214 828 8134, Fax +1 214 874–4538, E-Mail lopperman@bcd.tamhsc.edu

Rice DP (ed): Craniofacial Sutures. Development, Disease and Treatment.
Front Oral Biol. Basel, Karger, 2008, vol 12, pp 197–208

The Bmp Pathway in Skull Vault Development

Robert Maxson, Mamoru Ishii

Department of Biochemistry and Molecular Biology, Norris Comprehensive Cancer Center and Hospital, University of Southern California Keck School of Medicine, Los Angeles, Calif., USA

Abstract

The Bmp pathway is of critical importance in the development of the skull vault. Analysis of gain and loss of function phenotypes of Bmp pathway effectors, particularly *Msx* genes, has shown that the Bmp pathway functions in the growth of both mesodermal and neural crest-derived calvarial bones. It is required for the development of the frontal and parietal bones during the interval between the initial osteogenic mesenchymal condensations at E12.5 to the apposition of the paired frontal and parietal bones at E18.5. During postnatal development, forced expression of the Bmp inhibitor, noggin, maintains the patency of sutures, consistent with a role for the Bmp pathway in regulating suture development. The availability of conditional mutants of Bmp ligands, receptors and downstream effectors will make possible an increasingly high resolution analysis of precisely how the Bmp functions in these processes and how aberrations in its activity can contribute to pathological conditions such as familial parietal foramina and craniosynostosis.

Introduction

The skull is one of the most intricately patterned and evolutionarily plastic vertebrate organs. Understanding the relationship between its form and its function, as well as how, in molecular terms, its pattern arises during embryonic development are questions that resonate across the disciplines of developmental biology, functional morphology and evolutionary biology. The general picture of skull vault development is one of disparate mesenchymal cell populations migrating, undergoing specification to osteogenic lineages, and forming the components of the skull, including bones, cartilages, sutures, and dura. Thus, during skull vault development, mesenchymal cells of neural crest and mesodermal origin migrate to positions overlying the developing cerebral hemispheres. Controlled by signals from the dura, which is also of neural crest origin, they differentiate along an osteogenic pathway, forming the calvarial bones. In later stages, the bones of the skull vault are united by sutures, fibrous joints that serve as growth centers and allow the skull vault to grow in concert with the brain [1–3]. There are thus two phases in the morphogenesis of the skull vault, the first including the genesis, migration and initial specification of skeletogenic mesenchymal precursor cells, the second the differentiation of the skeletogenic mesenchyme and the ensuing appositional growth of the bones at the sutures.

Underlying the development of the skull vault is a complex series of signaling processes. These commence with the initial specification of neural crest and mesodermal precursors in the early embryo and continue through the appositional growth phase. Although these signaling processes are understood only in broad outline, findings from human genetics together with data from animal models and ex vivo approaches have shown that Fgf, Notch, TGF-β and Bmp pathways have prominent roles. In this review, we focus on the Bmp pathway.

Origins of the Calvarial Bones and the Establishment of Tissue Boundaries

Fate-mapping experiments have shown that the skull vault originates from neural crest and head mesoderm, though the relative contributions of these two cell lineages to the component bones has been controversial. Using an interspecies (quail-chick) transplantation approach as a means of following neural crest, Le Douarin and colleagues [4] have argued for an entirely neural crest origin for the calvaria, while Noden [5] has reached the conclusion that the calvarial bones are derived almost entirely from mesoderm, with only a small neural crest contribution to the frontal bone. In the mouse, Wnt1-Cre/R26R mapping experiments showed that the frontal bones are composed entirely of neural crest, the parietal bones of head mesoderm [6]. Neural crest-derived cells emigrate from the caudal forebrain, midbrain, and prorhombomere (pr) A of the hindbrain as a continuous population. PrA is the area between the midbrain and the preotic sulcus, which later separates into rhombomeres (r) 1 and 2. By E10.5, such cells form a condensed layer of skeletogenic mesenchyme beneath the surface ectoderm. The frontal and parietal bones thus develop from adjacent neural crest and mesodermal cell populations; from E9.5 through the remainder of embryonic development, the border between these populations is strikingly precise and there is little or no mixing [6]. What is most intriguing about this pattern is the sharpness of the border between mesoderm and neural crest. The establishment and maintenance of this border must involve mechanisms that produce precise sorting of cells.

Genetics of Skull Vault Development

The development of the skull vault provides a model of how mesenchymal populations produce patterned structures. It is also of interest because it is affected by a number of human diseases [1, 2, 7]. As discussed in detail elsewhere in this volume, anomalies in skull vault development are common in humans, occurring in as many as 1/2,500 live births [1]. Among these are craniosynostosis and persistent calvarial foramina. Craniosynostosis is the premature fusion of the calvarial bones at the sutures. Persistent calvarial foramina are defects in the ossification of bones of the skull vault. Several genes responsible for one or both of these defects have been identified [2, 7, 8]. These include FGF receptors 1, 2 and 3 [9–13], the basic hlh gene, *Twist* [2], and the homeobox genes *Msx2* and *Alx4* [7, 14]. A gain of function mutation in *Msx2* can cause craniosynostosis [15]. Heterozygous loss of *Msx2* function results in persistent foramina in the skull vault [16]. More recently haploinsufficiency for *Alx4* has been shown to cause calvarial foramina [17–19]. Intriguingly, heterozygous loss of *Twist* function can cause craniosynostosis, and, in a portion of affected individuals, calvarial foramina [20–23]. Thus, in humans, *Twist* is required both to prevent premature suture fusion, and for the normal growth of the calvarial bones. Similarly, *Msx2* is required for calvarial bone growth, and, when carrying a gain of function (p146h) mutation, can cause fusion of calvarial bones. Recently, mutations in *Jagged 1*, a gene encoding a ligand in the Notch signaling pathway, were shown to cause Alagille syndrome, demonstrating that the Notch pathway has a role in suture development [24]. Finally, mutations in *ephrinB1* were found to cause frontonasal dysplasia, a syndrome that includes craniosynostosis as a key feature [25].

Analysis of transgenic mice and targeted mouse mutants has provided results that parallel findings in humans. *Twist* mutant mice have synostosis of the coronal suture [20, 21, 26]. We showed that overexpression of *Msx2* under the control of its own promoter or heterologous promoters causes overgrowth of the bones of the skull vault, a phenotype that may mimic the early stages of synostosis [27]. Both *Msx1* and *Msx2* mutant mice exhibit calvarial foramina [28–30] (fig. 1). Several mutations affecting the Fgf pathway have been shown to reproduce some features of human craniosynostosis syndromes. These include insertion of a retrovirus between the *Fgf3* and *Fgf4* genes [31], a targeted deletion of an alternatively spliced exon of *Fgfr2*, which also gives rise to a phenotype resembling Pfeiffer syndrome [32], and a knock-in of the Pro250Arg mutation in

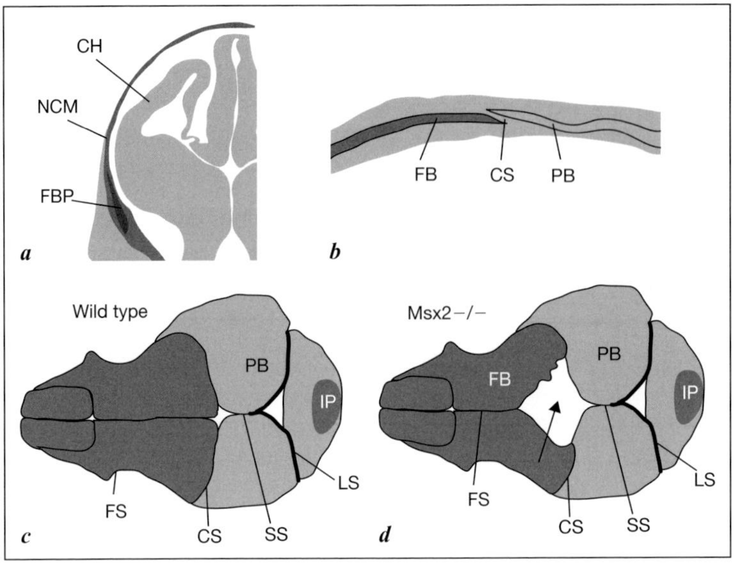

Fig. 1. Schematic diagrams showing stages of calvarial development. ***a*** Coronal section at level of frontal bone rudiment at E12.5. Neural crest-derived osteogenic mesenchyme (black) has migrated into positions surrounding the cerebral hemispheres. The frontal bone primordium, a crescent of ALP-positive cells has appeared and will elongate dorsally during subsequent development. ***b*** Longitudinal section of E14.5 embryo showing neural crest-derived frontal bone, mesoderm-derived parietal bone, and coronal suture. ***c***, ***d*** Dorsal views of newborn skulls showing distribution of neural crest-derived bone. ***d*** Large defect in posterior frontal bone and anterior parietal bone (arrow). CH = Cerebral hemisphere; NCM = neural crest-derived mesenchyme; FBP = frontal bone primordium; FB = frontal bone; CS = coronal suture; PB = parietal bone; FS = frontal suture; SS = sagittal suture; LS = lambdoid suture; IP = interparietal bone.

Fgfr1 (equivalent to the Pro252Arg mutation in *FGFR1*), which causes Pfeiffer syndrome [11]. In general, these mutations appear to cause upregulation of the osteoblast determinant, Runx2, findings that support the emerging hypothesis that the Fgf pathway functions to maintain a balance between proliferation and differentiation of osteogenic cells in the osteogenic fronts of sutures [14].

The BMP Pathway

BMPs are a large class of peptide ligands that function in a strikingly broad array of biological functions in embryonic development and homeostasis. They are key participants in the specification of embryonic axes, in inductive tissue interactions during organogenesis, and in the differentiation and proliferation of many embryonic cell types [33–35]. Moreover, BMPs can elicit changes in cell fate in a concentration-dependent manner, and thus can function as classical morphogens [36].

BMPs signal through serine-threonine kinase receptors [37, 38]. An active heterotetramer receptor complex forms upon interaction of ligand with type I and type II receptor dimers [33, 39, 40]. This leads to the phosphorylation of one or more members of the receptor-regulated Smad family (R-Smads) [41]. Smads are intracellular proteins related to the *Drosophila* Mad protein [42, 43]. Upon phosphorylation, R-Smads associate with Smad4 and translocate to the nucleus where they serve as effectors of transcription [44–46]. Smad1, 5 and 8 function in the BMP pathway and Smad2 and 3 in the activin and TGF-β pathway [33, 47–50]. Smad4 is common to all three branches of the TGF-β superfamily [34].

How Smads influence gene expression in vertebrate embryos remains unclear. Smads are capable of activating transcription, yet bind DNA weakly [51, 52]. From work on the activin and TGF-β-dependent Smads, it has become clear that Smads interact with certain sequence-specific transcription factors to modify their activity [38, 52–59]. There is relatively little information on transcription factors recruited to BMP-responsive promoters by BMP-dependent Smads [60–62]. One example is the DNA-binding transcription factor OAZ, which associates with Smad1 during BMP2-induced activation of the *X-vent* promoter in *Xenopus* [63]. In addition, the transcription factor Xvent-2 can act as a Smad1-specific coactivator during maintenance of its own transcriptional regulation [64].

We have identified a BMP-responsive element within the 560 fragments [65]. This element consists of a core sequence, required for BMP signaling in most sites of *Msx2* expression, and ancillary elements that mediate signaling in diverse developmental settings. Genetic fine structure analysis of the core element identified two classes of functional sites — four GCCG sequences related to the consensus binding site of Mad/Smad-related BMP signal transducers, and a single TTAATT sequence, matching the consensus site for Antennapedia superclass homeodomain proteins. ChIP, gel shift, and mutagenesis experiments suggest that the GCCG sites are direct targets of Smad1. Intriguingly, however, these sites are not sufficient for BMP responsiveness in mouse embryos; the TTAATT sequence is also required. Overlapping the TTAATT sequence are potential binding sites for paired-related homeodomain proteins and forkhead-related proteins [65].

The Role of the BMP Pathway in Skull Vault Development

Initial studies with Bmp ligands and receptors provided little information on the role of the Bmp pathway in skull vault development because embryos bearing mutations in these Bmp pathway components did not survive long enough to permit evaluation of skull development. However, analysis of gain and loss of function phenotypes of Bmp pathway effectors, particularly *Msx* genes, has been informative.

Loss of function of *Msx2* results in a frontoparietal defect similar to a defect present in humans with heterozygous loss of function of *MSX2* (fig. 1) [3, 28, 30]. Tracing this defect back in development, Ishii et al. [30] showed that it is first detectable between E11.5 and E12.5 in a crescent of osteogenic cells above the eye (fig. 1). These cells compose the frontal bone rudiment, which consists of neural crest-derived cells that migrate from the area of the midbrain. These cells are part of a capsule of osteogenic mesenchyme that surrounds the brain by around E11.5. Their differentiation begins with the appearance of Runx2-positive cells in the rudiment, and proceeds in a wave dorsally and posteriorly, ultimately resulting in a frontal bone delimited by the frontal and sagittal sutures. It remains unclear to what extent the appearance of differentiated osteogenic cells in the growing rudiment is driven by differentiation of preexisting ostoeblast precursors, migration of such precursors, or proliferation of osteogenic cells in the advancing fronts. There is evidence for all three mechanisms; thus each may contribute to frontal bone growth.

In *Msx2* mutant mice at E12.5, the frontal bone rudiment is reduced in size, as shown by a reduced number of alkaline phosphatase (Alp)- and Runx2-positive cells [30]. During subsequent stages of development, differentiation of the frontal bone osteogenic mesenchyme is retarded. By P21, a midline defect, representing approximately 20% of the area of the paired frontal bones, remains patent.

Msx1 mutant mice have a phenotype that closely resembles that of Msx2 mutants [Fu and Maxson, unpubl. data]. Further, compound *Msx1–2* mutants exhibit a foramen defect whose severity increases with decreasing Msx dosage [Ishii et al., unpubl. data]. At the extreme, in double homozygous null mutants, neural crest precursor cells migrate to the area of the frontal bone rudiment but fail to differentiate [Ishii and Maxson, unpubl. data]. Thus it appears that the key defect in *Msx* mutants is a failure of osteogenic lineage cells to proceed beyond the osteoprogenitor stage. The defect in osteogenesis is not confined to neural crest-derived bone: defects in the anterior and posterior portions of the parietal bone are evident in *Msx1–2* homozygote-heterozygote combinations.

It remains unclear what activates *Msx* genes in the frontal bone rudiment. Bmp2, Bmp4 and Bmp7 ligands are expressed in the rudiment, as well as in neural crest precursor populations, in the dura and in the brain [66; Sun and Maxson, unpubl. observations]. Thus it is likely that Bmps, acting at the rudiment stage or earlier, activate *Msx* gene expression and initiate progression to an osteogenic phenotype.

Intriguingly, a frontal foramen phenotype similar to that of *Msx2* mutant mice has been described in *Alx4* mutants [67]. Like *Msx2*, *Alx4* is regulated by Bmps [68]. Analysis of compound *Alx4-Msx2* mutants suggested that the two genes function additively in frontal bone development [67]. Epistasis analysis revealed that *Msx2* expression is reduced in the *Alx4* mutant, while *Alx4* expression is virtually unchanged in the *Msx2* mutant. Thus *Alx4* may lie upstream of *Msx2* in frontal bone development.

FoxC1, a forkhead-related transcription factor that is also Bmp-responsive, has a prominent role in skull vault development. *FoxC1−/−* mutant mice exhibit a severe skull vault defect that resembles that of *Msx1–2* compound mutants [68]: development of osteogenic mesenchyme fails to progress beyond the initial condensation phase. Consistent with the view that *FoxC1* may lie in the same pathway as *Msx2* are findings to the effect that *FoxC1* is required for Bmp-mediated activation of *Msx2* in cranial mesenchyme [68]. Moreover, *FoxC1* is also required for Bmp-mediated activation of *Alx4*. Thus *FoxC1* may function upstream of *Msx2* and *Alx4* in skull vault development.

Intriguingly, mice with heterozygous mutations in *Twist* exhibit a frontoparietal foramen similar to that of *Msx2* knockouts, but smaller [30]. This defect is substantially worse in *Msx2-Twist* double heterozygous embryos than in individual heterozygotes. Underlying this increase in the severity of skull vault defect are greater deficiencies in both the differentiation and proliferation of frontal bone skeletogenic mesenchyme. Genetic and molecular data both show that *Msx2* and *Twist* do not function in a simple, linear pathway but rather act in parallel [30].

These data led us to propose [30] that *Msx2*, a target of the Bmp pathway [69], and *Twist*, a target of the Fgf pathway [70], integrate inputs from these two pathways to cooperatively control the differentiation and proliferation of neural crest-derived skeletogenic mesenchyme and thus the patterning of the frontal bone. We suggested that in the frontal bone anlagen, *Msx2* and *Twist* act as a nexus for Fgf and Bmp signaling, and participate in the control of the identity and/or proliferation of the frontal bone skeletogenic mesenchyme. We envisaged a model analogous to a regulatory network documented in Drosophila, in which *msh*, together with *ladybird* and *even skipped*, regulate the identity of cardiac muscle progenitor cells [71]. Such a combinatorial interaction could maintain stringent control over the proliferation and differentiation of the skeletogenic mesenchyme, and thus serve as part of the mechanism that coordinates the growth of skull with that of the brain. Finally, we suggested that our results may have implications for the pathophysiology of familial parietal foramina, and possibly craniosynostosis. These results predict that in humans, *Twist* activity may influence the penetrance of calvarial defects caused by haploid loss of *Msx2* function. Reciprocally, *Msx2* activity may influence the penetrance of defects resulting from *Twist* mutations. The clinical manifestations in individuals affected with familial parietal foramina and Saethre-Chotzen syndrome may thus depend on the sum of the activity of these two gene products.

Finally, the few available results of targeting of genes encoding Bmp ligands suggest similar defects in frontal bone development. Homozygous mutants in Bmp7 exhibit a frontal foramen similar to that of Msx2 [Ishii et al., unpubl. data]. Similarly, the frontal bone rudiment is reduced in size in such mice, suggesting that the mechanistic basis of the phenotype is similar to that of Msx2. Conditional mutants of Bmp2 and Bmp4 are available [72, 73]. Conditional inactivation of Bmp4 in the neural crest by means of Wnt1-Cre produces a frontal foramen phenotype at the newborn stage, similar to *Msx* mutants [Maxson and Martin, unpubl. data], consistent with a role for the Bmp pathway in the differentiation of the cranial osteogenic mesenchyme.

A second major category of skull vault defects that can be traced to the Bmp pathway are those that affect the development of cranial sutures. A gain of function mutation in *MSX2* is associated with Boston-type craniosynostosis [15], and overexpression of *Msx2* in mice causes overgrowth of the parietal bones at the sagittal suture [39]. Further evidence that a gain of *Msx2* function has a role in craniosynostosis comes from the work of Merrill et al. [74] who showed that *Msx2* is ectopically expressed in *Twist* mutant mice in mesoderm-derived cranial mesenchyme adjacent to the coronal suture. This ectopic expression is required for the development of coronal synostosis. Thus *Msx2* appears to be negatively regulated by *Twist* and required downstream of *Twist* for the morphogenesis of the coronal suture.

Intriguingly, the Bmp inhibitor, *noggin*, is also overexpressed in this same mesodermal cell population adjacent to the coronal suture, suggesting that loss of Bmp signaling may activate *Msx2* and cause synostosis [Sun and Maxson, unpubl. observations]. If correct, this result would imply that *Msx2* is regulated positively by Bmp signaling in the developing frontal bone, but negatively in the mesoderm flanking the coronal suture.

In contrast to the idea that reduced Bmp signaling causes synostosis, Longaker and colleagues [75] have shown that forced expression of *noggin* prevents suture fusion in postnatal rats. Taken at face value these results suggest that the effect of Bmp signaling on suture development may depend on the identity of the suture and the developmental stage. In the coronal suture during embryonic development, reduced Bmp signaling may promote synostosis, while in the sagittal suture at postnatal stages, reduced Bmp signaling may promote suture patency.

In summary, the Bmp pathway is of critical importance in the development of the skull vault. It is required for the expansion of ossification centers, and possibly for their initial formation. It also has a key role in the development of cranial sutures. The availability of conditional mutants of Bmp ligands, receptors and downstream effectors will make possible an increasingly high-resolution analysis of precisely how the Bmp functions in these processes and how aberrations in its activity can contribute to pathological conditions such as familial parietal foramina and craniosynostosis.

Acknowledgments

This work was supported by NIH grants DE12941 and DE12450 to RM. We thank Hualin Fu, Jingjing Sun and Mandy Ting for helpful comments on the manuscript.

References

1 Cohen MM Jr, MacLean RE: Craniosynostosis: Diagnosis, Evaluation, and Management, ed 2. New York, Oxford University Press, 2000.
2 Wilkie AO: Craniosynostosis: genes and mechanisms. Hum Mol Genet 1997;6:1647–1656.
3 Wilkie AO, Tang Z, Elanko N, et al: Functional haploinsufficiency of the human homeobox gene MSX2 causes defects in skull ossification. Nat Genet 2000;24:387–390.
4 Couly GF, Coltey PM, Le Douarin NM: The triple origin of skull in higher vertebrates: a study in quail-chick chimeras. Development 1993;117:409–429.
5 Noden DM: Interactions and fates of avian craniofacial mesenchyme. Development 1988;103:121–140.
6 Jiang X, Iseki S, Maxson RE, Sucov HM, Morriss-Kay GM: Tissue origins and interactions in the mammalian skull vault. Dev Biol 2002;241:106–116.
7 Wilkie AO, Oldridge M, Tang Z, Maxson RE Jr: Craniosynostosis and related limb anomalies. Novartis Found Symp 2001;232:122–133.
8 Ornitz DM, Marie PJ: FGF signaling pathways in endochondral and intramembranous bone development and human genetic disease. Genes Dev 2002;16:1446–1465.
9 Meyers GA, Orlow SJ, Munro IR, Przylepa KA, Jabs EW: Fibroblast growth factor receptor 3 (FGFR3) transmembrane mutation in Crouzon syndrome with acanthosis nigricans. Nat Genet 1995;11:462–464.
10 Reardon W, Winter RM, Rutland P, Pulleyn LJ, Jones BM, Malcolm S: Mutations in the fibroblast growth factor receptor 2 gene cause Crouzon syndrome. Nat Genet 1994;8:98–103.
11 Muenke M, Schell U, Hehr A, et al: A common mutation in the fibroblast growth factor receptor 1 gene in Pfeiffer syndrome. Nat Genet 1994;8:269–274.
12 Wilkie AOW, Slaney SF, Oldridge M, Poole MD, Ashworth GJ, Hockley AD, Hayward RD, David DJ, Pulleyn LJ, Rutland P, Malcolm S, Winter RM, Reardon W: Apert syndrome results from localized mutations of FGFR2 and is allelic with Crouzon syndrome. Nat Genet 1995;9:165–172.
13 Jabs EW, Li X, Scott AF, Meyers G, Chen W, Eccles M, Mao J-I, Charnas LR, Jackson CE, Jaye M: Jackson-Weiss and Crouzon syndromes are allelic with mutations in fibroblast growth factor receptor 2. Nat Genet 1994;8:275–279.
14 Wilkie AO, Morriss-Kay GM: Genetics of craniofacial development and malformation. Nat Rev Genet 2001;2:458–468.
15 Jabs EW, Muller U, Li X, et al: A mutation in the homeodomain of the human MSX2 gene in a family affected with autosomal dominant craniosynostosis. Cell 1993;75:443–450.
16 Wuyts W, Reardon W, Preis S, et al: Identification of mutations in the MSX2 homeobox gene in families affected with foramina parietalia permagna. Hum Mol Genet 2000;9:1251–1255.
17 Wuyts W, Cleiren E, Homfray T, Rasore-Quartino A, Vanhoenacker F, Van Hul W: The ALX4 homeobox gene is mutated in patients with ossification defects of the skull (foramina parietalia permagna, OMIM 168500). J Med Genet 2000;37:916–920.

18 Wu YQ, Badano JL, McCaskill C, Vogel H, Potocki L, Shaffer LG: Haploinsufficiency of ALX4 as a potential cause of parietal foramina in the 11p11.2 contiguous gene-deletion syndrome. Am J Hum Genet 2000;67:1327–1332.
19 Mavrogiannis LA, Antonopoulou I, Baxova A, et al: Haploinsufficiency of the human homeobox gene ALX4 causes skull ossification defects. Nat Genet 2001;27:17–18.
20 el Ghouzzi V, Le Merrer M, Perrin-Schmitt F, et al: Mutations of the TWIST gene in the Saethre-Chotzen syndrome. Nat Genet 1997;15:42–46.
21 Howard TD, Paznekas WA, Green ED, et al: Mutations in TWIST, a basic helix-loop-helix transcription factor, in Saethre-Chotzen syndrome. Nat Genet 1997;15:36–41.
22 Thompson EM, Baraitser M, Hayward RD: Parietal foramina in Saethre-Chotzen syndrome. J Med Genet 1984;21:369–372.
23 Young ID, Swift PG: Parietal foramina in the Saethre-Chotzen syndrome. J Med Genet 1985;22:413–414.
24 Kamath BM, Stolle C, Bason L, et al: Craniosynostosis in Alagille syndrome. Am J Med Genet 2002;112:176–180.
25 Twigg SR, Kan R, Babbs C, et al: Mutations of ephrin-B1 (EFNB1), a marker of tissue boundary formation, cause craniofrontonasal syndrome. Proc Natl Acad Sci USA 2004;101:8652–8657.
26 Carver EA, Oram KF, Gridley T: Craniosynostosis in Twist heterozygous mice: a model for Saethre-Chotzen syndrome. Anat Rec 2002;268:90–92.
27 Liu YH, Tang Z, Kundu RK, et al: Msx2 gene dosage influences the number of proliferative osteogenic cells in growth centers of the developing murine skull: a possible mechanism for MSX2-mediated craniosynostosis in humans. Dev Biol 1999;205:260–274.
28 Satokata I, Ma L, Ohshima H, et al: Msx2 deficiency in mice causes pleiotropic defects in bone growth and ectodermal organ formation. Nat Genet 2000;24:391–395.
29 Satokata I, Maas R: Msx1 deficient mice exhibit cleft palate and abnormalities of craniofacial and tooth development. Nat Genet 1994;6:348–356.
30 Ishii M, Merrill AE, Chan YS, et al: Msx2 and Twist cooperatively control the development of the neural crest-derived skeletogenic mesenchyme of the murine skull vault. Development 2003;130:6131–6142.
31 Carlton MB, Colledge WH, Evans MJ: Crouzon-like craniofacial dysmorphology in the mouse is caused by an insertional mutation at the Fgf3/Fgf4 locus. Dev Dyn 1998;212:242–249.
32 Hajihosseini MK, Wilson S, De Moerlooze L, Dickson C: A splicing switch and gain-of-function mutation in FgfR2-IIIc hemizygotes causes Apert/Pfeiffer-syndrome like phenotypes. Proc Natl Acad Sci USA 2001;98:3855–3860.
33 Shi Y, Massague J: Mechanisms of TGF-beta signaling from cell membrane to the nucleus. Cell 2003;113:685–700.
34 Massague J, Chen YG: Controlling TGF-beta signaling. Genes Dev 2000;14:627–644.
35 Hogan BL: Bone morphogenetic proteins: multifunctional regulators of vertebrate development. Genes Dev 1996;10:1580–1594.
36 Gurdon JB, Bourillot PY: Morphogen gradient interpretation. Nature 2001;413:797–803.
37 ten Dijke P, Miyazono K, Heldin CH: Signaling via hetero-oligomeric complexes of type I and type II serine/threonine kinase receptors. Curr Opin Cell Biol 1996;8:139–145.
38 Massague J: TGF-beta signal transduction. Annu Rev Biochem 1998;67:753–791.
39 Liu YH, Kundu R, Wu L, et al: Premature suture closure and ectopic cranial bone in mice expressing Msx2 transgenes in the developing skull. Proc Natl Acad Sci USA 1995;92:6137–6141.
40 Nohno T, Ishikawa T, Saito T, et al: Identification of a human type II receptor for bone morphogenetic protein-4 that forms differential heteromeric complexes with bone morphogenetic protein type I receptors. J Biol Chem 1995;270:22522–22526.
41 Heldin CH, Miyazono K, ten Dijke P: TGF-beta signalling from cell membrane to nucleus through SMAD proteins. Nature 1997;390:465–471.
42 Raftery LA, Twombly V, Wharton K, Gelbart WM: Genetic screens to identify elements of the decapentaplegic signaling pathway in Drosophila. Genetics 1995;139:241–254.
43 Sekelsky JJ, McKim KS, Chin GM, Hawley RS: The Drosophila meiotic recombination gene mei-9 encodes a homologue of the yeast excision repair protein Rad1. Genetics 1995;141:619–627.

44 Kretzschmar M, Liu F, Hata A, Doody J, Massague J: The TGF-beta family mediator Smad1 is phosphorylated directly and activated functionally by the BMP receptor kinase. Genes Dev 1997;11:984–995.
45 Lagna G, Hata A, Hemmati-Brivanlou A, Massague J: Partnership between DPC4 and SMAD proteins in TGF-beta signalling pathways. Nature 1996;383:832–836.
46 Liu F, Pouponnot C, Massague J: Dual role of the Smad4/DPC4 tumor suppressor in TGFbeta-inducible transcriptional complexes. Genes Dev 1997;11:3157–3167.
47 Liu F, Hata A, Baker JC, et al: A human Mad protein acting as a BMP-regulated transcriptional activator. Nature 1996;381:620–623.
48 Hoodless PA, Haerry T, Abdollah S, et al: MADR1, a MAD-related protein that functions in BMP2 signaling pathways. Cell 1996;85:489–500.
49 Suzuki A, Ueno N, Hemmati-Brivanlou A: Xenopus msx1 mediates epidermal induction and neural inhibition by BMP4. Development 1997;124:3037–3044.
50 Wiersdorff V, Lecuit T, Cohen SM, Mlodzik M: Mad acts downstream of Dpp receptors, revealing a differential requirement for dpp signaling in initiation and propagation of morphogenesis in the Drosophila eye. Development 1996;122:2153–2162.
51 Shi Y, Wang YF, Jayaraman L, Yang H, Massague J, Pavletich NP: Crystal structure of a Smad MH1 domain bound to DNA: insights on DNA binding in TGF-beta signaling. Cell 1998;94: 585–594.
52 Wrana JL: Regulation of Smad activity. Cell 2000;100:189–192.
53 Chen H, Ovchinnikov D, Pressman CL, Aulehla A, Lun Y, Johnson RL: Multiple calvarial defects in lmx1b mutant mice. Dev Genet 1998;22:314–320.
54 Chen JN, van Eeden FJ, Warren KS, et al: Left-right pattern of cardiac BMP4 may drive asymmetry of the heart in zebrafish. Development 1997;124:4373–4382.
55 Chen Y, Bei M, Woo I, Satokata I, Maas R: Msx1 controls inductive signaling in mammalian tooth morphogenesis. Development 1996;122:3035–3044.
56 Hua X, Liu X, Ansari DO, Lodish HF: Synergistic cooperation of TFE3 and smad proteins in TGF-beta-induced transcription of the plasminogen activator inhibitor-1 gene. Genes Dev 1998;12:3084–3095.
57 Labbe E, Silvestri C, Hoodless PA, Wrana JL, Attisano L: Smad2 and Smad3 positively and negatively regulate TGF beta-dependent transcription through the forkhead DNA-binding protein FAST2. Mol Cell 1998;2:109–120.
58 Labbe E, Letamendia A, Attisano L: Association of Smads with lymphoid enhancer binding factor 1/T cell-specific factor mediates cooperative signaling by the transforming growth factor-beta and wnt pathways. Proc Natl Acad Sci USA 2000;97:8358–8363.
59 Germain S, Howell M, Esslemont GM, Hill CS: Homeodomain and winged-helix transcription factors recruit activated Smads to distinct promoter elements via a common Smad interaction motif. Genes Dev 2000;14:435–451.
60 Ionescu AM, Drissi H, Schwarz EM, et al: CREB cooperates with BMP-stimulated Smad signaling to enhance transcription of the Smad6 promoter. J Cell Physiol 2004;198:428–440.
61 Shi X, Yang X, Chen D, Chang Z, Cao X: Smad1 interacts with homeobox DNA-binding proteins in bone morphogenetic protein signaling. J Biol Chem 1999;274:13711–13717.
62 Shim S, Bae N, Han JK: Bone morphogenetic protein-4-induced activation of Xretpos is mediated by Smads and Olf-1/EBF associated zinc finger (OAZ). Nucleic Acids Res 2002;30:3107–3117.
63 Hata A, Seoane J, Lagna G, Montalvo E, Hemmati-Brivanlou A, Massague J: OAZ uses distinct DNA- and protein-binding zinc fingers in separate BMP-Smad and Olf signaling pathways. Cell 2000;100:229–240.
64 Henningfeld KA, Friedle H, Rastegar S, Knochel W: Autoregulation of Xvent-2B; direct interaction and functional cooperation of Xvent-2 and Smad1. J Biol Chem 2002;277:2097–2103.
65 Brugger SM, Merrill AE, Torres-Vazquez J, et al: A phylogenetically conserved *cis*-regulatory module in the Msx2 promoter is sufficient for BMP-dependent transcription in murine and Drosophila embryos. Development 2004;131:5153–5165.
66 Kim HJ, Rice DP, Kettunen PJ, Thesleff I: FGF-, BMP- and Shh-mediated signalling pathways in the regulation of cranial suture morphogenesis and calvarial bone development. Development 1998;125:1241–1251.

67 Antonopoulou I, Mavrogiannis LA, Wilkie AO, Morriss-Kay GM: Alx4 and Msx2 play phenotypically similar and additive roles in skull vault differentiation. J Anat 2004;204:487–499.
68 Rice R, Rice DP, Olsen BR, Thesleff I: Progression of calvarial bone development requires Foxc1 regulation of Msx2 and Alx4. Dev Biol 2003;262:75–87.
69 Vainio S, Karavanova I, Jowett A, Thesleff I: Identification of BMP-4 as a signal mediating secondary induction between epithelial and mesenchymal tissues during early tooth development. Cell 1993;75:45–58.
70 Rice DP, Kim HJ, Thesleff I: Apoptosis in murine calvarial bone and suture development. Eur J Oral Sci 1999;107:265–275.
71 Jagla T, Bidet Y, Da Ponte JP, Dastugue B, Jagla K: Cross-repressive interactions of identity genes are essential for proper specification of cardiac and muscular fates in Drosophila. Development 2002;129:1037–1047.
72 Ma L, Martin JF: Generation of a Bmp2 conditional null allele. Genesis 2005;42:203–206.
73 Jiao K, Kulessa H, Tompkins K, et al: An essential role of Bmp4 in the atrioventricular septation of the mouse heart. Genes Dev 2003;17:2362–2367.
74 Merrill AE, Bochukova EG, Brugger SM, et al: Cell mixing at a neural crest-mesoderm boundary and deficient ephrin-Eph signaling in the pathogenesis of craniosynostosis. Hum Mol Genet 2006;15:1319–1328.
75 Warren SM, Brunet LJ, Harland RM, Economides AN, Longaker MT: The BMP antagonist noggin regulates cranial suture fusion. Nature 2003;422:625–629.

Dr. Robert Maxson
Department of Biochemistry and Molecular Biology, Norris Comprehensive Cancer Center and Hospital, University of Southern California Keck School of Medicine
1441 Eastlake Avenue
Los Angeles, CA 90033 (USA)
Tel. +1 323 865 0633, Fax +1 323 865 0098, E-Mail maxson@usc.edu

Rice DP (ed): Craniofacial Sutures. Development, Disease and Treatment.
Front Oral Biol. Basel, Karger, 2008, vol 12, pp 209–230

Current Treatment of Craniosynostosis and Future Therapeutic Directions

Derrick C. Wan[a,b], *Matthew D. Kwan*[a,c], *H. Peter Lorenz*[a], *Michael T. Longaker*[a]

[a]Department of Surgery, Stanford University Medical Center, Stanford, Calif., [b]Department of Surgery, University of California, San Francisco, San Francisco, Calif., and [c]Department of Surgery, Temple University Hospital, Philadelphia, Pa., USA

Abstract

Normal craniofacial development is contingent upon coordinated growth between the brain and overlying calvaria. Craniosynostosis, the premature fusion of one or more cranial sutures, perturbs this natural framework, resulting in dramatic dysmorphology of the skull and face along with a multitude of associated functional abnormalities. Traditional approaches to the treatment of craniosynostosis have employed complex surgical remodeling of the skull vault and facial deformities all aimed at increasing the amount of intracranial volume and restoring a more normal craniofacial appearance. Significant morbidity and mortality, however, have plagued these procedures, driving dramatic evolution in our approach towards the treatment of pathologically fused sutures. Recent clinical and genetic studies have identified multiple forms of human craniosynostosis, each associated with mutations within various cytokine signaling pathways. Knowledge garnered from these investigations bear promise for the future development of alternative strategies to enhance or perhaps even replace contemporary approaches for the treatment of craniosynostosis.

Introduction

Craniosynostosis, the premature fusion of one or more cranial sutures, was first described by Otto [1] in 1830. Since that time, several theories have been forwarded to explain not only the pathogenesis of pathologic suture fusion, but also the multitude of accompanying calvarial and facial dysmorphisms observed. Studies by Virchow in the 1850s led to the proposal of calvarial growth in a plane parallel to that of the fused suture, with sagittal synostosis resulting in a scaphocephalic, or boat-shaped, skull secondary to compensatory growth in the anteroposterior axis [2]. Virchow, however, also attributed craniosynostosis to either cretinism or an inflammation of the meninges [2]. Subsequent work by Park and Powers [3] led to a conceptual revision in the 1920s, as congenital abnormalities in the suture mesenchyme became thought of as responsible for premature suture fusion. And in the 1950s, etiologic explanations for craniosynostosis once again changed, with studies by Moss [4] purporting aberrations in the basicranium altering transmission of force, via the dura mater, to the overlying cranial sutures ultimately effecting premature fusion. While recent genetic and mechanical studies have now supplanted this notion, investigations by Moss nonetheless engendered a radical shift in the surgical approach to craniosynostosis. Given the observation that suturectomy alone did not restore normal calvarial development, complex craniofacial procedures were also deemed necessary to allow for proper growth and cranial expansion [4]. Such realizations resulted in the pioneering work of Paul Tessier [5].

Contemporary studies have now led to the recognition that normal calvarial expansion is contingent upon coordinated growth between the brain and overlying skeletal elements. Allometric growth of the skull relies on an integration of complex interactions between the brain, dura mater, suture mesenchyme, and bone plates through multiple morphogenetic mechanisms, minor perturbations of which may result in pathologic development. Premature fusion of one or more cranial sutures results in restriction of the growing brain, with subsequent morphologic bony deformities due to specific patterns of compensatory growth. The most common type of craniosynostosis, whether isolated or part of a larger syndromic pattern, is sagittal synostosis, resulting in a scaphocephalic deformity [6]. Other notable forms include metopic, resulting in a trigonocephalic deformity, unilateral coronal, resulting in a plagiocephalic deformity, and bilateral coronal synostosis, resulting in a turribrachycephalic deformity. While lambdoid synostosis may also result in a plagiocephalic skull, this clinical entity has been infrequently encountered [6].

In addition to these calvarial dysmorphologies, premature pathologic suture fusion, as demonstrated by Moss, is also often associated with multiple craniofacial deformities [7]. Hypotelorism, upward slanting of the lateral canthi, palpebral fissure widening, displacement of the orbital rim and/or ear, and deviation of the nasal bone have all been commonly reported [8]. In syndromic forms of craniosynostosis, midface hypoplasia with a short and narrow palate can also be quite prominent, resulting in a class III malocclusion [8]. And in the extremities, syndactyly of both the hands and feet often accompanies some forms of syndromic craniosynostosis [8]. Each of these dysmorphisms, like the deformities in the skull, must be addressed by the clinician to allow for proper physical and psychological development of the child.

In addition to these morphologic abnormalities of the calvarial vault and craniofacial skeleton, several functional aspects of premature suture fusion also merit significant consideration. While still a contentious debate, concerns regarding elevations in intracranial pressure remain nonetheless exigent. Studies by Renier et al. [9] have suggested the risk for increase in intracranial pressure to be associated with multiple suture involvement, and that decreases in pressure measurements may follow surgical remodeling of the skull. Gault et al. [10], likewise, demonstrated high intracranial pressure to occur most frequently in children with multiple premature suture fusions. Considering the dramatic growth by the brain during the first 2 years of life, it would be reasonable to expect a mismatch in cranial volume to result in elevated pressures and possible mental retardation. Though this is not often the case, continued disquietude has often driven early surgical intervention.

Other functional considerations, in addition to intracranial pressure, have also been well described in association with craniosynostosis. With continued development in radiographic imaging, hydrocephalus has become an entity frequently observed in patients with both syndromic and nonsyndromic craniosynostosis. While this may often be secondary to elevations in intracranial pressure, ventriculomegaly may be more indicative of aberrant brain development, as can be seen in Apert's syndrome [11]. Visual disturbances are also commonly reported in those with premature pathologic suture fusion. Exorbitism and optic nerve atrophy can be readily attributed to abnormal craniofacial development [12]. In addition, stretching of the nerve, compression by carotid vessels, or secondary effects of increased intracranial pressure have also been associated with optic nerve dysfunction [8]. Finally, the risk for mental retardation has long been argued as a possible sequelae of craniosynostosis. Though the true incidence of mental retardation in patients with pathologic suture fusion is often argued, the general risk has routinely been cited as greater than that in the normal population [8]. Several studies have purported that despite no statistical difference in IQ scoring, patients with craniosynostosis may yet have immeasurable deficits in cognition which require more subtle forms of testing to fully elucidate [9, 13]. This concern has been best documented for premature fusion of the midline sagittal (SAG) and/or metopic suture. Collectively, these functional abnormalities represent a significant challenge in the treatment of craniosynostosis. Because the specter of irreparable neurologic damage is ever present, careful evaluation and follow-up have become the rule.

Dramatic advancements have occurred in our understanding of craniosynostosis and its etiopathogenesis over the past 2 centuries. Undoubtedly, however, the premature fusion of one or more cranial sutures still represents a potential harbinger for significant medical disability. Despite considerable evolution in our knowledge base, surgical intervention remains the best singular recourse for correction of the many morphologic and functional abnormalities seen with craniosynostosis. This chapter will further explore current approaches and philosophies for the treatment of premature suture fusion, as well as detail more recent investigations highlighting the potential for development of future targeted therapy.

Current Approaches and Treatment Philosophies

Surgical treatment of craniosynostosis found its origins in the late 1800s, when techniques such as fragmentation of the cranial vault and linear craniectomy were employed. These early procedures were accompanied by a high rate of reossification and poor esthetic outcomes, mandating multiple subsequent procedures [8]. Simple craniectomy, however, still finds limited use today for transient cranial decompression. These early procedures have now been supplanted by surgical remodeling of the affected area of the cranial vault and orbits. Surgery is generally performed at 6–9 months in order to take full advantage of the regenerative capacity of the skull at this age.

Preoperative Considerations

While premature suture fusion can begin in the prenatal period, diagnosis of craniosynostosis regularly does not occur until the early perinatal months. Persistent abnormality in cranial shape is usually noted by either the parents or pediatrician, prompting referral to a craniofacial surgeon/clinic [14]. Because suture synostosis may be part of a larger syndromic pattern involving cardiac, genitourinary, and musculoskeletal systems, detailed family history and maternal history are paramount. Physical examination of the child should include not only assessment of the head and neck, but also of the digits, toes, and spine. Furthermore, manual palpation of the skull allows for detection of abnormal ridging patterns, assessment of sutural patency, and evaluation of relative anterior and posterior fontanel fullness [14].

As compensatory growth of the calvaria occurs in directions less constrained, characteristic morphologic deformities arise which can assist in the determination of specific sutural involvement. Radiographic investigations, nonetheless, are still routinely employed to substantiate precise structural anatomy. Conventional views of the skull with anterior-posterior, lateral, and Towne's projections can collectively yield accurate information in the evaluation of craniosynostosis. Signs of suture fusion readily apparent on plain radiography include bony bridging with resultant heaping, sclerosis, straightening of the suture, and loss of suture clarity [15]. Specific limitations with this modality exist, however, in the identification of segmental involvement and in the differentiation between lambdoid synostosis and positional plagiocephaly [16]. Because of these shortcomings, computed tomography has become the definitive standard for the evaluation of suture anatomy [17]. Three-dimensional scans facilitate thorough definition of not only affected sutures, but also allow for evaluation of the skull base and aid in identifying signs of increased intracranial pressure. Such data have led to a refinement in preoperative planning and assessment of postoperative results [8]. Other forms of radiologic investigation, including ultrasonography and magnetic resonance imaging, have also been reported for the documentation of premature suture fusion [18, 19]. While less invasive, these modalities necessitate trained interpretation, and the incremental information derived from these studies has been subject to debate [14].

Following comprehensive description of sutural involvement, the need for intervention must be addressed on an individual basis. No consensus has been reached as to an optimal time for surgery, but multiple studies have suggested an association between delay of treatment and increased risk for elevated intracranial pressure [10]. Furthermore, uncorrected calvarial suture synostosis invariably exacerbates associated facial deformities. Secondary to these considerations, most craniofacial surgeons elect to begin surgical correction at 3–6 months of age, a time when children are generally capable of withstanding the physiologic stress of surgery [8]. Earlier intervention may be indicated, however, should evidence for elevated intracranial pressure or optic nerve dysfunction arise. Nevertheless, the goals of surgery are to exact volumetric gains within the calvaria, normalize calvarial shape, and alleviate pressure concerns while minimizing any long-term functional complications. Most craniofacial surgeons agree that surgery must be performed prior to 1 year of age to capitalize on the inherent malleability and regenerative capacity of the immature skull [14].

Surgical Treatment

Sagittal synostosis, characterized by compensatory growth in the anteroposterior direction resulting in an elongated 'boat'-shaped skull, is the most common form of craniosynostosis. Typically sporadic, only 2% of prematurely fused SAG sutures demonstrate a familial predisposition. In addition to the increased length and decreased width of the skull, sagittal synostosis also effects a distinctive frontal and occipital prominence, further complicating calvarial reconstruction. Early attempts at surgical correction focused solely on removal of the pathologic suture by strip craniectomy [20]. Refusion, however, invariably occurred, mitigating any gains made in the operating room [20]. More aggressive procedures have since evolved, encompassing remodeling of the entire calvarial vault in one sitting. Such procedures separate both the bifrontal and biparieto-occipital fragments to allow for recontouring using radial osteotomies, followed by wire or suture fixation back to a shortened midline parietal segment [8, 21]. Each parietal bone is also removed and remodeled to increase lateral convexity prior to reattachment with the underlying dura mater alone [21]. This approach not only releases the synostotic constraint, but also augments transverse width and improves calvarial contour. Finally, as an alternative, less invasive strategy, endoscopic extended strip craniectomy in conjunction with postoperative molding helmet therapy has recently been utilized for the correction of sagittal synostosis [22]. Retrospective studies have shown this approach to reduce mean operative time, estimated blood loss, hospital costs, and length of stay [23]. Outcome analyses 1 year following surgery, however, have suggested inadequate correction of cephalic index relative to more substantial procedures [24]. This may be attributed to limitations in opportunity for craniofacial surgeons to exact immediate and total remodeling of skull shape with the endoscopic technique [14]. Nonetheless, this technique continues to evolve, with some surgeons now incorporating additional parietal and occipital bone osteotomies.

In contrast to sagittal synostosis, metopic synostosis represents a significantly less common pathologic entity, accounting for just 10% of isolated, nonsyndromic craniosynostoses [25]. Premature metopic suture fusion results in retrusion of the lateral aspects of the frontal bone and the supraorbital ridge, with compensatory enlargement of parietal bones and anterior displacement of the coronal (COR) suture yielding a 'keel'-shaped skull [8]. Hypotelorism can also be quite prominent, with an accompanying upward slant of the lateral canthi and eyebrows. Treatment objectives for metopic synostosis include volumetric enlargement of the anterior cranial fossa, restoration of a normal shape to the frontal bones and supraorbital rim, and normalization of the interdacryon distance. Standard approaches employ a bifrontal craniotomy to remove the frontal and, occasionally, parietal bones, with remodeling accomplished through radial osteotomies and anterior advancement of the lateral supraorbital rims [21]. Resorbable plate fixation is then used to secure the anteriorly advanced supraorbital rims and remodeled forehead. Increase in the distance between the medial bony orbits is often achieved through incorporation of calvarial bone grafting with absorbable T plate fixation to the nasion [14].

Unilateral coronal synostosis is another uncommon disorder, with an incidence of 1 in 10,000 live births [26]. Unlike sagittal and metopic synostosis, unilateral coronal synostosis results in a pronounced, asymmetric calvarial and facial deformity. Premature COR suture fusion results in a single frontoparietal bone impairing ipsilateral expansion of the anterior cranial fossa while simultaneously deforming the middle cranial fossa through ventral bowing of the greater wing of the sphenoid. Compensatory growth in the periphery produces bulging of the temporal bone, widening of the palpebral fissure, displacement of the ipsilateral orbital rim and ear, and finally deviation of the chin and nasal root. Operative correction entails a unilateral or bilateral frontal craniotomy with total forehead reconstruction and supraorbital rim advancement. Rongeuring of the greater wing of the sphenoid back to the level of the lateral supraorbital fissure is also performed [8].

Bilateral coronal synostosis, frequently observed in Apert and Crouzon syndromes, represents an entirely distinct entity from that of unilateral coronal synostosis. Characterized by a towering, vertically elongated head, the calvarial vault becomes notably short in the anteroposterior direction and widened in the mediolateral direction [27]. Other associated deformities include recessed superior and lateral orbital rims and a flattened occiput [27]. Reduction in skull height and simultaneous lengthening in the anteroposterior direction require significant calvarial remodeling with particular attention paid to the maintenance of normal intracranial pressure. Bifrontal and biparieto-occipital osteotomies are made, leaving behind parietal bone struts used to relocate the cranial vertex posteriorly [21]. Excised calvarial bone grafts are then remodeled using controlled fractures and radial osteotomies to achieve a more conventional contour. And like other procedures described, treatment of bilateral coronal synostosis also requires superior and lateral orbital rim anterior advancement to correct the recessed fronto-orbital bar [14]. Postoperative molding helmet therapy is now routine in most centers for optimal molding of skull shape following surgery [8].

The least common form of craniosynostosis is isolated lambdoid synostosis [28]. Premature fusion of the lambdoid suture produces flattening of the occiput, deformation of the cranial base posteriorly, and frontal bossing [8]. The ipsilateral ear also becomes posteriorly displaced, allowing discrimination from pure positional (deformational) plagiocephaly in which the ear is typically positioned anteriorly [8]. The advent of high-resolution three-dimensional computed tomography has enabled more accurate distinction between these two divergent pathologies [28]. Surgical repair depends on the severity of deformity, but generally involves elevation of a parieto-occipital bone segment, remodeling through radial osteotomies, and dural plication prior to repositioning of the bone graft [21, 27]. In contrast, pure positional (deformational) plagiocephaly can be readily treated nonoperatively through head turning, helmet, and/or band therapy [28].

In the setting of syndromic forms of craniosynostosis, maxillary hypoplasia and class III malocclusion commonly occur. Thus, additional midface and orthognathic surgery may also be indicated. While the optimal age for correction of midface deformities has been debated, most centers wait until late childhood, unless severe exorbitism with exposure keratitis or airway obstruction dictates earlier intervention [8]. A subcranial approach for Le Fort III advancement is the most common procedure used; however, other techniques including monobloc with Le Fort III and frontal advancement are employed depending on the degree of forehead and facial deformity [8]. Despite appropriate treatment for midface retrusion, though, significant dentofacial deformities nonetheless arise. Correction of class III malocclusion is commonly performed once the patient has reached facial skeletal maturity and may entail either a Le Fort I maxillary advancement or two-jaw (maxillary and mandibular) surgery [8]. Osseous genioplasty is routinely performed as an adjunctive cosmetic procedure. With these considerations in mind, current approaches for the correction of facial dysmorphology in syndromic craniosynostoses have yielded promising results, demonstrating dramatic improvement in both morphologic and functional outcomes.

Complications

Considering the extensive nature of procedures aimed at remodeling the calvarial vault, complications can occur following surgical therapy for craniosynostosis. While many series have reported a mortality rate as high as 2.3%, most international figures fall in the range of 1.5–2% [8]. Evaluating experiences at 6 major centers with a combined 793 craniofacial operations, Whitaker et al. [29] noted 13 deaths, constituting a 1.6% mortality rate. Overall, complications occurred in 16.5% of cases, including infections in 4.4% [29]. Most deaths were attributed to hemorrhagic complications, but a variety of other causes have also been reported including air emboli, cerebral edema, and respiratory infections [30]. Deaths were also more common in the treatment of syndromic compared to nonsyndromic isolated craniosynostosis. Attention to intraoperative hemodynamics and careful postoperative ICU monitoring is therefore critical to best minimize overall morbidity and mortality. And beyond the immediate perioperative period, long-term complications such as suture refusion remain incontrovertibly extant. Clinically significant suturectomy site reossification rates have been reported as high as 20%, making reoperation, despite all its attendant risks, an intervention which must often be considered [31].

Operative blood loss can be either insidious or overt, and considering the relative blood volume in pediatric patients, continuous minor hemorrhage may nevertheless represent a significant hemodynamic stress [29]. Iatrogenic injury to any of the major dural sinuses can result in dramatic bleeding, necessitating prompt compression and immediate repair [8]. In most cases, however, the actual amount of blood loss can be much more deceptive. Gradual, persistent hemorrhage from cut bone may cumulatively necessitate transfusion. Furthermore, bleeding into the subgaleal space may be pronounced and should be considered in the postoperative period [29]. Ultimately, most patients undergoing calvarial vault remodeling require packed red blood cell transfusions, often in conjunction with fresh frozen plasma. Like hemorrhage, infection is another significant concern following calvarial remodeling; current figures suggest an incidence of 2.5–4.4% [29, 32]. While some studies have documented a declining rate, infectious sequelae can still be potentially catastrophic [29, 32]. Most infections involve either the meninges or devitalized calvarial bone grafts [8]. Resultant swelling, erythema, tenderness, or purulent drainage may be noted postoperatively. Irrespective of the cause, infections must be treated aggressively with antibiotics capable of crossing the blood-brain barrier and potential debridement or removal of the infected bone [8, 32]. Lastly, neurologic complications, including cerebrospinal fluid leak and seizures secondary to intracerebral contusion/bleeding, are salient considerations which must be recognized. Careful identification and repair of dural tears along with close monitoring of postoperative electrolyte levels can minimize these concerns.

As the number of craniofacial procedures performed annually has steadily increased over the past 2 decades, efforts have been made to identify contributing factors for the reduction of morbidity and mortality following complex calvarial remodeling. With increasing experience and improved techniques, faster operating times have indubitably resulted in decreased infection rates [32]. Furthermore, the common implementation of a short 24- to 48-hour postoperative antibiotic course has likely led to a decline in infectious complications [32]. Finally, the shift towards a centralization of these procedures in children's hospitals equipped with proper facilities and specialized anesthesia/intensive care expertise has without question resulted in reduced morbidity and mortality [14]. Such centers have reported extremely low complication rates, especially when treating nonsyndromic craniosynostoses [8].

Molecular Genetics and Future Targeted Therapy

Despite dramatic advancements in the surgical treatment of premature suture fusion and the continued efforts at minimizing morbidity and mortality, complications remain nonetheless exigent with significant potential for disability. And considering the frequent need for subsequent procedures, whether secondary to postoperative refusion or to correct accompanying facial dysmorphologies, the biomedical burden of craniosynostosis continues to be high [31]. With a more comprehensive understanding of molecular mechanisms guiding both normal and pathologic suture fusion, the promise exists for development of novel therapeutic strategies designed to either complement or even replace surgical therapy. While the etiology of craniosynostosis remains largely unknown, increasing insight has been garnered through clinical genetic studies and the use of murine models for cranial suture fusion. Integrating these findings, multiple targets for future therapy have emerged.

Genetics of Craniosynostosis

Several investigations have been performed evaluating the roles of growth factors and various cytokines in governing suture fate. The importance of fibroblast growth factors (FGFs) has been particularly evident, as mutations in their receptors have been implicated in a multitude of craniosynostosis syndromes. Of the four known FGF receptors (FGFRs), mutations in three have been associated with premature pathologic suture fusion [33–35]. Considering these findings, a large body of work has been dedicated to the elucidation of their function with respect to suture development. FGFR gain-of-function mutations identified with human craniosynostosis have been primarily localized to the IgII-IgIII linker region, with resultant stabilization of ligand-receptor interactions and enhanced receptor dimerization. X-ray crystallographic analysis has demonstrated additional intermolecular contacts between FGF ligands and their receptors, providing a structural basis for increased receptor activity [33, 34, 36]. Well-recognized mutations include the FGFR2 Ser252Trp and Pro253Arg substitutions associated with Apert syndrome and the analogous Pro252Arg mutation in FGFR1 associated with Pfeiffer syndrome [33]. Similar mutations in FGFR3 have also been noted in patients with Muenke syndrome and type I thanatophoric dysplasia [37, 38].

As gain-of-function FGFR mutations have been clearly implicated in the pathogenesis of human craniosynostosis, extensive research using the murine model has further focused on defining the interplay between the FGF ligands and their receptors. In rats and mice, the posterior frontal (PF) suture fuses in a predictable manner, whereas both the SAG and the COR sutures remain perpetually patent [39]. This differential suture fate has been exploited by researchers as a model to elucidate underlying molecular mechanisms guiding suture fusion or the maintenance of patency. Most studies have specifically focused on FGF2 and its receptor interactions in view of the fact that FGF2 has been shown to be an abundant ligand with potent mitogenic and osteoinductive capacity [35, 40]. Studies by Moore et al. [41] have demonstrated reduction in FGF2 activity, through introduction of neutralizing antibodies, to limit both proliferation and osteoblast differentiation. Evaluating expression specifically within the suture complex, FGF2 has been found to be notably elevated in the PF dura mater at times just before and during the period of expected fusion [42–44]. In contrast, minimal expression of FGF2 has been noted in both the patent SAG and COR sutures at similar time points [42, 43]. Ectopic FGF2 expression within the COR suture, however, was found to induce pathologic suture fusion in mice [45, 46]. Collectively, these data suggest a facilitatory role for FGF2 in the process of physiologic murine PF suture fusion. Furthermore, the upregulation of FGF2 activity in fusing sutures, along with abnormal suture fusion in the setting of ectopic FGF2 expression, provides an elegant corollary to the gain-of-function FGFR mutations observed in human craniosynostosis.

Extending these findings, transgenic mice have recently been reported with similar FGFR mutations to those noted in human craniosynostosis syndromes. Analogous to the FGFR1 Pro252Arg mutation in Pfeiffer syndrome, Zhou et al. [47] have demonstrated mice carrying the FGFR1 Pro250Arg mutation to exhibit pathologic SAG and COR suture fusion, marked facial asymmetry, and hypoplasia of the midface. Further analyses have shown these mice to also upregulate runx2/cbfa1, osteopontin, and osteocalcin, suggesting this gain-of-function FGFR1 mutation precipitates premature suture fusion through the promotion of osteoblast differentiation and bone formation [47]. Parallel studies have also been conducted with transgenic mice carrying an FGFR2 Ser250Trp mutation orthologous to that observed in Apert syndrome [48]. But while these mice also demonstrate premature COR suture fusion with secondary skull distortion, in vitro studies on harvested osteoblasts have revealed increased bax expression, suggesting a possible role for programmed cell death in craniosynostosis [48]. These findings thus raise the possibility that different gain-of-function FGFR mutations may employ disparate molecular mechanisms toward a similar end of pathologic suture fusion. In addition, they also highlight the significance of FGFs and their receptors in the pathogenesis of craniosynostosis and suggest a possible target for future therapeutic strategies.

While multiple studies have endeavored to better define the role FGFs play in suture synostosis, recent investigations have demonstrated MSX2 and Twist to be potential downstream modulators of FGF activity [49–51]. Associated with Boston-type craniosynostosis, the homeobox-containing msx2 gene has been shown to be upregulated in response to increased FGF signaling [49]. Exogenous FGF2 delivery to mice calvariae was found to enhance Msx2 expression, along with the osteogenic differentiation markers runx2/cbfa1, osteopontin, and osteocalcin [49]. Interestingly, examination of the skull revealed pathologic obliteration of the COR suture in regions of greatest msx2 upregulation [49]. These observations have been further supported by studies on msx2 gain-of-function transgenic mice, which demonstrate enhanced parietal bone growth and pathologic SAG suture fusion [50, 51]. Like msx2, twist may be another gene potentially involved in the direction of downstream cellular response secondary to FGF signaling. Heterozygous mutations or deletions in twist have been associated with Saethre-Chotzen syndrome, an autosomal dominant human craniosynostotic syndrome [52, 53]. Furthermore, haploinsufficiency of this basic helix-loop-helix transcription factor in mice has also been shown to precipitate COR suture fusion [54]. Experiments with human osteoblasts have suggested twist to attenuate cellular responses to FGF ligand, with overexpression resulting in a downregulation of early growth response element-1, a known mediator of FGF signaling, and maintenance of an undifferentiated, spindle-shaped phenotype [55]. Twist may therefore be critical for the perpetuation of a slowly dividing, osteoprogenitor state, facilitating continued suture patency. And like MSX2, perturbations in Twist may result in dysregulated FGF signaling, with premature osteoblast differentiation and subsequent pathologic suture fusion.

In contrast to the strong demonstration of altered FGF signaling and its downstream modulators effecting changes in osteoblast biology and premature human synostosis, clinical genetics has yet to uncover a categorical form of craniosynostosis unconditionally associated with mutations in the transforming growth factor (TGF)-β pathway. Despite its ubiquity in bone and skeletal biology, only recently has an autosomal dominant gain-of-function mutation in TGF-β receptors (TGF-βR) been reported in conjunction with a variable craniosynostotic phenotype [56]. Nonetheless, multiple investigations in both humans and rodents have suggested specific TGF-β isoforms to be important in suture development and maintenance of patency. Analysis of synostotic suture samples from 10 infants revealed a relative increase of the TGF-β_2 isoform immunoreactivity in actively fusing sutures when compared to control patent sutures [57]. Observations by Opperman in rats have likewise confirmed a differential upregulation of TGF-β_2 within the PF suture complex, implicating this growth factor in the process of fusion [58]. Conversely, immunohistochemical studies have localized the TGF-β_3 isoform to osteogenic fronts of patent sutures, suggesting a role in the maintenance of patency [57, 59]. Furthermore, as a more potent competitor for membrane receptors, TGF-β_3 may thus preferentially bind to shared TGF-βRI, thereby downregulating the pro-osteogenic effects of TGF-β_2 [60]. Findings from human craniosynostotic samples, in combination with those derived from the murine model, therefore strongly implicate TGF-β signaling in the regulation of suture fate. Irrespective of the fact that mutations within the TGF-β pathway have only recently become identified with clinical craniofacial pathology, the distinct presence of various TGF-β isoforms during the process of suture development strongly suggests these growth factors to be a potential target in the genesis of future therapeutics.

Bone morphogenetic proteins (BMPs), additional members of the TGF-β superfamily, have also received similar attention in the regulation of suture fusion. Originally identified by their ability to promote ectopic bone formation, unopposed BMP activity has been purported to result in the absence of joint specification with resultant bony fusion in extremities of transgenic mice [61]. Investigations on murine cranial sutures, however, have suggested that antagonists of BMP signaling, and not the BMP molecules themselves, may be the critical effectors of differential suture fate. Abundant levels of BMPs have been demonstrated in both fusing PF and patent SAG sutures of mice, suggesting suture-specific regulation of BMP activity to mediate observed patterns of suture fate [45]. Interestingly, the expression of specific BMP antagonists has been directly linked to relative levels of FGF2 activity. In situ hybridization studies revealed transcripts for noggin to be prevalent within both the SAG and COR sutures of mice; in contrast, noggin was conspicuously absent in the PF suture throughout the entire period of expected fusion [45]. In vitro osteoblast studies have further supported the notion that high FGF2 activity within the PF suture complex elicits a downregulation in the expression of noggin, leaving endogenous BMP activity unopposed [45]. Such unabated BMP signaling, like that observed in the extremities, may thus result in suture synostosis.

Similar to Noggin, other BMP antagonists have also emerged with potential roles in the determination of suture fate. Microarray analyses have particularly demonstrated BMP3 to possess an expression profile highly suggestive of an osteogenic antagonist [62]. Initially purified from bone, rhBMP3, like Noggin, was found to inhibit embryonic ventralization, implying a similar regulatory role for BMP signaling [63]. Unlike Noggin, however, BMP3 does not temper ligand-receptor interaction [64]. Rather, BMP3 exerts its antagonistic function through activin receptor activation and competition for shared downstream SMAD effectors [65]. Importantly, gene analysis has revealed increased BMP3 expression in patent rat calvarial sutures, potentially implicating this gene in the maintenance of suture patency [66]. Unfortunately, generation of BMP3 null transgenic mice has provided little additional information, as no significant abnormalities have yet to be noted in their calvarial development [65]. Further studies are therefore requisite before clinical considerations can be made as to the potential value of this therapeutic target.

Among other classes of molecules, abnormalities in Nell-1 and Ephrin-B1 have also been noted in cases of human craniosynostosis. Nell-1, an 810-amino acid polypeptide with six epidermal growth factor-like repeats and a hydrophobic amino terminus, was originally identified by differential-display PCR to be distinctly upregulated in synostosed human COR suture samples [67]. Overexpression in transgenic mice has been reported to promote apoptosis within cells along the osteogenic front and obliteration of the COR suture, implicating enhanced programmed cell death as an alternative mechanism resulting in pathologic suture fusion [68]. Recent studies have also identified Ephrin-B1 to be associated with coronal synostosis [69]. As a member of the Ephrin family of transmembrane ligands for the tyrosine kinase Eph receptor, heterozygous loss-of-function mutations in Eprhin-B1 have been observed in an X-linked craniofacial disorder with COR synostosis as a feature in females [69, 70]. Interestingly, males with this same mutation do not exhibit pathologic suture fusion and are generally not as severely affected as females. While the functional role of Ephrin-B1 and how it may result in suture synostosis remains largely undefined, murine studies have suggested this molecule to be involved in the delineation of suture boundaries [69]. Characterization of molecular interactions that determine tissue patterning and ultimate fate in the skull will thus undoubtedly assist in our understanding of these genes.

Collectively, the integration of data from both clinical and rodent investigations has provided a glimpse into the biomolecular mechanisms underlying the process of suture fusion. Investigators have identified several factors, including members of the FGF, TGF-β, and BMP families which may work alone or in concert to ultimately orchestrate suture fate. In addition, a growing number of other genes have been recently reported which may also assist in the modulation of responses to these various signaling pathways. But while the multitude of growth factors, cytokines, and transcription factors described speaks to the complexity of calvarial suture development, they nevertheless afford a wealth of imaginable approaches for the future treatment of craniosynostosis.

Development of Targeted Therapy

The body of knowledge garnered from both clinical genetic and murine model investigations has provided an ample stage for the development of future therapeutic strategies. Prior attempts at modulating prospective suture fate following suturectomy have employed various schemes of barrier interposition to minimize osteogenic obliteration of the intervening mesenchyme. Early studies applied a silicon membrane to COR suturectomy sites in an experimental rabbit model for craniosynostosis [71]. While this resulted in a general maintenance of suture patency and abatement of significant skull deformity, progressive bone formation was observed, likely deposited from surrounding periosteum and dura mater [71]. Subsequent studies have used Gore-Tex, with a smaller pore size in the range of 20–40 μm, to prevent osteoblast migration into the operative site [72]. Suturectomy edges wrapped with Gore-Tex have been observed to maintain patency, thereby improving secondary craniofacial morphology [72]. In the short term, this allowed for normal allometric calvarial expansion, but as the resultant inhibition in suturectomy site osteogenesis was found to be persistent, reoperative removal of the Gore-Tex implant was eventually necessary to allow for long-term defect repair. With these considerations in mind, and with the inherent complications of long-lasting foreign-body implantation (i.e. infection), alternative strategies employing cytokine therapy have thus become increasingly attractive.

Given the strong association between dysregulated FGF signaling and pathologic fusion, downregulation of either membrane receptors or the inhibition of downstream signaling events may be potential approaches to effect alterations in suture fate. Investigations have demonstrated FGF signal transduction to occur via ligand-induced receptor homo- and heterodimerization resulting in phosphorylation of intracellular tyrosine residues [73]. Ultimate activation of protein kinase C and/or the Ras/MAP kinase pathways transpires through Src-homology 2 domain-containing proteins, leading to changes in the transcriptional profile of the cell [73]. Ueno et al. [74] have demonstrated a truncated form of FGFR1, lacking its cytoplasmic domain, to inhibit signal transduction by each of three different wild-type FGFR1, 2 and 3, the same isoforms implicated in human craniosynostosis. Rat calvarial osteoblasts expressing this same truncated receptor have been found to display less phosphorylated early response kinase (ERK)-1 and -2 in response to rhFGF2 stimulation, intimating a reduction in cytoplasmic signaling within the MAP kinase pathway [46]. Resultant expression of collagen I, an early marker for bone formation, was also diminished, suggesting impaired osteogenic differentiation in these cells [46]. And when dominant-negative FGFRs were transfected in utero into the PF suture of fetal rats, postnatal suture fusion was found to be interrupted [46]. These findings highlight the potential therapeutic implications for FGF signal modulation. In the presence of a gain-of-function FGFR mutation, genetic manipulation with suture-targeted induction of a truncated receptor may allow for downregulation of both ligand-independent and ligand-dependent FGF signaling. Such a perturbation may thus engender a more physiologic level of FGF activity, thereby effecting a change in the course of syndromic craniosynostosis.

As an alternative modality to dominant-negative gene transfection, endogenous instruments of cellular defense could likewise be exploited to achieve a reduction in the level of protein receptors themselves. RNA interference, with its high degree of specificity, has already been employed in multiple disease models to suppress particular proteins with encouraging results. Continuous intrathecal infusion of siRNA constructs targeting the pain-related cation-channel $P2X_3$ in rats was found to result in a diminished pain response when compared to missense siRNA-treated or untreated controls [75]. Sequential intravenous injections of Fas-directed constructs were also shown to limit in vivo liver fibrosis following treatment of mice with canavalin A [76]. While both of these investigations clearly underscore the potential utility of RNA interference in the treatment of disease, they also, unfortunately, highlight the inherent instability of siRNA constructs, with multiple, potentially costly, administrations requisite to obtain a transient result at best. Recent studies have employed chemical modifications in the siRNA structure to achieve more lasting results, showing detectable levels of apoB-targeted constructs 24 h following a single intravenous administration in mice [77]. Concomitant reduction in total cholesterol levels was also observed over this same time interval [77].

Considering the natural development of human brains, however, with a doubling in volume over the first 2 years of life, much more durable suppression of the overactive FGFR would be necessary to potentially maintain suture patency throughout this period of growth [78]. Nonetheless, the specificity and general efficiency of gene suppression confers great promise for the use of RNA interference in the future treatment of pathologic suture fusion secondary to FGFR gain-of-function mutations.

Downstream from the level of ligand-receptor interactions, multiple opportunities also exist for targeted downregulation of the FGF signal transduction machinery. Investigations using microarray gene analysis of Apert syndrome osteoblasts have identified enhanced expression of interleukin-IL (IL-1α) and RhoA, among other genes, when compared to control osteoblasts lacking the Ser252Trp FGFR2 mutation [79]. Treatment of these Apert osteoblasts with either SB203580, a specific inhibitor of p38 mitogen-activated protein kinase (MAPK), or PD98059, a specific inhibitor of MAPK kinase (MEK), resulted in reduced IL-1α and RhoA expression, thereby antagonizing the effects of aberrant FGF signaling [79]. SB203580 has also been shown to impede osteogenic differentiation, as demonstrated by a reduction in alkaline phosphatase activity [80]. And in similar fashion, U0126, an alternative MEK inhibitor, has been reported to reduce rhFGF2-mediated changes in the osteoblastic expression of BMP2 [81]. Such findings therefore reveal the utility of these compounds to engender changes in the cellular biology and bone-forming capacity of osteoblasts. From the perspective of cranial development, inhibitors of the MAPK pathway have also been observed to alter the process of suture fusion. Direct application of PD98059 to cultured mouse calvariae was found to dampen not only osteopontin expression, but also FGF2-accelerated cranial suture closure [82]. Collectively, these data thus demonstrate the efficacy of MAPK inhibitors in the modulation of FGF signaling and osteoblast biology. As an alternative or adjunct to the targeting of gain-of-function receptors, these compounds may therefore find use in the future treatment of syndromic craniosynostosis.

While studies continue to investigate the therapeutic potential of FGF downregulation, manipulations in the TGF-β signaling pathway may likewise yield efficacious designs. As elevated levels of TGF-β_2 have been noted in cranial sutures undergoing both physiologic and premature fusion, strategies have employed neutralizing antibodies in an attempt to delay or prevent osseous sutural obliteration [59]. Opperman et al. [59] have shown that the application of TGF-β_2 antibodies to an ex vivo rat calvarial organ culture system could rescue sutures from expected fusion. Similarly, subperiosteal delivery of TGF-β_2 antibodies within a collagen gel to rat PF sutures in culture could likewise result in a significant reduction of sutural bridging when compared to controls [83].

In contrast to suppression of TGF-β_2, upregulation of TGF-β_3 has also been explored as an alternative strategy to hinder the process of suture fusion. Given the expression pattern of TGF-β_3 suggesting its potential implication in the maintenance of patency, studies have hypothesized that this isoform may be capable of preventing or rescuing fusing sutures [58]. Delivery of exogenous TGF-β_3 to the COR suture in a delayed-onset synostotic rabbit model has been proven to result in significantly greater width between osteogenic fronts when assessed 2 months postoperatively [84]. Furthermore, while a dose-dependent effect has been reported for sutural response to exogenous TGF-β_3, as little as 3 ng has been shown to delay in vivo rat PF osteogenic obliteration [85]. With these promising results, manipulation of TGF-β signaling may very well become a prominent modality to clinically tailor the process of suture fusion. Whether through application of neutralizing TGF-β_2 antibodies or the administration of exogenous TGF-β_3, therapeutic modulation of this cytokine axis may one day plausibly allow for the prevention of both primary and postoperative cranial suture synostosis.

As a final approach for potential cytokine-based treatment of pathologic suture fusion, investigators have focused on the BMP signaling pathway and reported antagonists to the pro-osteogenic effects of BMP ligands. Studies have already demonstrated Noggin upregulation to result in impaired osteoblast differentiation and reduced bone formation in vivo [86]. U-33 preosteoblastic cells overexpressing noggin were found to exhibit defective maturation, with a resultant decrease in runx2/cbfa1, osteopontin, and osteocalcin transcript levels [86]. Transgenic mice with this same overexpression of noggin were also observed to have a dramatic decrease in bone formation and mineral density [86]. A precise balance between BMP agonists and antagonists such as noggin therefore indubitably exists, regulating the pro-osteogenic effects of BMP ligands and subsequent bone formation. Translating this notion to calvarial sutures, an upregulation of antagonists like noggin may thus result in diminished bone formation with resultant impairment in the process of suture fusion. Using a mouse model, Warren et al. [45] have already demonstrated that forced Noggin expression through an adenoviral vector could result in maintenance of patent PF sutures. In addition, exogenous Noggin protein delivered within a slow release collagen vehicle has been shown to limit suture resynostosis following COR suturectomy in rabbits. These findings therefore suggest that Noggin-based therapy may have the potential to prevent postoperative refusion in children undergoing calvarial reconstruction. And as BMP3 functions in likewise fashion antagonizing the osteoinductive effects of BMP ligands, similar use of this cytokine to impair osteogenesis may lend toward the future treatment of craniosynostosis.

Conclusion

Since its first description nearly 200 years ago, significant refinement in the clinical approach and pathogenetic understanding of craniosynostosis has transpired. While the multitude of morphologic and functional disabilities associated with premature suture fusion have driven the evolution of surgical practice, children still face complex and challenging procedures aimed at increasing cranial volume while reconstructing both the skull vault and facial deformity. With inherent concerns regarding hemorrhage and infection, neurologic deficit, and postoperative refusion, alternative and/or adjunctive therapeutic approaches have been sought to improve outcomes. Recent advances in developmental biology and genetics have elucidated some of the events governing suture fate, highlighting multiple axes of cellular signaling with potential for clinical manipulation. Investigations employing various animal models have identified downregulation of FGF signaling, modulation of relative TGF-β isoforms, and perturbations in the balance between BMP agonists and antagonists as promising strategies to effect changes in suture fate. Such knowledge and comprehension may therefore one day facilitate therapeutic translation, ultimately enhancing or perhaps even replacing contemporary modalities of craniosynostosis treatment.

Acknowledgments

This work was supported by National Institutes of Health grant R01 DE13194 and the Oak Foundation to Michael T. Longaker and the Ethicon-SUS Research Fellowship to Derrick C. Wan.

References

1 Otto AW: Lehrbuch der Pathologischen Anatomie. Berlin, Rucher, 1830.
2 Virchow R: Über den Cretinismus, namentlich in Franken, und über pathologische Schädelformen. Verh Phys Med Gesellsch Würzburg 1851;2:231–271.
3 Park EA, Powers GF: Acrocephaly and scaphocephaly with symmetrically distributed malformations of the extremities. Am J Dis Child 1920;20:235–315.
4 Moss ML: The pathogenesis of premature cranial synostosis in man. Acta Anat 1959;37:351–370.
5 Tessier P: Total facial osteotomy. Crouzon's syndrome, Apert's syndrome: oxycephaly, scaphocephaly, turricephaly (in French). Ann Chir Plast 1967;12:273–286.
6 Posnick JC: Craniofacial syndromes and anomalies; in Posnick JC (ed): Craniofacial and Maxillofacial Surgery in Children and Young Adults. Philadelphia, Saunders, 2000, vol 1, pp 391–527.
7 Moss ML: Experimental alteration of sutural area morphology. Anat Rec 1957;127:569–589.
8 Grabb WC, Smith JW, Aston SJ: Plastic Surgery, ed 4. Boston, Little, Brown, 1991.

9 Renier D, Sainte-Rose C, Marchac D, Hirsch JF: Intracranial pressure in craniostenosis. J Neurosurg 1982;57:370–377.
10 Gault DT, Renier D, Marchac D, Jones BM: Intracranial pressure and intracranial volume in children with craniosynostosis. Plast Reconstr Surg 1992;90:377–381.
11 Kreiborg S, Cohen MM Jr: The infant Apert skull. Neurosurg Clin North Am 1991;2:551–554.
12 Newman SA: Ophthalmic features of craniosynostosis. Neurosurg Clin North Am 1991;2: 587–610.
13 Marchac D, Renier D: The 'floating forehead'. Early treatment of craniofacial stenosis (in French). Ann Chir Plast 1979;24:121–126.
14 Panchal J, Uttchin V: Management of craniosynostosis. Plast Reconstr Surg 2003;111:2032–2049.
15 Benson ML, Oliverio PJ, Yue NC, Zinreich SJ: Primary craniosynostosis: imaging features. AJR Am J Roentgenol 1996;166:697–703.
16 Aviv RI, Rodger E, Hall CM: Craniosynostosis. Clin Radiol 2002;57:93–102.
17 Panchal J, Marsh JL, Park TS, Kaufman B, Pilgram T: Photographic assessment of head shape following sagittal synostosis surgery. Plast Reconstr Surg 1999;103:1585–1591.
18 Blaumeiser B, Loquet P, Wuyts W, Nothen MM: Prenatal diagnosis of Pfeiffer syndrome type II. Prenat Diagn 2004;24:644–646.
19 Robson CD, Barnewolt CE: MR imaging of fetal head and neck anomalies. Neuroimaging Clin North Am 2004;14:273–291, viii.
20 Kaufman BA, Muszynski CA, Matthews A, Etter N: The circle of sagittal synostosis surgery. Semin Pediatr Neurol 2004;11:243–248.
21 Persing JA, Edgerton MT, Jane JA: Scientific Foundations and Surgical Treatment of Craniosynostosis. Baltimore, Williams & Wilkins, 1989.
22 Jimenez DF, Barone CM: Endoscopic craniectomy for early surgical correction of sagittal craniosynostosis. J Neurosurg 1998;88:77–81.
23 Barone CM, Jimenez DF: Endoscopic craniectomy for early correction of craniosynostosis. Plast Reconstr Surg 1999;104:1965–1973.
24 Panchal J, Marsh JL, Park TS, Kaufman B, Pilgram T, Huang SH: Sagittal craniosynostosis outcome assessment for two methods and timings of intervention. Plast Reconstr Surg 1999;103: 1574–1584.
25 Albin RE, Hendee RW Jr, O'Donnell RS, Majure JA: Trigonocephaly: refinements in reconstruction. Experience with 33 patients. Plast Reconstr Surg 1985;76:202–211.
26 Hansen M, Mulliken JB: Frontal plagiocephaly. Diagnosis and treatment. Clin Plast Surg 1994;21:543–553.
27 Persing JA, Jane JA: Treatment of syndromic and nonsyndromic bilateral coronal synostosis in infancy and childhood. Neurosurg Clin North Am 1991;2:655–663.
28 Ellenbogen RG, Gruss JS, Cunningham ML: Update on craniofacial surgery: the differential diagnosis of lambdoid synostosis/posterior plagiocephaly. Clin Neurosurg 2000;47:303–318.
29 Whitaker LA, Munro IR, Salyer KE, Jackson IT, Ortiz-Monasterio F, Marchac D: Combined report of problems and complications in 793 craniofacial operations. Plast Reconstr Surg 1979;64: 198–203.
30 Davies DW, Munro IR: The anesthetic management and intraoperative care of patients undergoing major facial osteotomies. Plast Reconstr Surg 1975;55:50–55.
31 McCarthy JG, Epstein F, Sadove M, Grayson B, Zide B: Early surgery for craniofacial synostosis: an 8-year experience. Plast Reconstr Surg 1984;73:521–533.
32 Fearon JA, Yu J, Bartlett SP, Munro IR, Chir B, Whitaker L: Infections in craniofacial surgery: a combined report of 567 procedures from two centers. Plast Reconstr Surg 1997;100:862–868.
33 Wilkie AOM, Slaney SF, Oldridge M, Poole MD, Ashworth JG, Hockley AD, Hayward RD, David DJ, Pulleyn LJ, Rutland P, et al: Apert syndrome results from localized mutations of FGFR2 and is allelic with Crouzon syndrome. Nat Genet 1995;9:165–171.
34 Muenke M, Schell U, Hehr A, Robin NH, Losken HW, Schinzel A, Pulleyn LJ, Rutland P, Reardon W, Malcolm S, et al: A common mutation in the fibroblast growth factor receptor 1 gene in Pfeiffer syndrome. Nat Genet 1994;8:269–274.
35 Wilkie AOM, Morriss-Kay GM, Jones EY, Heath JK: Functions of fibroblast growth factors and their receptors. Curr Biol 1995;5:500–507.

36 Ibrahimi OA, Eliseenkova AV, Plotnikov AN, Yu K, Ornitz DM, Mohammadi M: Structural basis for fibroblast growth factor receptor 2 activation in Apert syndrome. Proc Natl Acad Sci USA 2001;98:7182–7187.
37 Bellus GA, Gaudenz K, Zackai EH, Clarke LA, Szabo J, Francomano CA, Muenke M: Identical mutations in three different fibroblast growth factor receptor genes in autosomal dominant craniosynostosis syndromes. Nat Genet 1996;14:174–176.
38 Tavormina PL, Shiang R, Thompson LM, Zhu YZ, Wilkin DJ, Lachman RS, Wilcox WR, Rimoin DL, Cohn DH, Wasmuth JJ: Thanatophoric dysplasia (types I and II) caused by distinct mutations in fibroblast growth factor receptor 3. Nat Genet 1995;9:321–328.
39 Warren SM, Longaker MT: New directions in plastic surgery research. Clin Plast Surg 2001;28:719–730.
40 Nakamura T, Hanada K, Tamura M, Shibanushi T, Nigi H, Tagawa M, Fukumoto S, Matsumoto T: Stimulation of endosteal bone formation by systemic injections of recombinant basic fibroblast growth factor in rats. Endocrinology 1995;136:1276–1284.
41 Moore R, Ferretti P, Copp A, Thorogood P: Blocking endogenous FGF-2 activity prevents cranial osteogenesis. Dev Biol 2002;243:99–114.
42 Mehrara BJ, Mackool RJ, McCarthy JG, Gittes GK, Longaker MT: Immunolocalization of basic fibroblast growth factor and fibroblast growth factor receptor-1 and receptor-2 in rat cranial sutures. Plast Reconstr Surg 1998;102:1805–1820.
43 Most D, Levine JP, Chang J, Sung J, McCarthy JG, Schendel SA, Longaker MT: Studies in cranial suture biology: up-regulation of transforming growth factor-beta1 and basic fibroblast growth factor mRNA correlates with posterior frontal cranial suture fusion in the rat. Plast Reconstr Surg 1998;101:1431–1440.
44 Gosain AK, Recinos RF, Agresti M, Khanna AK: TGF-beta1, FGF-2, and receptor mRNA expression in suture mesenchyme and dura versus underlying brain in fusing and nonfusing mouse cranial sutures. Plast Reconstr Surg 2004;113:1675–1684.
45 Warren SM, Brunet LJ, Harland RM, Economides AN, Longaker MT: The BMP antagonist noggin regulates cranial suture fusion. Nature 2003;422:625–629.
46 Greenwald JA, Mehrara BJ, Spector JA, Warren SM, Fagenholz PJ, Smith LE, Bouletreau PJ, Crisera FE, Ueno H, Longaker MT: In vivo modulation of FGF biological activity alters cranial suture fate. Am J Pathol 2001;158:441–452.
47 Zhou YX, Xu X, Chen L, Li C, Brodie SG, Deng CX: A Pro250Arg substitution in mouse Fgfr1 causes increased expression of Cbfa1 and premature fusion of calvarial sutures. Hum Mol Genet 2000;9:2001–2008.
48 Chen L, Li D, Li C, Engel A, Deng CX: A Ser250Trp substitution in mouse fibroblast growth factor receptor 2 (Fgfr2) results in craniosynostosis. Bone 2003;33:169–178.
49 Ignelzi MA Jr, Wang W, Young AT: Fibroblast growth factors lead to increased Msx2 expression and fusion in calvarial sutures. J Bone Miner Res 2003;18:751–759.
50 Liu YH, Tang Z, Kundu RK, Wu L, Luo W, Zhu D, Sangiorgi F, Snead ML, Maxson RE: Msx2 gene dosage influences the number of proliferative osteogenic cells in growth centers of the developing murine skull: a possible mechanism for MSX2-mediated craniosynostosis in humans. Dev Biol 1999;205:260–274.
51 Liu YH, Kundu R, Wu L, Luo W, Ignelzi MA Jr, Snead ML, Maxson RE Jr: Premature suture closure and ectopic cranial bone in mice expressing Msx2 transgenes in the developing skull. Proc Natl Acad Sci USA 1995;92:6137–6141.
52 el Ghouzzi V, Le Merrer M, Perrin-Schmitt F, Lajeunie E, Benit P, Renier D, Bourgeois P, Bolcato-Bellemin AL, Munnich A, Bonaventure J: Mutations of the TWIST gene in the Saethre-Chotzen syndrome. Nat Genet 1997;15:42–46.
53 Howard TD, Paznekas WA, Green ED, Chiang LC, Ma N, Ortiz de Luna RI, Garcia Delgado C, Gonzalez-Ramos M, Kline AD, Jabs EW: Mutations in TWIST, a basic helix-loop-helix transcription factor, in Saethre-Chotzen syndrome. Nat Genet 1997;15:36–41.
54 Carver EA, Oram KF, Gridley T: Craniosynostosis in Twist heterozygous mice: a model for Saethre-Chotzen syndrome. Anat Rec 2002;268:90–92.
55 Lee MS, Lowe GN, Strong DD, Wergedal JE, Glackin CA: TWIST, a basic helix-loop-helix transcription factor, can regulate the human osteogenic lineage. J Cell Biochem 1999;75:566–577.

56 Loeys BL, Chen J, Neptune ER, Judge DP, Podowski M, Holm T, Meyers J, Leitch CC, Katsanis N, Sharifi N, et al: A syndrome of altered cardiovascular, craniofacial, neurocognitive and skeletal development caused by mutations in TGFBR1 or TGFBR2. Nat Genet 2005;37:275–281.
57 Roth DA, Gold LI, Han VK, McCarthy JG, Sung JJ, Wisoff JH, Longaker MT: Immunolocalization of transforming growth factor beta 1, beta 2, and beta 3 and insulin-like growth factor I in premature cranial suture fusion. Plast Reconstr Surg 1997;99:300–309.
58 Opperman LA, Nolen AA, Ogle RC: TGF-beta 1, TGF-beta 2, and TGF-beta 3 exhibit distinct patterns of expression during cranial suture formation and obliteration in vivo and in vitro. J Bone Miner Res 1997;12:301–310.
59 Opperman LA, Chhabra A, Cho RW, Ogle RC: Cranial suture obliteration is induced by removal of transforming growth factor (TGF)-beta 3 activity and prevented by removal of TGF-beta 2 activity from fetal rat calvaria in vitro. J Craniofac Genet Dev Biol 1999;19:164–173.
60 Opperman LA, Galanis V, Williams AR, Adab K: Transforming growth factor-beta3 (Tgf-beta3) down-regulates Tgf-beta3 receptor type I (Tbetar-I) during rescue of cranial sutures from osseous obliteration. Orthod Craniofac Res 2002;5:5–16.
61 Brunet LJ, McMahon JA, McMahon AP, Harland RM: Noggin, cartilage morphogenesis, and joint formation in the mammalian skeleton. Science 1998;280:1455–1457.
62 Nacamuli RP, Fong KD, Lenton KA, Song HM, Fang TD, Salim A, Longaker MT: Expression and possible mechanisms of regulation of BMP3 in rat cranial sutures. Plast Reconstr Surg 2005;116:1353–1362.
63 Takao M, Hino J, Takeshita N, Konno Y, Nishizawa T, Matsuo H, Kangawa K: Identification of rat bone morphogenetic protein-3b (BMP-3b), a new member of BMP-3. Biochem Biophys Res Commun 1996;219:656–662.
64 Groppe J, Greenwald J, Wiater E, Rodriguez-Leon J, Economides AN, Kwiatkowski W, Baban K, Affolter M, Vale WW, Belmonte JC, et al: Structural basis of BMP signaling inhibition by Noggin, a novel twelve-membered cystine knot protein. J Bone Joint Surg Am 2003;85-A(suppl 3):52–58.
65 Daluiski A, Engstrand T, Bahamonde ME, Gamer LW, Agius E, Stevenson SL, Cox K, Rosen V, Lyons KM: Bone morphogenetic protein-3 is a negative regulator of bone density. Nat Genet 2001;27:84–88.
66 Nacamuli RP, Song HM, Fang TD, Fong KD, Mathy JA, Shi YY, Salim A, Longaker MT: Quantitative transcriptional analysis of fusing and nonfusing cranial suture complexes in mice. Plast Reconstr Surg 2004;114:1818–1825.
67 Ting K, Vastardis H, Mulliken JB, Soo C, Tieu A, Do H, Kwong E, Bertolami CN, Kawamoto H, Kuroda S, et al: Human NELL-1 expressed in unilateral coronal synostosis. J Bone Miner Res 1999;14:80–89.
68 Zhang X, Carpenter D, Bokui N, Soo C, Miao S, Truong T, Wu B, Chen I, Vastardis H, Tanizawa K, et al: Overexpression of Nell-1, a craniosynostosis-associated gene, induces apoptosis in osteoblasts during craniofacial development. J Bone Miner Res 2003;18:2126–2134.
69 Twigg SR, Kan R, Babbs C, Bochukova EG, Robertson SP, Wall SA, Morriss-Kay GM, Wilkie AO: Mutations of ephrin-B1 (EFNB1), a marker of tissue boundary formation, cause craniofrontonasal syndrome. Proc Natl Acad Sci USA 2004;101:8652–8657.
70 Tang XX, Biegel JA, Nycum LM, Yoshioka A, Brodeur GM, Pleasure DE, Ikegaki N: cDNA cloning, molecular characterization, and chromosomal localization of NET(EPHT2), a human EPH-related receptor protein-tyrosine kinase gene preferentially expressed in brain. Genomics 1995;29:426–437.
71 Antikainen T: Silicon membrane interpositioning for the prevention of skull deformity following experimental craniosynostosis. Childs Nerv Syst 1993;9:321–324.
72 Stelnicki EJ, Vanderwall K, Harrison MR, Longaker MT, Kaban LB, Hoffman WY: The in utero correction of unilateral coronal craniosynostosis. Plast Reconstr Surg 1998;101:287–296.
73 Powers CJ, McLeskey SW, Wellstein A: Fibroblast growth factors, their receptors and signaling. Endocr Relat Cancer 2000;73:165–197.
74 Ueno H, Gunn M, Dell K, Tseng A, Williams L: A truncated form of fibroblast growth factor receptor 1 inhibits signal transduction by multiple types of fibroblast growth factor receptors. J Biol Chem 1992;267:1470–1476.

75 Dorn G, Patel S, Wotherspoon G, Hemmings-Mieszczak M, Barclay J, Natt FJ, Martin P, Bevan S, Fox A, Ganju P, et al: siRNA relieves chronic neuropathic pain. Nucleic Acids Res 2004;32:e49.
76 Song E, Lee SK, Wang J, Ince N, Ouyang N, Min J, Chen J, Shankar P, Lieberman J: RNA interference targeting Fas protects mice from fulminant hepatitis. Nat Med 2003;9:347–351.
77 Soutschek J, Akinc A, Bramlage B, Charisse K, Constien R, Donoghue M, Elbashir S, Geick A, Hadwiger P, Harborth J, et al: Therapeutic silencing of an endogenous gene by systemic administration of modified siRNAs. Nature 2004;432:173–178.
78 Enlow DH: Facial Growth, ed. Philadelphia, Saunders, 1990.
79 Lomri A, Lemonnier J, Delannoy P, Marie PJ: Increased expression of protein kinase Calpha, interleukin-1alpha, and RhoA guanosine 5′-triphosphatase in osteoblasts expressing the Ser252Trp fibroblast growth factor 2 receptor Apert mutation: identification by analysis of complementary DNA microarray. J Bone Miner Res 2001;16:705–712.
80 Luo XH, Guo LJ, Yuan LQ, Xie H, Zhou HD, Wu XP, Liao EY: Adiponectin stimulates human osteoblasts proliferation and differentiation via the MAPK signaling pathway. Exp Cell Res 2005;309:99–109.
81 Spector JA, Mathy JA, Warren SM, Nacamuli RP, Song HM, Lenton K, Fong KD, Fang DT, Longaker MT: FGF-2 acts through an ERK1/2 intracellular pathway to affect osteoblast differentiation. Plast Reconstr Surg 2005;115:838–852.
82 Kim HJ, Lee MH, Park HS, Park MH, Lee SW, Kim SY, Choi JY, Shin HI, Ryoo HM: Erk pathway and activator protein 1 play crucial roles in FGF2-stimulated premature cranial suture closure. Dev Dyn 2003;227:335–346.
83 Moursi AM, Winnard PL, Fryer D, Mooney MP: Delivery of transforming growth factor-beta2-perturbing antibody in a collagen vehicle inhibits cranial suture fusion in calvarial organ culture. Cleft Palate Craniofac J 2003;40:225–232.
84 Chong SL, Mitchell R, Moursi AM, Winnard P, Losken HW, Bradley J, Ozerdem OR, Azari K, Acarturk O, Opperman LA, et al: Rescue of coronal suture fusion using transforming growth factor-beta 3 (Tgf-beta 3) in rabbits with delayed-onset craniosynostosis. Anat Rec A Discov Mol Cell Evol Biol 2003;274:962–971.
85 Opperman LA, Moursi AM, Sayne JR, Wintergerst AM: Transforming growth factor-beta 3(Tgf-beta3) in a collagen gel delays fusion of the rat posterior interfrontal suture in vivo. Anat Rec 2002;267:120–130.
86 Wu XB, Li Y, Schneider A, Yu W, Rajendren G, Iqbal J, Yamamoto M, Alam M, Brunet LJ, Blair HC, et al. Impaired osteoblastic differentiation, reduced bone formation, and severe osteoporosis in noggin-overexpressing mice. J Clin Invest 2003;112:924–934.

Michael T. Longaker, MD, MBA
Department of Surgery, Stanford University Medical Center
257 Campus Drive West
Stanford, CA 94305-5148 (USA)
Tel. +1 650 736 1707, Fax +1 650 736 1705, E-Mail longaker@stanford.edu

Author Index

Subject Index